NEW DRUGS
Third Edition

NEW DRUGS

Third Edition

edited by

JOHN FEELY MD FRCPI

Professor of Pharmacology and Therapeutics,
Trinity College, and Consultant Physician,
St James's Hospital, Dublin

Published by the BMJ Publishing Group
Tavistock Square, London WC1H 9JR

Second edition 1991
Third edition 1994

ISBN 0 7279 0821 9

Made and printed in England by
Latimer Trend & Company Ltd, Plymouth

Contents

Generic (pharmacopoeial, approved, or non-proprietary) drug names are used throughout the book, including the index. When proprietary names are included they appear in parentheses after the generic names. In the index they are also cross referenced to the generic names.

1 Drug handling and response

JOHN FEELY, MARTIN J BRODIE

Over 500 pharmacological agents have come on to the market in the past 25 years, and more than 100 are currently being developed. The production of hormones and regulatory peptides through recombinant DNA (deoxyribonucleic acid) technology heralds another therapeutic revolution. Despite the increasing adoption of postmarketing surveillance, we rely heavily on perceptive observations by practising doctors not only for the early detection of adverse events but also for the recognition of unanticipated additional benefits that come to be regarded as secondary indications—for example, intraocular β blockers for glaucoma, topical minoxidil for baldness.

An increasing amount of assessment of new drugs will be undertaken by family doctors. This development is important, as many drugs are used almost entirely in general practice. In the final analysis the prescriber has to judge from available information whether or not to try a new treatment for the patient. For many, the interpretation of the clinical data, often presented in indigestible pharmacokinetic terms and as complicated clinical trials, is hindered by a lack of familiarity with the jargon and methods. This and the next chapter will consider some basic principles in clinical pharmacology, an appreciation of which will facilitate better use of the available drugs and proper evaluation of newly introduced therapeutic agents.

Pharmacokinetics

Pharmacokinetics, or how the body handles drugs, is the quantitative study of the time course of drug absorption, distribution, metabolism, and excretion and is by necessity a mathematical description. Some of the terms seem at first sight to have little relevance to everyday clinical practice, but they can enhance

1

prescribers' abilities to recognise the causes of therapeutic problems and to alter dosage schedules in a wide variety of clinical settings.

ABSORPTION

The absorption of most orally administered drugs takes place in the upper gastrointestinal tract, by and large, by passive diffusion. We are particularly interested in the extent to which a drug is absorbed. This is sometimes referred to as bioavailability, which also takes into account presystemic elimination or first pass metabolism. The speed of drug absorption, expressed as T_{max} (see fig 1.2), may be important when a rapid effect is needed—for example with analgesics and antibiotics. The rate is not a critical factor in long term treatment provided that a consistent amount of drug is absorbed from each dose to maintain adequate steady state concentrations.

A delay in absorption may result from concomitant disease (for example, migraine) or drug administration (for example, narcotic

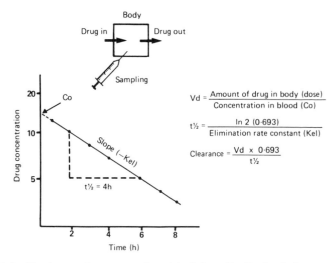

FIG 1.1—Simple one compartmental model of drug distribution in humans and concentration–time curve in plasma. Volume of distribution (Vd) is calculated from extrapolated concentration at time 0 (Co), assuming homogeneous and instantaneous mixing of drug. Elimination half life ($t\frac{1}{2}$) may be "eyeballed" from curve or derived mathematically from its slope. Relation between clearance, $t\frac{1}{2}$, and Vd is shown.

2

analgesics), which reduce transit time through the gastrointestinal tract. The effect of food is complex. As a general rule the absorption of lipid soluble drugs will be enhanced by a meal, but this is of marginal benefit as, for most of these, the process is rapid and complete. A few drugs such as captopril, digoxin, and rifampicin are better absorbed on an empty stomach. Gastric irritants, such as non-steroidal anti-inflammatory agents and iron, should be taken with a meal. Capsules and tablets should be washed down with a glass of water with the patient in an upright position, sitting or standing, as this enhances passage into the stomach and more rapid dissolution. Giving drugs orally to a recumbent patient should be avoided if possible, particularly agents that have the potential to damage the oesophageal mucosa—for example, tetracyclines, iron salts, and slow release potassium preparations.

DISTRIBUTION

After absorption a drug passes via the circulation into body water and into cells. The extent of this distribution is largely determined by the physicochemical characteristics of the compound. Drugs that are highly soluble in lipid—the vast majority—tend to have large volumes of distribution (Vd (see fig 1.1), measured in hundreds of litres), whereas those that are highly protein bound, such as warfarin, remain largely within the plasma and have a volume similar to that of the vascular compartment—about 7l.

Although the simplest model of distribution assumes the body to be a single homogeneous compartment (fig 1.1) most drugs are best described by a two compartmental system (fig 1.2). The drug initially enters a central compartment (V_1), primarily the circulation and highly vascular organs, where rapid diffusion leads to a sharp decline in drug concentration (α phase). A larger peripheral compartment (V_2) incorporates many tissues, including muscle, fat, bone, et cetera. Although drugs do pass between these compartments, entry and elimination is through the central one only. Concentrations decrease more slowly in the elimination (β) phase owing to irreversible removal by hepatic metabolism or renal excretion, or both.

When the apparent volume of distribution seems to exceed the total volume of body water (about 42l)—for example, with tricyclic antidepressants—there is substantial uptake and binding within tissues, such as muscle or brain, where the concentration may be

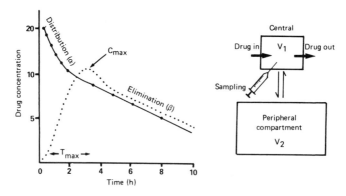

FIG 1.2—Typical two compartmental model (——) after intravenous administration of a drug. Profile after a single oral dose (. . . .) is also shown. C_{max} = Maximum concentration; T_{max} = time to achieve C_{max}.

considerably higher than that in plasma. Drugs that have a large volume of distribution and a long elimination half life—for example, digoxin—may be given initially in a loading dose to saturate these tissue binding sites. The maintenance dose will then depend on the rate of elimination.

HALF LIFE

The elimination half life of a drug is the time taken for the circulating concentration to fall by half (fig 1.1). For most drugs the rate of decline in plasma concentration is constant and directly proportional to the amount present (first order kinetics), with progressively more being removed at higher concentrations. This exponential decay, when plotted on a logarithmic scale, produces a straight line whose slope represents the rate of elimination. When there is a particularly good relation between concentration and effect the half life may be useful in predicting a drug's duration of action. The half life in this case may also help to determine the appropriate frequency of dosing—for example, twice a day for a drug with an elimination half life of about 12h. For most drugs, however, the half life does not easily equate with response, as there is substantial accumulation in tissues and avid binding to receptor sites. The presence of active metabolites may also alter the time course of the effect. Some drugs act by influencing biological systems, such as enzymes or cell membranes, that have their own inherent duration of action.

4

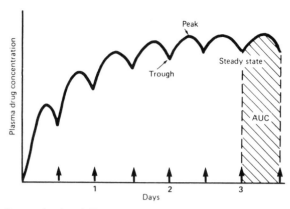

FIG 1.3—Repeated twice daily oral dosing of a drug with half life (t½) of 12 h showing concentration–time curve to steady state. ▨ = Area under plasma concentration–time curve (AUC) after one dose. This can be used to calculate clearance (administered dose/AUC).

The half life can be used to predict the time to achieve the steady state concentration in the circulation. It takes around five half lives to achieve equilibrium, when the amount of drug eliminated is equivalent to that absorbed (fig 1.3). The half life can be used in the same way to calculate the time required for the drug concentration to decrease to a desired concentration or to be cleared almost completely from the circulation—again five half lives.

CLEARANCE

Clearance denotes the volume of blood or plasma from which the drug is completely removed per unit time. Most drugs are biodegraded through the action of liver enzymes to produce more water soluble metabolites. A few are excreted unchanged into the urine. Doctors are familiar with the concept of clearance regarding renal function. If the renal clearance of a water soluble drug is about 120 ml/min this suggests that the glomerular filtration rate is the main limiting factor. Additional tubular secretion of the drug can be assumed to be occurring when clearance is more rapid than this. Information on the kinetics of such a drug is required for patients whose renal function can be expected to be altered—for example, in the newborn, elderly, or patients who have renal disease.

Clearance of some drugs after intravenous dosing is equivalent to blood flow through the liver (500–1500 ml/min)—for example, lignocaine and morphine. The liver is so efficient at extracting

5

these drugs from the blood that the rate of delivery to that organ is the rate limiting factor in their metabolism. Occasionally the calculated clearance after oral administration of a drug is even greater than the blood flow through the liver—for example, 2–5 l/min for propranolol and tricyclic antidepressants—suggesting that there is appreciable presystemic metabolism in the gut wall or liver, or both. Such an occurrence may be confirmed when the clearance value is lower after an intravenous dose (systemic clearance) than that obtained after oral administration, as is the case with verapamil and salbutamol.

A few drugs (notably ethanol, phenytoin, and theophylline) do not obey simple first order kinetic laws. For these the rate of elimination at high concentrations is independent of the drug concentration and is described by "zero order" (or saturation) kinetics, in which a constant amount is cleared per unit time. Thus first order kinetics apply at lower doses and zero order metabolism takes over at higher concentrations, which explains why increments need to be progressively reduced with increasing dosage.

DRUG METABOLISM

Most lipid soluble compounds are metabolised in the liver to products that are more water soluble. This is often a two phase process, with initial oxidation carried out primarily by a family of enzymes (mono-oxygenase or mixed function oxidases) found in the endoplasmic reticulum of hepatocytes. Their cellular content can be measured in vitro as cytochrome P450 because of the production of a characteristic wave band at 450 nm on spectrophotometry. Many drugs also undergo a second step (phase 2) by conjugation, in which an endogenous substance such as glucuronic acid or sulphate is attached to the drug or its metabolite. Larger molecules are then eliminated in the bile, whereas smaller ones (molecular weight less than 300) are excreted through the kidney.

Although most lipid soluble drugs are rendered inactive by metabolism, a few prodrugs are activated by oxidative processes—for example, cyclophosphamide, sulindac, and enalapril. Some metabolites are of interest because they have a longer duration of action than the parent compound (for example, those from flurazepam and clorazepate). Paracetamol hepatotoxicity is produced by an evanescent oxidative metabolite that binds irreversibly to liver cell macromolecules. In an overdose the normal cellular defensive mechanism of conjugation with glutathione is overwhelmed.

A large variety of endogenous substances, exogenous toxins, and lipid soluble drugs are metabolised in the liver by a few enzyme systems. The rate at which drugs are metabolised depends on a combination of interlinked factors—the genetically determined enzyme complement, the physiological and pathological state of the major organs, and environmental factors including the presence of other drugs, alcohol consumption, and cigarette smoking (fig 1.4). The variability in enzyme content and the differential effect of those genetic and environmental factors makes a single dosage regimen with a lipid soluble drug unrealistic.

Initial estimates of drug clearance and half life are usually derived from studies in healthy subjects, often young men because of the possibility of teratogenesis if administered to women of child bearing age. Metabolism is less efficient in patients, particularly those with liver disease or cardiac failure, and in the elderly. In some conditions such as burns several systems are affected, and profound and sometimes opposing changes occur in oxidative and conjugative metabolism, drug binding, and renal elimination. Unfortunately the influences on metabolism are too diverse and

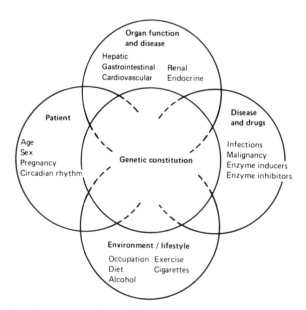

FIG 1.4—Overlapping variables that influence rate and extent of drug metabolism in the liver.

7

unpredictable to allow precise recommendations for dosage to be adjusted in individual patients. They do, however, help to explain the considerable variability seen in response to treatment and allow general predictions of the probable effects of aging, organ failure, and concomitant drug treatment. This background knowledge, combined with a careful appraisal of efficacy and toxicity, will facilitate drug use in these groups of patients at high risk.

PHARMACOGENETICS

There is increasing recognition of the potentially pivotal role of genetics in determining the rate at which drugs are metabolised. Several primary routes of metabolism such as acetylation and hydroxylation are subject to strong genetic control. This may explain individual or ethnic susceptibility to enhanced toxicity or poor efficacy with particular agents. About 8% of the European population show a reduced capacity to oxidise certain drugs. A poor capacity for hydroxylation helps to explain why some patients develop profound hypotension with debrisoquine and considerable β blockade with metoprolol and why phenformin and perhexiline were withdrawn from clinical practice because they produced lactic acidosis and hepatotoxicity, respectively, in an unacceptable proportion of patients. Genetic polymorphism of drug metabolism is an important determinant in the responses, beneficial or toxic, to newer antiarrhythmics such as encainide, flecainide, and propafenone and possibly to most tricyclic antidepressants.

Throughout the world there is a much larger variation in acetylation among ethnic groups. Fast acetylators make up 90% of Eskimos, 40% of Europeans, but only about 20% of Egyptians: such people are less likely to be cured of tuberculosis by the intermittent administration of isoniazid. Slow acetylators more often develop peripheral neuropathy when treated with isoniazid and systemic lupus erythematosus when treated with procainamide and hydralazine. Similarly, evidence is accumulating that the serious "idiosyncratic" toxicity (blood dyscrasias, rash, and nephrotic syndrome) seen after treatment with penicillamine and gold is more common in patients whose ability to sulphoxidate is comparatively low. The metabolism of certain environmental toxins may be associated with metabolic polymorphisms—for example, primary liver cancer in Nigerians is predominantly seen in fast hydroxylators, and bladder cancer in people who work with dye is more commonly found in slow acetylators.

STEREOISOMERISM

Many pharmaceuticals, perhaps one quarter, exist in mirror image forms as optically active stereoisomers (or enantiomers). The drug on the market is often a racemate, or equal mixture of left (L or S) and right (R or D) isomers. Isomers may differ in metabolism, pharmacological effect, and toxicity. For example, propranolol is marketed as the racemate DL, but only L-propranolol is responsible for the β blockade—D-propranolol has little activity. Other β blockers such as timolol and sotalol and the calcium antagonist verapamil also show stereoselective differences in drug action. These isomers may be cleared by the body at different rates.

One of the better known examples concerns warfarin. Most pharmacological activity resides within the s isomer, whose clearance is faster than that of R-warfarin. Interactions with other drugs such as sulphinpyrazone and co-trimoxazole show stereoselective inhibition of the s enantiomer only. Phenylbutazone inhibits the breakdown of the s isomer and induces the metabolism of R-warfarin. The result is potentiated anticoagulation with no change in total warfarin concentrations. The commercial production of individual isomers could result in more specific and safer drugs. One isomer of thalidomide, for example, is hypnotic while the other is teratogenic.

DRUG BINDING TO PLASMA PROTEIN

Drugs may be bound to several proteins in the circulation, particularly albumin and the acute phase reactant α_1 acid glycoprotein. In general, acidic and neutral drugs bind to albumin, and basic drugs bind to α_1 acid glycoprotein. Low concentrations of albumin—for example, in the nephrotic syndrome or hepatic cirrhosis—or increased α_1 acid glycoprotein concentrations—for example, in rheumatoid arthritis or Crohn's disease—will alter the binding of drugs such as warfarin and lignocaine, respectively. As the free (unbound) fraction is pharmacologically active, such a change may affect distribution and accessibility to hepatic metabolic sites and renal excretion mechanisms. The free component is the one that is transferred into the cerebrospinal fluid, transplacentally to the fetus, and into breast milk.

Alterations in binding are likely to be of clinical relevance only for drugs that are more than 90% protein bound. A decrease of 1%

in warfarin binding (normally 99% bound) will result in a 100% increase in concentrations of the free drug. The effect of this will be offset by increased hepatic metabolism (first order process). The result is a more subtle variation in the concentration–time curve— that is, higher peaks and lower troughs but a similar steady state. For the same reason drug interactions caused by the displacement of binding sites on circulating proteins are not regarded as a great cause of toxicity (see chapter 4).

RENAL ELIMINATION

The kidney is responsible for excreting water soluble drugs and metabolites. Lipid soluble substances are also filtered by the glomerulus, but these will diffuse back into the circulation further down the nephron. The extent of back diffusion is less for drugs that are highly ionised or dissociated. This situation can be exploited in the management of overdose, when the rates of renal excretion may be substantially increased by altering urinary pH— for example, alkalinisation in overdose of aspirin and barbiturates, acidification in overdose of amphetamines.

The tubules actively secrete several weak acids such as penicillin, cephalosporins, salicylates, probenecid, and thiazides and bases such as amiloride, cimetidine, and procainamide by two separate systems. Interactions may occur because of competition between drugs for these sites of tubular transport. Thus probenecid has been useful for many decades to increase circulating concentrations of penicillin. Some drugs, including digoxin and aminoglycosides, are excreted unchanged by the kidney, and information on their handling in patients who have disorders of renal function is of obvious importance. Unfortunately, serum concentrations of urea, which are largely determined by protein intake, and of creatinine, which reflect formation in muscle, are not sufficiently sensitive indices to assess changes in the glomerular filtration rate and renal drug clearance. Measuring creatinine clearance provides the most accurate guideline for adjusting dosage. This can be estimated from a simple equation such as:

creatinine clearance (ml/min) = ((140 − age) × weight (kg))/ plasma creatinine concentration (μmol/l).

Although this calculation may overestimate creatinine clearance in grossly overweight or oedematous patients and when serum creatinine concentration is rising rapidly, it is accurate enough for most patients whose renal function is stable. Patients who have renal failure require lower doses of water soluble drugs, often at extended intervals.

Pharmacodynamics

Pharmacodynamics is the description of the pharmacological properties of a drug. Many drugs depend for their action on binding to a receptor protein in the cell or its membrane to produce a direct effect (agonist) or to block the effect of an endogenous agonist (antagonist).

A number of highly specific receptors have been identified—for example, for

- adrenaline;
- acetylcholine;
- histamine;
- dopamine;
- opioids;
- benzodiazepines.

Subclasses of most receptors—for example, $\beta_1 - \beta_2$ adrenoceptors—have been recognised. A few drugs have been shown to be partial agonists (antagonists at low concentrations and agonists at high)—for example, buprenorphine and pindolol. Drugs may act on more than one receptor site, particularly in the central nervous system. Some influence the transduction process (or coupling) between receptor occupancy and drug effect, which is usually mediated by an internal energy releasing system such as cyclic adenosine monophosphate. Others affect general processes such as nerve conduction or muscle contraction.

Receptors exist in a dynamic state. Their number and functional state—the avidity with which they will bind agonists—vary with disease state and drug treatment. Continued exposure to an agonist leads to the internalisation of receptors, thus limiting or reducing efficiency ("down regulation"). This may be seen with the long term use of a selective β_2 agonist in asthma. Tolerance, or decreased responsiveness, may develop when an increased dose is required to produce the same effect. This may be a consequence of the down regulation of receptors, a homoeostatic adaptive response, or the stimulation of the drug's metabolism. Tolerance to the antianginal effect of nitrates has been explained by a deficiency

11

of reduced sulphydryl groups that nitrates induce in vascular smooth muscle. Intermittent treatment may allow replenishment and restore efficacy. In some disease processes, such as insulin resistance, defects exist not only at the receptor but also within the mechanism of coupling or at a postreceptor site.

Long term treatment with an antagonist will lead to an increase in receptor binding sites ("up regulation"). This phenomenon may explain the syndrome associated with the rapid withdrawal of some drugs—for example, rebound angina after withdrawing propranolol. The sensitivity of patients to low doses of a particular drug may be a consequence of age, concomitant renal or hepatic disease, or the type and severity of the underlying condition. Thus the pathophysiology of the disorder—for example, renal hypertension or coronary artery spasm—may determine the extent of response to various antihypertensive or antianginal drugs. The sensitivity of the central nervous system to benzodiazepines and narcotic analgesics in patients who have hepatic encephalopathy is largely a pharmacodynamic process.

The homoeostatic and biochemical milieu may also influence the response to treatment—for example by altering the electrolyte balance. A depletion of sodium predisposes a patient to lithium toxicity and hypokalaemia to digoxin toxicity. Synergism of drugs with similar pharmacodynamic properties may be beneficial, as with the antibiotic components of co-trimoxazole or with combined levodopa and selegiline (selective monoamine oxidase inhibitor) treatment in Parkinson's disease.

VARIATION IN RESPONSE

Variation in response to the same dose of drug is the rule rather than the exception in clinical practice. Assuming that a patient is compliant and that there are no pharmaceutical problems, the main reasons for this variability include a combination of pharmacokinetic and pharmacodynamic factors. A multifactorial situation therefore exists, the individual factors of which may be difficult to dissect. An understanding of the probable components, however, will allow the prescriber to make adjustments when something goes wrong. A lack of pharmacological effect or the development of toxicity may warrant an alteration in dosage or substitution of another drug.

Several issues need to be considered when assessing the choice of treatment. Information on efficacy and the magnitude of risk–

benefit ratio are important, particularly when deciding between comparable drugs. Potency—the relation between dose (concentration) and effect—is of little clinical relevance. The therapeutic ratio, or the closeness of the relation between the dose producing the pharmacological or beneficial effect and that associated with toxicity, is critical in risk–benefit analysis. For drugs with a low or narrow therapeutic ratio—for example, digoxin, warfarin, and phenytoin—increments of dosage should be small and the response or concentration, or both, reviewed frequently. Another problem, long recognised but poorly studied, is the placebo effect, or how patients' perceptions of treatment influence their responses. In some organic disorders a substantial proportion of patients respond satisfactorily to placebo—for example, 40% who have peptic ulcer or angina. A new treatment must be shown to be at least as good as standard treatment and, whenever possible, better than placebo.

Compliance

Despite evidence to the contrary, most prescribers generally assume that patients take their drugs as directed. The incidence of non-compliance is difficult to estimate, but studies show that 20–30% of patients receiving short term curative treatment and up to half of those taking long term prophylactic treatment do not comply fully. The impact of incomplete compliance on outcome will depend on the drug and the disease as well as on the extent to which the drug is not taken. Some patients adjust their compliance in line with the side effects they experience. This information may be withheld to avoid upsetting the doctor! A few patients take (almost) none of the treatment prescribed. Some doctors are not fully aware of what drugs their patients are taking, particularly when patients are attending hospital clinics as well as the general practitioner's surgery. Confusion with generic and proprietary names can occur, and combination preparations—for example, a β blocker and a thiazide diuretic—may not be recognised as such.

About 70% of the population receives at least one prescription a year; this use of drugs is even greater in the elderly. Most patients also buy non-prescription drugs. Compliance can be improved by minimising the number of drugs prescribed and the frequency of their administration. Such rationalisation should be accompanied

13

by discussing with the patient the expected benefits and possible side effects of the treatment. A realistic expectation of outcome must be shared by the doctor and the patient.

The pharmaceutical industry goes to considerable lengths to produce drugs to be taken once a day, slow release formulations, calendar packs, and other reminders, often without supportive evidence that these more expensive presentations actually do increase compliance. Doctors should assess compliance regularly, particularly when treatment seems not to be working (or toxic). This should include objectively assessing drug effect whenever possible, inquiring about common side effects, counting residual tablets, and measuring drug concentration when appropriate.

Alvan G, Balant LP, Bechtel PR, Boobis AR, Gram LF, Pithan K, eds. *European Consensus Conference on Pharmacogenetics: European cooperation in the field of scientific and technical research*. Luxembourg: Office for Official Publications of the European Communities, 1990. (Comprehensive series of papers on all aspects of this topic.)

Bonate PL. Pathophysiology and pharmacokinetics following burn injury. *Clin Pharmacokinet* 1990;**18**:118–30.

Brodie MJ, Harrison I. *Practical prescribing*. Edinburgh: Churchill Livingstone, 1986. (Simple and readable introduction directed at the general practitioner. Drug information, side effects, and adverse interactions is tabulated for easy access.)

Clark DWJ. Genetically determined validity in acetylation and oxidation: therapeutic implications. *Drugs* 1985;**29**:342–75.

Evans WE, Schentag JJ, Jusko WJ, eds. *Applied pharmacokinetics. Principles of therapeutic drug monitoring*, Spokane: Applied Therapeutics, 1987. (Detailed assessment of bespoke prescribing.)

Grahame-Smith DG, Aronson JK. *Oxford textbook of clinical pharmacology and drug therapy*. 2nd ed. Oxford: Oxford Medical Publications, 1992. (Excellent undergraduate textbook that covers the general principles and includes a useful pharmacopoeia.)

Laurence DR, Bennet PN. *Clinical pharmacology*. 7th ed. London: Churchill Livingstone, 1992. (Standard inexpensive undergraduate textbook that is both interesting and useful.)

O'Connor P, Feely J. Clinical pharmacokinetics and endocrine disorders: therapeutic implications. *Clin Pharmacokinet* 1987;**13**:345–64.

Reidenberg MM. Kidney function and drug action. *N Engl J Med* 1985;**313**:816–8.

Speight TM, ed. *Avery's drug treatment. Principles and practice of clinical pharmacology and therapeutics*. Auckland: Adis Press, 1987. (Comprehensive but digestible treatise on applied clinical pharmacology. The appendices give detailed pharmacokinetic data, including a guide to drug dosage in renal and liver failure.)

Wilkinson GR. Clearance approaches in pharmacology. *Pharmacol Rev* 1987;**39**:1–47.

Williams K, Lee E. Importance of drug enantiomers in clinical pharmacology. *Drugs* 1985;**30**:333–54.

2 Therapeutic drug monitoring and clinical trials

MARTIN J BRODIE, JOHN FEELY

Monitoring drug concentrations

The idea of using a measured concentration to help decide the optimum dose of a drug and consequently derive the maximum therapeutic benefit with the minimum risk of side effects is a seductive concept. Unfortunately the ability of the biochemist to measure the concentration of a wide variety of pharmacological agents quickly and cheaply has outstripped the doctor's ability to apply these concentrations clinically. Only a few drugs are appropriate for routine monitoring, and these have a narrow therapeutic ratio and show a good relation between concentration and efficacy or toxicity.

Despite the absence of much supportive data a "therapeutic range" has been enthusiastically espoused and adopted for many drugs. This terminology assumes unequivocal benefit and bestows an inflated validity on a single measurement of the drug. Additionally, the calculations leading to the range are obtained from population kinetics and are not applicable to a substantial minority of patients. A "target range" of concentrations, around which clinical improvement might be expected without toxicity, provides a more appropriate starting point and avoids the pitfalls implicit in the term "therapeutic."

A drug concentration should not be considered in isolation but must help to answer a clinical question. Knowledge of the circulating concentration of a drug is useful only when it is considered in the context of the patient's symptoms and signs. It is important to ensure that a steady state concentration has been attained (five half lives after starting treatment or changing dose) and to standardise the sampling time in relation to the dose, particularly for drugs with a short elimination half life.

ANTICONVULSANTS

Despite "optimum" treatment with the antiepileptic drugs that are currently available, more than one fifth of epileptic patients will continue to have seizures. Moreover, there is little evidence that treatment with two drugs has an advantage over one used properly. The prescriber who fails to appreciate these points may condemn patients who have intractable epilepsy to a lifetime of polypharmacy with two, three, or even four drugs, with a resultant increased likelihood of metabolic and central nervous toxicity. The target range of concentrations (table 2.1) must be regarded only as a guide around which to alter the dose either upwards or downwards depending on the clinical response or the development of unacceptable side effects. The patient, not the biochemist, will report whether the anticonvulsant concentration is therapeutic or toxic. It is essential that the prescriber ensures that the dosage is adjusted according to the clinical state of the patient and resists the temptation to make changes in line with his own (or the biochemist's) interpretation of the clinical relevance of a high or low circulating concentration.

With this in mind the predictive value of anticonvulsant monitoring depends on the closeness of the relation among concentration, effect, and toxicity for each drug. This relation is closest with phenytoin, intermediate with carbamazepine, and poor with ethosuximide, phenobarbitone, primidone, and sodium valproate. A lower than expected concentration of all these drugs, however, will identify, at the very least, patients whose poor control of seizures is likely to be a consequence of poor compliance rather than failure of treatment.

Phenytoin

Phenytoin is one of the few drugs for which measurement of concentration is essential. Complete control is most often achieved with steady state concentrations of 40–80 µmol/l (10–20 mg/l). Nevertheless, some patients remain free of seizures with concentrations well below 40 µmol/l (10 mg/l), and others will tolerate more than 120 µmol/l (30 mg/l) with improved control and without developing neurotoxicity. Side effects that depend on concentration (including sedation, headache, dysarthria, nystagmus, and ataxia) usually but by no means invariably develop at concentrations of about 80 µmol/l (20 mg/l). The hepatic metabolism of

TABLE 2.1—*Drugs routinely available for monitoring concentration*

	Elimination half life (h)	Route of elimination	Target range of concentrations*		Clinical value
			Molar	Metric	
Amikacin	2–3	Renal	—	Trough <10 mg/l peak 20–30 mg/l	+++
Carbamazepine	25–45 (single) 8–24 (chronic)	Hepatic	17–42 µmol/l	4–10 mg/l	++
Digoxin	24–48	Renal	1–2·6 nmol/l	0·8–2 ng/ml	++
Ethosuximide	30–60	Hepatic	280–700 µmol/l	40–100 mg/l	+
Gentamicin	2–3	Renal	—	Trough <2·5 mg/l peak 5–10 mg/l	+++
Lithium	7–35	Renal	0·7–1·3 mmol/l (acute mania) 0·4–0·8 mmol/l (prophylaxis)	—	+++
Netilmicin	2–3	Renal	—	Trough <2·5 mg/l peak 5–10 mg/l	+++
Phenobarbitone	72–144	Hepatic/renal	40–172 µmol/l	10–40 mg/l	+
Phenytoin	9–40	Hepatic	40–80 µmol/l	10–20 mg/l	+++
Primidone	4–12	Hepatic	23–55 µmol/l	5–12 mg/l	+
Tobramycin	2–3	Renal	—	Trough <2·5 mg/l peak 5–10 mg/l	+++
Sodium valproate	7–17	Hepatic	347–693 µmol/l	50–100 mg/l	+
Theophylline	3–13	Hepatic	55–110 µmol/l	10–20 mg/l	++

* To convert metric to molar concentrations multiply by 1000 and divide by the molecular weight.
Clinical value of monitoring concentration: + = little, + + + = great.

phenytoin is saturable, so at higher concentrations a small increment in dose will produce a disproportionately large and unpredictable increase in concentration (fig 2.1). In these circumstances accurate tailoring of the dose can be undertaken only with the help of concentration monitoring. In no instance should the dose be increased by more than 100 mg at a time. If the plasma concentration is 32–48 µmol/l (8–12 mg/l) dosage increments should be limited to 50 mg; above 48 µmol/l (12 mg/l) increments should be limited to 25 mg. Toxicity is diagnosed on clinical grounds (sedation, nystagmus, or ataxia) and, as with all anticonvulsants, a drug concentration in itself cannot be considered to be "toxic". Because phenytoin has a long half life a single daily dose may be used, and the timing of sampling for monitoring concentration is not critical.

Carbamazepine

Carbamazepine's elimination half life may be as long as 48 h after a single dose but drops to 12 h or fewer during the first few weeks of treatment as a consequence of the autoinduction of metabolism. The subsequent decrease in circulating concentration after an increase in dose averages 30% and can occasionally result in a breakthrough of seizures (fig 2.2). On first exposure to the drug many patients develop mild neurotoxic side effects (nausea, headache, drowsiness, diplopia, nystagmus, or ataxia) at concentrations of around 34 µmol/l (8 mg/l), and a slow build up in dosage is

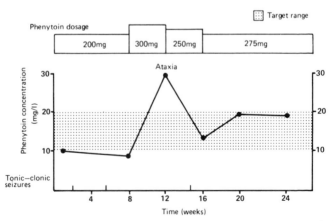

FIG 2.1—Effect of saturation of metabolism on the relation between phenytoin dose and concentration.

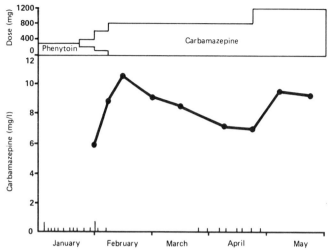

FIG 2.2—Deteriorating control of seizures in patient receiving fixed dose of carbamazepine with decreasing plasma concentrations attributable to autoinduction of metabolism. | = Generalised seizure; | = partial seizure. (Taken from Macphee GJA, Brodie MJ. Carbamazepine substitution in severe partial epilepsy: implications of autoinduction of metabolism. *Postgrad Med J* 1985;**61**:783–99.)

recommended. Tolerance develops rapidly, allowing much higher concentrations to be achieved without sedation in most patients. The target range of 17–42 µmol/l (4–10 mg/l) is wide but higher concentrations are often required in patients who have partial seizures and for whom the drug can be particularly effective. As there is substantial variation in concentration during the interval between doses, ideally a trough concentration sample taken just after a dose and a peak concentration sample taken 4 h later should be measured. When a single measurement is used in the surgery or the outpatient clinic the drug should be assayed at the same interval after the dose on each occasion, especially in patients receiving a twice daily dosage regimen.

Carbamazepine concentrations can be used to provide a baseline at which seizures are completely controlled in case of later problems and may also help to identify the concentration at which unacceptable side effects develop once maximum induction and tolerance have taken place. To offset the headache and diplopia associated with a high peak concentration the number of doses may be increased to three or four without altering the total daily intake of the drug. The recently introduced controlled release formulation of carbamazepine reduces the fluctuations between doses by about half and improves the value of a single estimation of serum carbamazepine concentration. Poorly compliant patients may take two doses a day of this new preparation, instead of three or more.

Sodium valproate

Sodium valproate is the third of the triumvirate of first line anticonvulsants. In contrast with phenytoin and carbamazepine the correlation between valproate concentration and efficacy is extremely poor. A tentative target range of 347–693 µmol/l (50–100 mg/l) has been suggested (table 2.1). Adverse reactions are more common at concentrations above this but, as with the other drugs, concentrations associated with the desired pharmacological response and those complicated by the development of unwanted side effects vary substantially among patients. Measuring concentrations can be helpful, however, in deciding whether to persevere with sodium valproate treatment in the face of continuing seizures. As concentrations rise above 1040 µmol/l (150 mg/l) it becomes increasingly appropriate to change to another drug rather than to try a further increment.

Ethosuximide

The use of ethosuximide is confined largely to treating absence seizures in children. It can be prescribed safely and effectively without recourse to monitoring, as the dose usually correlates well with the circulating concentration. Side effects that limit doses, however, do not readily correlate with high blood concentrations and are usually volunteered by patients. Measuring serum ethosuximide concentrations may be useful in distinguishing patients who are resistant to the pharmacological effect of the drug from those who have low concentrations as a consequence of incomplete compliance or rapid metabolism.

Phenobarbitone

The use of phenobarbitone as an anticonvulsant has declined since it was recognised as producing widespread and often subtle cognitive and psychomotor impairment. The value of measuring the circulating concentration is limited, as the concentration associated with good control varies considerably between patients. In addition, the development of tolerance to its effects on the central nervous system makes the toxic threshold imprecise. Nevertheless, in individual patients an unexpectedly high concentration may explain undue sedation and help in adjusting the dosage.

Primidone

Primidone is biotransformed in the liver to two active metabolites, one of which is phenobarbitone, so it is possible to provide polypharmacy with this single agent. A poor correlation exists between plasma concentration of the parent drug and anticonvulsant efficacy. When monitoring is undertaken phenobarbitone is usually measured to try to confirm clinical toxicity. An occasional patient, however, will show a high concentration of primidone with little detectable phenobarbitone.

Lamotrigine and vigabatrin

The value of monitoring the concentrations of these drugs has not been established (see chapter 25).

DIGOXIN

Digoxin is still widely prescribed despite the continuing controversy about its indications and its value as maintenance treatment. The usefulness of monitoring is compromised by the number of common factors that alter myocardial sensitivity to the drug (table 2.2). Unequivocal digoxin toxicity, including nausea, vomiting, and cardiac arrhythmias, can occur at concentrations well within the target range, particularly in the presence of hypokalaemia. Conversely, a high plasma concentration can only confirm but not diagnose toxicity, as some patients show increasing benefit without side effects at concentrations up to 3·8 nmol/l (3 ng/ml).

Circulating concentrations of digoxin are unrepresentative of tissue content during absorption and distribution, so samples should always be taken at least 6h after the last dose. Indications

TABLE 2.2—*Factors affecting tissue response to digoxin*

Increase response	Decrease response
Hypokalaemia	
Hypomagnesaemia	
Hypercalcaemia	Hypocalcaemia
Hypothyroidism	Hyperthyroidism
Old age	Infancy
Hypoxia	

for monitoring include assessing compliance and confirming clinical toxicity and suspected drug interactions. In particular, antiarrhythmics such as amiodarone, quinidine and verapamil increase digoxin concentrations. Occasionally measurement will be useful: when there is a poor initial response to treatment, when the drug history is uncertain, or when the clinical state (particularly renal function) is fluctuating—for example, after a myocardial infarction. Most authorities agree that if the serum digoxin concentration is found to be <1 nmol/l (<0.8 ng/ml) the drug may usually be stopped without ill effect.

LITHIUM

Lithium remains the paradigm of a drug whose efficacy and safety have been transformed by monitoring its concentration. Because the drug is excreted unchanged in the kidney, toxic concentrations result in a spiralling cycle of damage to the renal and nervous systems. Drug assay is essential in all patients at the start of treatment and at regular intervals thereafter. Samples should be taken in the morning $12 (\pm \frac{1}{2})$ h after the previous dose, preferably of a slow release preparation. During the start of treatment the first sample should be checked after 48–72 h to identify patients who develop toxic concentrations at a comparatively low dosage. The concentration should be measured again twice during the following week and at weekly intervals for the first month and then monthly for the next 6 months. To anticipate the possibility of gradual impairment in renal function, lithium should then be monitored every third month of regular treatment, with simultaneous measurement of serum creatinine concentration. The procedure should be repeated if the dose is altered or if an alternative formulation is introduced. A higher target range has been suggested for treating acute mania than for prescribing prophylactically (table 2.1).

In cases of suspected intoxication, whether after an acute overdose or during long term treatment, estimating lithium concentration should be requested as an emergency if permanent renal or neurological damage is to be avoided. When the concentration exceeds 2.5 nmol/l further measurements will be necessary. When haemodialysis is used, a repeat measurement 4–6 h later will detect rebound toxicity after redistribution within the body. Other indications for monitoring include potential drug interactions (thiazide diuretics and non-steroidal anti-inflammatory drugs are most dangerous), during dieting and intercurrent illness, and monthly throughout pregnancy. Lithium should not be prescribed if facilities for monitoring concentration are not available.

THEOPHYLLINE

A narrow therapeutic index together with substantial variation in metabolism among patients make theophylline a difficult drug to use well without monitoring its concentration. There is a linear relation between forced expiratory volume and the logarithm of circulating theophylline concentration within a range of 27·5–110 µmol/l (5–20 mg/l). Clinical evidence suggests that 55 µmol/l (10 mg/l) may usefully be regarded as the lower end of the target range for most asthmatic patients, though a few will show a satisfactory response at concentrations below this (fig 2.3). Agitation and tachycardia become apparent at concentrations of about 110 µmol/l (20 mg/l), though 5% of patients develop unacceptable

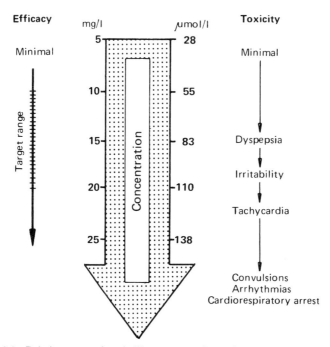

FIG 2.3—Relation among theophylline concentration, efficacy, and toxicity. (Taken from Brodie MJ, Hallworth MJ. Therapeutic monitoring of theophylline. *Hosp Update* 1988;**14**:1208–21.)

gastrointestinal distress at concentrations below 82·5 μmol/l (15 mg/l).

After an oral dose, timing of sampling is not critical if a sustained release preparation is used. Nevertheless, repeat measurements should be performed at the same interval after each dose. Monitoring should take place at least 72 h after any change in dose to ensure that steady state concentrations have been reached. When symptoms of theophylline intoxication are present measuring the concentration will confirm the diagnosis and facilitate the decision whether to stop the drug or merely to reduce the dose. As the drug may undergo saturable hepatic metabolism at the higher reaches of the target range, serious side effects can occur suddenly. Monitoring is therefore advisable whenever concentrations exceed 55 μmol/l (10 mg/l). Several commonly used drugs such as cimetidine, propranolol, verapamil, ciprofloxacin, and erythromycin inhibit the metabolism of theophylline and so can precipitate toxicity.

A measurement of the baseline concentration on admission is essential for every patient in whom intravenous aminophylline is being considered if there is any likelihood that the patient has been prescribed an oral preparation. Patients receiving a continuous infusion should be monitored after 12 h and then daily while the drug is being administered. Ideally the infusion should be stopped for 15 min before sampling to allow equilibration into the extravascular space.

AMINOGLYCOSIDES

Aminoglycosides are large molecules with short elimination half lives, and indications for their use are confined to serious infection. The main problems with this important group of antibiotics are concentration dependent ototoxicity and nephrotoxicity, which can be avoided by monitoring trough concentrations (for example, < 2·5 mg/l for gentamicin). Knowledge of the peak concentration is helpful in ensuring that tissue concentrations are likely to be inhibitory to the infecting organism (for example, 5–10 mg/l for gentamicin). As these drugs are excreted unchanged by the kidney, peak and trough concentrations should be measured routinely in all patients who have renal impairment and when the course of treatment exceeds 7 days. Concentration may be tailored by altering the dose or the dosage interval. Thus if the peak concentration is too low the dose should be increased: a high trough concentration can be corrected by widening the dosage interval. A judicious combination of both procedures is often necessary.

Clinical trials

The assessment and acceptance of a new treatment is critically dependent on well designed clinical trials that examine not only the drug's efficacy but also its potential for toxicity. The data produced should allow the prescriber to perform a precise benefit–risk analysis for an individual patient. Unfortunately many doctors do not view trials critically enough, and some pharmaceutical companies advertise results in a biased manner. Concern has been expressed about the conduct of "postmarketing surveillance" trials, some of which are largely marketing exercises. Guidelines have now been agreed between the industry and the medical profession. Whereas articles in the main medical journals have been subjected to stringent peer review and statistical assessment, those published in supplements and proceedings of sponsored meetings are often unrefereed. Accordingly, the list of references accompanying the promotional literature for a new agent should be scrutinised carefully.

In assessing the protocols or reports of trials it is essential to ensure that the design of the study is appropriate to providing clearly defined objectives (end points) that should answer specific clinical questions in an unequivocal manner. The experimental methods should identify the population of patients under study and state how they were selected. An examination of the criteria for entry and exclusion will show whether a representative sample of the population at whom the drug is targeted has been included. The numbers must be sufficient to allow appropriate statistical analysis of the results. An identical control population (matched for age, sex, severity of disease, and so on) receiving standard treatment in comparable dosage (or receiving placebo if no standard treatment exists) should be enrolled, and there should be unbiased randomisation of patients to either group. All patients should subsequently be accounted for and their compliance with the protocol ensured.

With chronic stable disorders such as hypertension or arthritis patients can serve as their own control (within subject trial) and so reduce the numbers required. A "run in" period of observation is often advised to show the stability of the disease. After this, patients may receive both forms of treatment (cross over) in random order. This is a less powerful comparative method than a "between subject" trial, in which patients receiving one form of treatment are compared directly with those receiving another treatment. Randomisation is necessary in both forms of trial—in between-subject trials to avoid observer bias and in within-subject trials to reduce any residual effect of the first form of treatment (carry over effect).

In evaluating response greater reliance is placed on objective (hard) data, preferably independent and sensitive measures of response to the drug such as blood pressure, blood glucose concentrations, or endoscopic evidence of ulcer healing. Although an assessment of the patient's quality of life is important, caution should be paid to studies "to try out" a drug that use subjective (soft) measures such as a value judgement of reported symptoms ("better"; "much better") or only acceptability to patients. This often represents a marketing, impressionistic approach rather than a scientific exercise. The presentation of the response of individual patients should be in real clinical terms rather than as a mean or percentage change. The same criteria should be applied to the incidence of side effects, which should be rigorously and specifically sought. Again, a real attempt should be made to obtain objective data.

The number of patients included in a trial is often too small to permit definitive statements about benefits, even when a significant result is found or when there seems to be no improvement. A common reason for finding "no significant difference," which is often erroneously presented as showing that both forms of treatment are equal, is too few patients in the study: an important benefit could possibly have been detected by a larger trial (type II error). The degree of uncertainty around the observed difference should be reported as confidence intervals, usually 95%. This gives the range from the smallest to the largest possible effect of treatment with which the trial data would be consistent. Such intervals are wide in small trials and are particularly important when assessing non-significant differences. The power of a study, or the probability that the investigation will identify the smallest difference of clinical importance—say 90% at the 5% level of significance—can be determined in advance to calculate the minimum number of patients required.

Statistical advice at the outset obviates the tendency for "data dredging" and a final statistical message with muddy conclusions. The degree of blindness—namely, single (either patient or observer) or double (both)—enhances the credibility of the results and avoids bias by the patient or the observer. Nevertheless, the use of a double blind technique is no guarantee of valid results in an otherwise poorly designed trial.

In assessing the outcome of a study one must be certain that the data justify the conclusions. The much sought after "significant" result, at the very least $p < 0.05$, means that there is a one in 20 statistical likelihood of the difference having arisen by chance and does not in itself imply biological or clinical relevance. An increase in serum potassium concentration of 0.1 mmol/l induced by a drug in all patients may be highly significant statistically but is of doubtful biological importance if it occurs within the normal range and is of lesser magnitude than the day to day variation. A new antibiotic, though showing a statistically significant lower mean inhibitory concentration against certain organisms in microbiological samples, is not necessarily an advance over established treatment in the absence of any change in the incidence of disease and death in patients. Sound common sense is required in assessing whether the reported benefits and safety margin of one drug over another are likely to be relevant in treating similar patients. In these straitened times cost must also come into the equation.

Anon. Reading between the lines in clinical trials. I. Design. *Drug Ther Bull* 1985;**23**:1–3.

Anon. Reading between the lines in clinical trials. II. Analysis. *Drug Ther Bull* 1985;**23**:5–7.

Aronson JK. Indications for the measurements of plasma digoxin concentrations. *Drugs* 1983;**26**:230–42.

Aronson JK, Hardman M. ABC of monitoring drug therapy: measuring plasma drug concentrations. *BMJ* 1992;**305**:1078–80.

Beghi EG, Mascio R, Tognini G. Adverse effects of anticonvulsant drugs—a critical review. *Adverse Drug Reactions and Acute Poisoning Review* 1986; **2**:63–86.

Brodie MJ. Established anticonvulsants and treatment of refractory epilepsy. *Lancet* 1990; **336:** 350–4.

Brodie MJ, Hallworth MJ. Therapeutic drug monitoring of carbamazepine. *Hosp Update* 1987;**13**:57–63.

Brodie MJ, Hallworth MJ. Therapeutic monitoring of digoxin. *Hosp Update* 1987;**13**:612–24.

Brodie MJ, Hallworth MJ. Therapeutic monitoring of theophylline. *Hosp Update* 1988;**14**:1208–21.

Brodie MJ, Hallworth MJ. Therapeutic monitoring of sodium valproate and ethosuximide. *Hosp Update* 1989;**15**:351–64.

Brodie MJ, McIntosh ME, Hallworth MJ. Therapeutic drug monitoring—the need for audit? *Scott Med J* 1985;**30**:75–82.

Burley DM, Binns TB, eds. *Pharmaceutical medicine*. London: Edward Arnold, 1985.

Chadwick DW. Overuse of monitoring of blood concentrations of antiepileptic drugs. *BMJ* 1987;**2**:723–4.

Florey C du V. Sample size for beginners, *BMJ* 1993;**306**:1181–4.

Glenny H, Nelmes P, eds. *Handbook of clinical drug research*. Oxford: Blackwell, 1986.

Gore SM. *Statistics in practice*. London: British Medical Association, 1984.

Hallworth MJ, Brodie MJ. Therapeutic monitoring of phenytoin. *Hosp Update* 1987;**13**:830–42.

Hallworth MJ, Brodie MJ. Therapeutic monitoring of lithium. *Hosp Update* 1988;**14**:1617–25.

Hallworth MJ, Brodie MJ. Therapeutic monitoring of aminoglycoside antibiotics. *Hosp Update* 1989;**15**:847–55.

Hill AB. *A short textbook of medical statistics*. 11th ed. London: Hodder and Stoughton, 1984.

Joint Committee of ABPI, BMA, CSM, and RCGP. Guidelines on postmarketing surveillance. *BMJ* 1988;**296**:399–400.

Phillips I. Good antimicrobial prescribing: aminoglycosides. *Lancet* 1982;**ii**:311–5.

Reynolds EH. Serum levels of anticonvulsant drugs: interpretation and clinical use. *Pharmacol Ther* 1980;**8**:217–35.

Schobben F, van der Kleijn E, Vree TB. Therapeutic drug monitoring of valproic acid. *Ther Drug Monit* 1980;**2**:61–71

Swinscow TDV. *Statistics at square one*. 9th ed. London: British Medical Association, 1989.

Thomson AH, Brodie MJ. Pharmacokinetic optimisation of anticonvulsant therapy. *Clin Pharmacokinet* 1992;**23**:216–30.

Tyrer SP. Lithium in the treatment of mania. *J Affect Disord* 1985;**8**:251–7

Widdop B, ed. *Therapeutic drug monitoring*. Edinburgh: Churchill Livingstone, 1985.

Woodbury DM, Penry JK, Pippenger CE, eds. *Antiepileptic drugs*. 2nd ed. New York: Raven Press, 1982.

Woodcock AA, Johnson MA, Geddes DM. Theophylline prescribing, serum concentrations and toxicity. *Lancet* 1983;**ii**:610–2.

3 Adverse reactions to drugs

DN BATEMAN, S CHAPLIN

At the beginning of the twentieth century syphilis was the great mimic of systemic disorders. Later, tuberculosis took over this role. Both of these diseases have been tamed by chemotherapy and now 'drugs' head the list of disease simulators.
Committee on Safety of Medicines, 1985[1]

Adverse drug reactions are a great concern of the general public, the pharmaceutical industry, the regulatory authorities, and the professions. It is only recently, however, that the concept that the use of drugs carries a variable but finite risk has become widely accepted. The evaluation of this risk and its relation to the benefits of treatment determine not only whether a drug is developed and licensed but also how widely it will be used. An understanding of the ways in which drug safety is assessed is therefore important in understanding the available information and assessing the risk to individual patients. This chapter reviews the current methods of monitoring adverse reactions and how they have contributed to detecting drug toxicity in recent years.

Classifying adverse reactions

Although several classifications of adverse reactions have been proposed, most are too complex for routine use. The suggestion by Rawlins and Thompson that adverse reactions can be divided into only two categories[2] is therefore welcome and provides a pragmatic basis for understanding drug toxicity.

Adverse reactions may present as an augmented but qualitatively normal response to a drug (type A) or as a bizarre, unexpected response (type B).

TYPE A

Type A reactions occur in patients who are unusually susceptible to the pharmacological action of the drug—examples include

29

- postural hypotension with antihypertensive agents;
- gynaecomastia with dopamine antagonists; and
- diarrhoea with broad spectrum antibiotics.

These reactions are fairly common, have higher incidences at higher doses, and can be predicted from a knowledge of the drug's actions. A reduction in dose will ameliorate the symptoms, which are not usually severe and seldom cause death.

TYPE B

By contrast, type B reactions are usually severe and proportionately more often fatal. They are not related to the drug's known pharmacological effects and do not moderate when the dose is reduced—the drug must be withdrawn. These reactions are often immunologically mediated (for example, anaphylactic shock) or may have a genetic basis (for example, malignant hyperpyrexia and possibly halothane hepatitis), and they are very rare. None the less, the detection of type B reactions often results in the withdrawal of a drug from general use; examples include

- benoxaprofen (hepatorenal syndrome);
- zomepirac (anaphylaxis); and
- zimeldine (adverse neurological effects).

Some well established adverse reactions do not fall easily into this classification because of the severity of the reaction (for example, blood dyscrasias caused by cytotoxic drugs are potentially fatal and severe but are common and dose dependent) or because the mechanism of the reaction has been explained by the pharmacology of the drug (for example, thrombosis induced by oral contraceptives). None the less, the type A-type B classification fits well with the way in which adverse reactions are detected during the development and clinical use of a drug.

Evaluation before marketing

ANIMAL STUDIES

Although it is difficult to draw direct parallels between toxicity in animal models and potential risks to humans, long term animal studies are used to screen for toxicity, carcinogenicity, and teratogenicity. These studies produce an overall picture of the toxicology of a drug and show which organs are at greatest risk of damage induced by drugs. This is linked with pharmacokinetic data to estimate the risk in humans. Mutagenicity studies are completed at an early stage in drug development, but because drugs may also "promote" neoplasms carcinogenicity studies are of long duration (24 months).

Animal studies may occasionally show toxicity at a late stage in a drug's development. For example, proxicromil, under development for the treatment of asthma, was abandoned in 1981 only 10 months before the anticipated marketing date after tests in animals had shown "unexpected findings." Many older drugs were marketed at a time when these studies were not routinely performed. Subsequent investigation may then show—as in the case of the laxative danthron—that the drug is potentially carcinogenic.

VOLUNTEER STUDIES AND CLINICAL TRIALS

By the time a drug is marketed it will usually have been given to fewer than 3000 people, usually in small studies of 100–200 subjects each. This limited experience provides an estimate of the most appropriate dose range, balancing greatest efficacy with the lowest incidence of type A adverse reactions. Subgroups who are particularly at risk are occasionally identified. For example, the elderly were found to have higher blood concentrations of the non-steroidal anti-inflammatory drug, nabumetone, and the maximum daily dose for this group of patients has been set at 1 g. In other cases unexpected but common adverse reactions are identified, and a suitable warning can be included in the data sheet. Nausea and vomiting typically occur in a small proportion of subjects in clinical trials, but almost one third of patients given fluvoxamine developed this reaction.

By the time a drug becomes available for widespread use there is usually no indication of the nature of its type B toxicity. These reactions, which may have an incidence of one in 10 000 or fewer, occur so occasionally during clinical trials that their occurrence may be coincidental and unrelated to drug treatment. It is therefore only after much wider use that very serious adverse reactions to most drugs are detected, and several methods of surveillance after marketing are currently in use.

Surveillance after marketing

There are several methods of monitoring safety when a drug is in general use. Each has its faults and cannot alone fulfil all the

31

requirements of a monitoring system. These can be summarised as:

- speed (detecting new adverse reactions rapidly and responding rapidly when appropriate);
- sensitivity (sufficient to detect rare adverse reactions but not to be overwhelmed by common reactions); and
- scope (of a size that will enable the risk to be measured—for example, by estimating incidence).

CASE REPORTS

The publication of reports of isolated adverse reactions in medical journals has proved to be an important means of detecting new and serious type B toxicity. This method of reporting should allow a quick response, as the reaction is notified very soon after its detection. As Venning has pointed out, however, such reports have not always been assiduously dealt with by regulatory authorities and may remain unvalidated after several years' further use of the drugs.[3]

The sensitivity of case reports is inherently high, as the reporting doctor does not usually have to pick out an important new reaction from among several others. The doctor must, however, recognise that the symptoms are induced by the drug rather than by other factors. The publication of case reports is invariably followed by reports of similar cases, to both the Committee on Safety of Medicines and to the publishing journal, as doctors are alerted about the reaction. This further emphasises the causal—rather than coincidental—link between drug and symptoms, but it confounds the estimation of the incidence of the reaction. Case reports alone provide no information about the population exposed to the drug; at present only correlation with national data on prescribing or sales figures gives an estimate of the risk. It is also difficult to identify from case reports which subgroups of patients are at risk, as even the existence of a few common characteristics in a small sample can bias the data.

Case reports have none the less been the first means by which some of the main type B adverse reactions in recent years have been identified.[3] Practolol was firmly assocated with dermatitis, keratoconjunctivitis, and sclerosing peritonitis 5 years after its introduction in 1970 by letters to the *Lancet* and the *British Medical Journal*. The Committee on Safety of Medicines issued a regulatory warning in 1975, and the drug was withdrawn in 1976. The first case report of part of this syndrome had been published in 1972.[4]

Benoxaprofen, a non-steroidal anti-inflammatory drug, was first marketed in 1980. Clinical trials in nearly 1700 patients had not indicated that the drug was exceptionally toxic, though photosensitivity and onycholysis had been reported in 9% of patients.[5] In 1982 two reports in the *British Medical Journal* highlighted the adverse effects that would eventually result in the drug's withdrawal. Photosensitivity induced by benoxaprofen was found to be due to phototoxicity rather than allergy and was dose dependent:[6] the reaction would therefore occur in all patients given sufficient drug and sunshine, and the true incidence would therefore be greater than the 10% estimated from studies performed before marketing. By this time eight cases of fatal cholestatic jaundice in elderly women had been reported.[7 8] The half life of benoxaprofen was known to be greater in the elderly, and this prompted the Committee on Safety of Medicines initially to vary the product licence to permit a reduced dose in the elderly. Subsequently, however, the large number of case reports in the medical press and to the Committee on Safety of Medicines led to the suspension of the product licence. By this time there were over 3500 reports to the Committee on Safety of Medicines, of which 61 were of fatal reactions.

The publication of case reports is therefore an important alerting system for type B reactions, but publications require validation—preferably but not essentially by controlled studies—to discriminate between coincidence and causality.

COHORT STUDIES

The influence of bias may be minimised by monitoring drugs prospectively and noting the incidence of disease and death in a group of patients treated with drugs compared with that in a control group. Such studies must be large, and they must be continued for many years if they are to detect less common adverse reactions. They are therefore expensive to conduct, and it may be unrealistic to expect that they can be carried out for all drugs. Prescription event monitoring is a type of cohort study that is considered separately below.

The cohorts of patients in these studies may be randomised or non-randomised. In non-randomised studies a treated group is

33

compared with a non-treated "control" population who do not have the condition for which the target drug is indicated. Two of the best known cohort studies of this type are the multicentre cimetidine surveillance study and the Royal College of General Practitioners' oral contraceptives study.

The cimetidine study started in 1978 with a grant from the drug's manufacturers, recruiting almost 10 000 patients and 10 000 controls by identifying prescriptions for cimetidine in four centres in the United Kingdom. Its results have largely substantiated the safety of cimetidine in routine use but have done little to resolve the controversy surrounding the drug's association with impotence.[9 10] This is because the detection of reactions depends on the general practitioner detecting and recording the event in the notes, whereas there is some evidence that men do not readily complain of impotence.[11] This study does not seem to have detected any new adverse reactions to cimetidine.

The Royal College of General Practitioners study began in 1968, recruiting 46 000 women and 1400 general practitioners. Again the detection of reactions depends on symptoms being reported to the doctor and might therefore underestimate the incidence of symptoms about which patients might be sensitive (for example, the effects on libido). This study has, however, quantified the risk of many serious type B adverse effects, notably cardiovascular disease[12] and higher than normal death rate.[13]

Cohort studies may also be randomised, when the drug under investigation is also indicated in the control population but they receive a placebo instead. The best known example of this approach is the World Health Organization's study of the prevention of ischaemic heart disease by clofibrate.[14] This trial identified 47% more deaths during treatment in the group given clofibrate, but this increased death rate disappeared when the drug was withdrawn.[15] The suspicion that treatment with clofibrate directly caused these deaths is therefore strong, though the mechanism remains unclear.

Cohort studies are therefore an excellent—if slow and expensive—method of measuring and, in some cases, identifying the more common types of drug toxicity. Although they show an association between a drug and symptoms, they do not necessarily prove a causal link, and most are too small to detect type B reactions reliably.

PRESCRIPTION EVENT MONITORING

This method of detecting adverse reactions, developed by the Drug Surveillance Research Unit in Southampton, differs from other systems of surveillance after marketing but is a type of cohort study. Patients who have received specific drugs are identified from prescriptions supplied by the Prescription Pricing Authority. Each general practitioner is then asked to report (on a form provided) any adverse events that were detected (that is, warranted an entry in the patient's notes) while the drug was being taken. The response rates of general practitioners have been between 50 and 75%.

Two advantages are claimed for prescription event monitoring over other surveillance methods. Firstly, the emphasis on detecting "events" rather than "reactions" obviates the need for judgement by the general practitioner about a causal link between drug and effect. This ought to enhance the detection of new adverse reactions and of diseases that are only rarely associated with drugs, and it should favour the detection of type B reactions. Secondly, the incidence of events can be calculated, as the number of prescriptions and events is known accurately. This method estimates the incidence of all events in the cohort of identified patients, but these data must be compared with those from a matched control group before the incidence of the events that are actually induced by the drug can be estimated reliably. Reports of prescription event monitoring suggest that patients are being used as their own controls by comparing the incidence of events during and after treatment with the drug.[16–18] This method, however, means that intercurrent illness or treatment with other drugs confounds interpretation of the data.

The system is claimed to be capable of detecting events that have an incidence of one in 5000, a sensitivity between that of clinical trials and the yellow card system (see below). As most cohorts have contained 10 000–15 000 patients, however, the detection of an excess of two to three cases above the normal incidence of symptoms is difficult. The duration of monitoring individual drugs by prescription event monitoring may also be too short to identify some type B reactions. For example, the average duration of treatment with benoxaprofen was $8\frac{1}{2}$ months in patients who developed the hepatorenal syndrome, whereas treatment in those monitored by prescription event monitoring lasted for 7 months.[19]

More recently prescription event monitoring identified a new event associated with enalapril.[20] In a population of 12 500 patients monitored for 1 year 19 patients developed deafness. This is in excess of the five patients who were expected to develop deafness (though a control group was not defined). This has not been validated by other work.

CASE-CONTROL STUDIES

When a type B adverse reaction has been identified its association with a drug is often investigated by a case-control study. In this retrospective method patients who have the identified disease—for example, breast cancer—are matched with a control group who are similar in potentially confounding factors (for example, smoking and parity) but who do not have the disease. The drug histories of the two groups are compared, and a significant excess of drug takers in the group with the disease may be evidence for a causal link with the drug.

Case-control studies have been used widely in evaluating the link between oral contraceptives and various cancers. This method is ideal under these circumstances because, like other type B reactions, cancer induced by drugs is rare, and huge numbers would have to be recruited to a cohort study to provide meaningful data. Further, cancer induced by drugs takes many years to become apparent, and the expense of a cohort study would be considerable. By contrast, the case-control study is relatively quick to carry out and much cheaper.

The findings of some case-control studies have, however, been controversial and contradictory. Some show an association between oral contraceptives and breast cancer,[21 22] whereas others consistently do not.[23 24] Different conclusions have been formed depending on the age of the patients recruited; some methods of identifying controls (for example, by random telephone dialling) have been criticised; and attempts to analyse the risks of different doses of hormones have been unsuccessful. There is less disagreement over the results of some other studies. The association between oral contraceptives and cervical cancer is now accepted, though the level of risk is still not clear, and the apparent protective effects against endometrial and ovarian cancer seem to be undisputed.

The association between aspirin and Reye's syndrome has been explored by no fewer than five case-control studies in the United

States, and each has shown a consistent association between the drug and the syndrome. Although design and conduct of these studies have been criticised, the consensus of their conclusions has provided good evidence for a rare but serious adverse reaction to aspirin that occurs in only a subgroup of the population.[25] A prospective study in the United Kingdom suggests that the epidemiology of Reye's syndrome in this country differs from that in the United States, but these studies formed the basis of the Committee on Safety of Medicines' recommendation to prohibit paediatric formulations of aspirin.[26]

Case-control studies therefore provide valuable information about the incidence of type B adverse reactions and the association between drugs and disease. There are, however, important problems in their interpretation that require careful consideration.

YELLOW CARDS

Spontaneous reporting of adverse reactions to drugs to a central body was introduced in the United Kingdom in 1964 after the establishment of the Dunlop Committee, later the Committee on Safety of Medicines. This scheme is familiar to most doctors and dentists in the United Kingdom, but fewer than 20% have ever completed a yellow card, and it is estimated that only about 10% of serious and fatal adverse reactions are reported to the Committee on Safety of Medicines. Despite these problems the yellow card system has provided some important data about drug safety and toxicity.

The principle of the system is that doctors will report suspected, not necessarily proved, adverse reactions to the Committee on Safety of Medicines. For older drugs the Committee is particularly interested in severe, usually type B, reactions, but for newly introduced drugs (marked with a ▼ in the *British National Formulary*) doctors are asked to report all suspected adverse reactions. The yellow cards therefore provide a large database of case reports drawn from the population of the country, and the system can detect both type A and B reactions.

The yellow card system has the potential to record unusual, unexpected, adverse effects not detected in clinical trials and, by correlation with prescribing data, to estimate the incidence of these reactions. Thus in the case of the angiotensin converting enzyme inhibitors captopril and enalapril, the yellow card system identified the risk of urticaria and confirmed the occurrence of cough, which had first been documented in case reports.

The system can also be used to examine the epidemiology of adverse reactions. It has to be assumed that the reporting rate does not differ for different subgroups of patients, and additional data on prescribing patterns are also required, usually from a commercial source. The population at risk is usually estimated from the number of prescriptions but this is an inaccurate denominator, making no distinction between "first" and "repeat" prescriptions. Furthermore, reporting rates tend to decline the longer a drug has been on the market, and comparisons among drugs must be made using data drawn from a comparable period, usually the first 5 years of marketing. This information is none the less valuable in formulating the Committee's recommendations on the regulation of drugs to the licensing authority.

An example of the use of these data to make regulatory decisions is the assessment of the risk of toxicity of non-steroidal anti-inflammatory drugs. The decisions to suspend the product licences of osmosin and benoxaprofen were based partly on the very high number of reports of type A and type B reactions per million prescriptions for these drugs compared with other drugs in this class. It is also possible to establish which drug in a therapeutic group is the least toxic. For example, ibuprofen seems from the data from yellow cards to be the safest anti-inflammatory drug, and the decision to license it as an over the counter medicine was based largely on these data.

The information from yellow cards can also be used to examine the risks of subsets of the population. By this method the elderly were identified as being particularly at risk of bone marrow toxicity from co-trimoxazole but not from other antibiotics.[27] By contrast, the young, and girls in particular, are at greatest risk of acute dystonic reactions to the dopamine receptor antagonists metoclopramide, prochlorperazine, and haloperidol.[28 29] This finding prompted a prospective study which showed that the risk with metoclopramide was greater than with prochlorperazine in adults.

The yellow card system is relatively inexpensive in terms of the data it generates. Its success depends on the cooperation of doctors and dentists. Attempts to improve reporting rates have included the introduction of yellow cards into the *British National Formulary* and FP10 prescribing pads. The Committee on Safety of Medicines are currently evaluating reporting by hospital pharmacists in a pilot scheme. The yellow cards seem likely to remain the most cost effective method of detecting unusual adverse reactions to drugs.

OTHER TECHNIQUES

Other methods of surveillance after marketing that are under investigation in the United Kingdom include record linkage, in which the health records of a defined population (for example, within a health authority district) can be correlated with data on the use of drugs.

National data on incidence of disease and death can also be scrutinised for trends that may be associated with changes in drug use. Changes in numbers of deaths from asthma in the United Kingdom in the 1960s highlighted the risk of inhalers containing adrenaline. This technique is not very sensitive compared with other methods, but can generate hypotheses for further investigation.

The evaluation of drug safety is complex, and there are many methods by which adverse reactions are detected. Each of these has advantages and failings, and no single system can offer the security that the community now demands.

1 Committee on Safety of Medicines. CSM update. *BMJ* 1985; **291**:46.
2 Rawlins MD, Thompson JW. Pathogenesis of adverse drug reactions. In: Davies DM, ed. *Textbook of adverse drug reactions*. Oxford: Oxford University Press, 1977:10–31.
3 Venning GR. Identification of adverse reactions to new drugs. II. How were 18 important adverse reactions discovered and with what delays? *BMJ* 1983;**286**:289–92.
4 Rowland MGM, Stevenson CJ. Exfoliative dermatitis and practolol. *Lancet* 1972;**ii**: 1130.
5 Mikulaschek WM. Long-term safety of benoxaprofen. *J Rheumatol* 1980; suppl 6:100–8.
6 Hindson C, Daymond T, Diffey B, Lawlor F. Side effects of benoxaprofen. *BMJ* 1982;**284**:1368–9.
7 Goudie BM, Birnie GF, Watkinson G *et al*. Jaundice associated with the use of benoxaprofen. *Lancet* 1982;**i**:959
8 Taggart HMcA, Alderdice JM. Fatal cholestatic jaundice in elderly patients taking benoxaprofen. *BMJ* 1982;**284**:1372.
9 Colin-Jones DG, Langman MJS, Lawson DH, Vessey MP. Post-marketing surveillance of the safety of cimetidine: twelve-month morbidity report. *Q J Med* 1985;**215**:253–68.
10 Colin-Jones DG, Langman MJS, Lawson DH, Vessey MP. Postmarketing surveillance of the safety of cimetidine: mortality during second, third, and fourth years of follow up. *BMJ* 1985;**291**:1084–8.

11 Peden NR, Cargill JM, Browning MCK, Sanders JHB, Wormsley KG. Male sexual dysfunction during treatment with cimetidine. *BMJ* 1979;**i**:659.

12 Layde PM, Ory HW, Beral V, Kay CR. Incidence of arterial disease among oral contraceptive users. *J R Coll Gen Pract* 1983;**33**:75–82.

13 Layde PM, Beral V, Kay CR. Further analyses of mortality in oral contraceptive users. *Lancet* 1981;**i**:541–6.

14 Committee of Principal Investigators. A co-operative trial in the prevention of ischaemic heart disease using clofibrate. *Br Heart J* 1978;**40**:1069–118.

15 Committee of Principal Investigators. WHO cooperative trial on primary prevention of ischaemic heart disease with clofibrate to lower serum cholesterol: final mortality follow-up. *Lancet* 1984;**ii**:600–4.

16 Drug Surveillance Research Unit. *PEM News*. Vol 1. Southampton: University of Southampton, 1983.

17 Drug Surveillance Research Unit. *PEM News*. Vol 2. Southampton: University of Southampton, 1984.

18 Drug Surveillance Research Unit. *PEM News*. Vol 3. Southampton: University of Southampton, 1985.

19 Rawlins MD. Postmarketing surveillance of adverse reactions to drugs. *BMJ* 1984;**288**:879–80.

20 Inman WHW, Rawson NSB. Deafness with enalapril and prescription event monitoring. *Lancet* 1987;**i**:872.

21 Pike MC, Henderson BE, Krailo MD, Duke A, Roy S. Breast cancer in young women and use of oral contraceptives: possible modifying effect of formulation and age. *Lancet* 1983;**ii**:926–30.

22 Meirik O, Lund E, Adami H-O, Bergstrom R, Christofferson T, Bergsjo P. Oral contraceptive use and breast cancer in young women. *Lancet* 1986;**ii**:650–4.

23 Centers for Disease Control Cancer and Steroid Hormone Study. Long-term oral contraceptive use and the risk of breast cancer. *JAMA* 1983;**249**:1591–5.

24 Cancer and Steroid Hormone Study of the Centers for Disease Control and the National Institute of Child Health and Human Development. Oral contraceptive use and the risk of breast cancer. *N Engl J Med* 1986;**315**:405–11.

25 Smith JM. Aspirin and Reye's syndrome. *Pharm J* 1986;**236**:250–1.

26 Goldberg A. *Letter to doctors, dentists and pharmacists*. London: Committee on Safety of Medicines, 1986.

27 Committee on Safety of Medicines. Deaths associated with co-trimoxazole, ampicillin and trimethoprim. *Curr Probl* 1985;**15**.

28 Bateman DN, Rawlins MD, Simpson JM. Extrapyramidal reactions with metoclopramide. *BMJ* 1985;**291**:930–2.

29 Bateman DN, Rawlins MD, Simpson JM. Extrapyramidal reactions to prochlorperazine and haloperidol in the United Kingdom. *Q J Med* 1986;**59**:549–56.

4 Adverse drug interactions

MARTIN J BRODIE, JOHN FEELY

Adverse drug interactions represent a great "growth industry" in medical publishing. Only a small proportion of reported problems have predictable clinical repercussions, but these still represent more than can be kept readily in mind. In addition, new interactions are being constantly uncovered. An appreciation of the risky drugs, the vulnerable patients, and the pharmacological mechanisms occurring will allow safe navigation through the maze of effective prescribing and will avoid iatrogenic disasters. Some knowledge of the clinical pharmacology of the drugs commonly used is essential. Such information is now readily accessible to all.

Harmful combinations

The prime concern of the prescriber is to treat disease and improve the quality and quantity of life. The past 20 years have witnessed a substantial boom in the development of powerful pharmacological agents that have the potential for harm as well as benefit. In many instances drug combinations will enhance efficacy or limit toxicity. Particular concern has, however, emerged regarding the problem of adverse interactions in which the concerted effects of two therapeutic agents are unintentionally greater or less than the sum of their individual actions. The increasing use of drugs in an aging population that has various degenerative disorders demands a good understanding of pharmacological properties. It is now possible to anticipate many adverse interactions of drugs and to recognise others early before patients suffer from serious toxicity.

Anecdotal case reports and studies in healthy volunteers have shown that many drugs interact. The variability of response among patients will fortunately ensure that only a handful of interactions result in important adverse effects. As no one can be completely familiar with all such eventualities, some selective

41

approach must be used to ensure that major interactions are avoided without precluding the safe and beneficial use of drug combinations. This can be made easier by appreciating the type of drug most likely to cause problems and by identifying patients at greatest risk.

Drugs at risk of interaction

Many of the most effective drugs in clinical practice have a narrow therapeutic ratio. These often affect a vital process such as blood pressure, respiration, or coagulation and have a steep dose-response curve, which ensures that an increase in dose is associated with a similar increment in effect. Others, depending on concentration, produce great toxic effects that may be life threatening—for example, aminoglycosides, cyclosporin, digoxin, lithium, and methotrexate. For a few the more important concern will be reduced efficacy—for example, corticosteroids and cardiac anti-arrhythmics. Phenytoin and theophylline are particularly susceptible to inhibitory interactions, as their metabolic breakdown in the liver is saturable. Table 4.1 lists several categories of risky drugs; many drugs fall into one or more of these categories.

TABLE 4.1—*Drugs at risk of interaction*

Type of effect	Examples of drugs
Major effect on a vital process	Warfarin, chlorpromazine, morphine
Steep dose response curve	Verapamil, levodopa, chlorpropamide
Concentration dependent toxicity	Digoxin, lithium, aminoglycosides, methotrexate
Loss of effect leads to breakthrough of disease	Quinidine, prednisolone, sodium valproate
Patient dependent on prophylactic drug action	Oral contraceptive, cyclosporin
Saturable hepatic metabolism	Phenytoin, ethanol, theophylline

Vulnerable patients

The clinical state of the patient is of paramount importance in anticipating the development of a serious adverse interaction (see table 4.2). Those at greatest risk are the elderly, who are extremely susceptible to the side effects of drugs, particularly those that affect the cardiovascular and central nervous systems. Elderly patients'

TABLE 4.2—*Patients particularly susceptible to drug interactions*

Elderly patients receiving many drugs

Patients who have acute illness—for example, severe anaemia, left ventricular failure, status asthmaticus, pneumonia

Patients who have unstable disease—for example, epilepsy, diabetes mellitus, cardiac arrhythmia, dementia

Patients dependent on drug treatment—for example, transplant recipients or those with connective tissue disorder or Addison's disease

Patients who have considerable renal or hepatic impairment—for example, cirrhosis, congestive cardiac failure, uraemia

Patients who have more than one prescribing doctor

comprehension is often poor, and many take several drugs. Many have degenerative disorders affecting several systems and have impaired compensatory homoeostatic mechanisms.

Most patients who are severely ill receive several drugs, and it may be difficult to distinguish iatrogenic toxicity from the symptoms and signs of the underlying disease. Patients who have cardiac failure, severe anaemia, hepatic precoma, or early dementia may have little leeway for further deterioration if a new clinical problem develops. Unstable conditions such as paroxysmal cardiac arrhythmias, brittle diabetes, or intractable epilepsy may be exacerbated by an adverse interaction that would have minimal consequences in another less vulnerable patient.

A reduced therapeutic effect of concurrent treatment may be of particular concern if a dangerous pathological process such as malignancy or vasculitis is being suppressed. Similarly, the patient's health may depend on uninterrupted steady state drug concentrations—for example, hydrocortisone or oral contraceptives. A disease affecting the liver or kidneys, the main organs responsible for eliminating drugs from the body, will increase the likelihood of drug interaction. Intercurrent viral hepatitis or pneumonic illness may also increase the susceptibility of a patient to adverse effects from a combination of drugs previously well tolerated.

When a patient's clinical condition changes, particularly if he or she is severely ill or elderly, all drug treatment should be reviewed as a matter of course. Some doctors are unaware of the totality of their patients' treatment, particularly when there is more than one potential prescriber—for example, the hospital clinic and the general practitioner. Patients should be questioned carefully about all the drugs they are taking, including those bought over the counter, herbal remedies, and alcohol consumption.

Mechanisms of drug interaction

The impossibility of remembering all the clinically important interactions may be considerably offset by appreciating the mechanisms by which drugs can interact. Link this to a basic knowledge of the pharmacology of the commonly prescribed drugs, and most known interactions may be predicted or recognised and new ones anticipated. Such an understanding will also facilitate the correct clinical decision when a problem does arise. Adverse drug interactions may be subdivided conveniently into those caused by the pharmacokinetics of the affected drug and those influencing the pharmacodynamic response to it.

PHARMACOKINETIC INTERACTIONS

Pharmacokinetic interactions may take place at any stage of absorption, distribution, metabolism, or excretion. Those caused by drug formulations or parenteral incompatibilities are outside the scope of this chapter. Because of the considerable variation among patients in the extent of change in drug concentrations, only a small proportion of patients receiving the combination are likely to suffer serious clinical consequences.

Absorption

Most drug interactions in the gut lumen result in decreased absorption. Antacids containing divalent or trivalent cations will form insoluble complexes with some drugs such as tetracycline, iron, and prednisolone. The anion exchange resin cholestyramine binds acidic drugs such as digoxin, thyroxine, and warfarin. Iron salts can interfere with the absorption of penicillamine, and sucralfate has been shown to reduce the bioavailability of phenytoin. These interactions depend on the simultaneous presence of both drugs in the stomach and can be avoided by separating doses by at least 2 h.

As most drugs are maximally absorbed in the upper small bowel, anticholinergics, tricyclic antidepressants, and opioids will delay gastric emptying and thus will reduce the time to and extent of the peak plasma concentration of a drug given concurrently. This is clinically relevant only if a rapid high peak concentration is important—for example, as with analgesics and antibiotics. Drugs that damage the mucosa—for example, cytotoxic agents—may reduce the absorption of phenytoin and digoxin. A few women who take a low dose combination oral contraceptive may be put at risk of pregnancy by concurrent administration of a broad spectrum antibiotic such as ampicillin or tetracycline (but not co-trimoxazole). The mechanism is thought to include disruption of the enterohepatic cycling of the oestrogenic component by removing the bacteria in the gut responsible for its deconjugation. Erythromycin increases the absorption of cyclosporin, the bioavailability of which is almost doubled. The mechanism is not known.

Enzyme induction

A few therapeutic agents bind to intracellular receptors in several organs—most importantly the liver—to stimulate the production of enzymes that metabolise drugs (see table 4.3). As protein synthesis is required, the maximum effect is not seen for up to 3 weeks. This results in accelerated metabolism of the induced drug, with a reduction in its circulating concentration and a probable weakening of the pharmacological effect. The most powerful inducers in widespread clinical use are the antibiotic

TABLE 4.3—*Some enzyme inducers and inhibitors in clinical use*

Inducers	Inhibitors	
Barbiturates	Allopurinol	Miconazole
Carbamazepine	Amiodarone	Nortriptyline
Dichloralphenazone	Azapropazone	Oral contraceptives
Ethanol (chronic)	Chloramphenicol	Oxyphenbutazone
Glutethimide	Chlorpromazine	Perphenazine
Griseofulvin	Cimetidine	Phenylbutazone
Meprobamate	Ciprofloxacin	Primaquine
Phenobarbitone	Dextropropoxyphene	Propranolol
Phenytoin	Diltiazem	Quinidine
Primidone	Disulfiram	Sodium valproate
(phenobarbitone)	Ethanol (acute)	Sulphinpyrazone
Rifampicin	Erythromycin	Sulphonamides
Sulphinpyrazone	Fluconazole	Tamoxifen
	Imipramine	Thioridazine
	Isoniazid	Trimethoprim
	Ketoconazole	Verapamil
	Metoprolol	Viloxazine
	Metronidazole	

rifampicin and the anticonvulsants phenobarbitone, phenytoin, carbamazepine, and primidone (metabolised in part to phenobarbitone). Lipid soluble drugs whose effects are essential for the patient's continued well being are the prime target for such interactions. Examples include oral contraceptives, warfarin, corticosteroids, and cyclosporin (fig 4.1).

Induction interactions have been reported with many other drugs, and these are eminently predictable, and thereby avoidable, problems. When an inducing agent is withdrawn the process goes into reverse, with a decline in the number of enzymes and a gradual increase in the drug concentration if dosage is not altered. This is the explanation for haemorrhage in patients treated with warfarin and in whom treatment with an enzyme inducer has just been stopped.

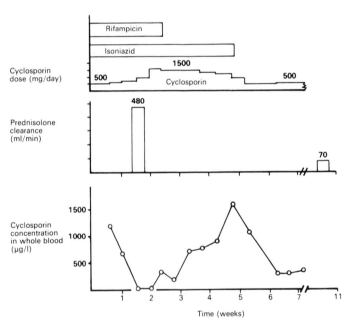

FIG 4.1—Effect of treatment with rifampicin on prednisolone metabolism and circulating cyclosporin concentrations in a patient with a transplanted kidney. (Taken from Langhoff E, Madsen S. Rapid metabolism of cyclosporin and prednisone in kidney transplant patients on tuberculostatic treatment. *Lancet* 1983;**ii**:1303.)

Enzyme inhibition

Most inhibitory interactions also affect hepatic enzymes. Many compounds have the potential for interfering with the metabolism of other drugs, usually by competing for binding sites on the appropriate enzymes (see table 4.3). Because this is a direct effect the time course is usually faster than for enzyme induction. A new steady state concentration of the inhibited drug will be achieved after five half lives, though side effects may be apparent before then. The most dangerous inhibitors are likely to be prescribed for ill patients who have intercurrent problems and who are already receiving other powerful drugs capable of causing concentration dependent toxic effects. These include antibiotics such as erythromycin and co-trimoxazole, cimetidine, and dextropropoxyphene (in co-proxamol). Commonly affected drugs are warfarin, phenytoin, carbamazepine, theophylline, and the sulphonylureas.

A more specific interaction is seen with inhibition by allopurinol of the xanthine oxidase enzymes responsible for most of the metabolism of azathioprine and 6-mercaptopurine. Sulphinpyrazine has the peculiar property of inhibiting the metabolism of some drugs—for example, phenytoin and warfarin—while inducing that of others such as theophylline. When an inhibitor is withdrawn the circulating concentration of the affected drug will decrease, with a potential loss of therapeutic efficacy (fig 4.2). Although less predictable than induction interactions, problems with metabolic inhibition can also be readily recognised and appropriate action taken.

First pass metabolism

A few drugs are biodegraded extensively as they pass through the gut wall and liver. Less than 30% of a dose reaches the systemic circulation as, for example, with propranolol, amitriptyline, chlorpromazine, and verapamil. These drugs may compete for binding sites on metabolic enzymes and increase each other's bioavailability—for example, chlorpromazine and propranolol. The best example of an interaction resulting from interference with first pass metabolism concerns the inhibition of tyramine breakdown in the gut wall by non-selective monoamine oxidase inhibitors such as phenelzine and tranylcypromine. The resultant severe hypertension, initially known as the "cheese reaction," was responsible for several fatal cases of cerebral haemorrhage in the

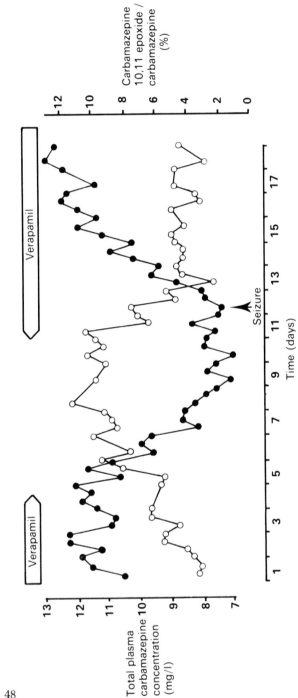

FIG 4.2—Serial plasma carbamazepine concentrations (●) and carbamazepine-10,11 epoxide:carbamazepine ratios (○) in a patient with refractory epilepsy during verapamil withdrawal and restoration. (Taken from Macphee GJA, McInnes GT, Thompson GG, Brodie MJ. Verapamil potentiates carbamazepine neurotoxicity: a clinically important inhibitory interaction. *Lancet* 1986;i:700–3.)

1960s. Monoamine oxidase inhibitors also reduce the metabolism of noradrenaline in the nervous system, further potentiating the sympathetic overactivity responsible for the symptoms and signs. The newer, more selective monoamine oxidase inhibitors such as selegiline are not implicated in this type of interaction.

Displacement of protein binding

When a drug is displaced from its binding sites on plasma proteins there is a transient increase in free concentration, which is offset almost immediately by distribution among the tissues. A compensatory increase in metabolism or excretion ensures that the new steady state free concentration differs little from that before the displacing drug was added. The total drug concentration decreases to accommodate the increase in the free fraction. The overall pharmacological effect is minimal unless the displacement is accompanied by metabolic inhibition. This double mechanism explains why phenylbutazone potentiates the anticoagulation effect of warfarin and why the addition of sodium valproate can produce phenytoin toxicity.

Renal excretion interactions

Only a few drugs are sufficiently soluble in water to rely on renal excretion as their main mode of elimination. Interference with this process is particularly well described for interactions that affect digoxin and lithium. Quinidine, verapamil, and amiodarone may all as much as double the serum concentration of digoxin. Thiazide diuretics and to a lesser extent frusemide and bumetanide reduce the excretion of lithium by increasing its reabsorption from the proximal tubules. Non-steroidal anti-inflammatory drugs (except for aspirin and sulindac), and angiotensin converting enzyme inhibitors hinder the excretion of lithium and so increase the circulating concentration. These are potentially dangerous interactions, as the nephrotoxicity produced may further reduce the elimination of lithium, and a spiralling cycle can result in life threatening intoxication.

Weak acids and bases compete for separate renal tubular transport systems. This is the basis for the use of probenecid to increase circulating concentrations of a penicillin or cephalosporin. Probenecid also potentiates methotrexate toxicity, and cimetidine reduces the excretion of procainamide in the same way. Aspirin also reduces the excretion of methotrexate.

PHARMACODYNAMIC INTERACTIONS

Pharmacodynamic interactions are less readily classified than those affecting drug concentrations, but they are in the main more predictable from the pharmacological actions of the drugs affected. They often provide fascinating and unexpected insights into the mode of action of a drug or the pathophysiology of a disease state. Several overlapping mechanisms may operate.

Synergism

The most common type of interaction is synergism between two drugs acting on the same system, organ, cell, or enzyme. All drugs that have a depressant function on the central nervous system—for example, ethanol, antihistamines, benzodiazepines, phenothiazines, methyldopa, clonidine, et cetera—may accentuate each other's sedative action. All non-steroidal anti-inflammatory agents reduce the adhesiveness of platelets and may potentiate the anticoagulation effects of warfarin. They can also provoke bleeding in the stomach. This interaction is not related to the inconsequential displacement of protein binding, which is often blamed. The antihistamines terfenadine and astemizole may rarely cause arrhythmias. This tendency is greatly enhanced when used with other arrhythmogenic drugs such as antiarrhythmics, antipsychotics and tricyclic antidepressant drugs. Potassium supplements can cause dangerous hyperkalaemia in patients already treated with potassium sparing diuretics, such as amiloride and spironolactone, or angiotensin converting enzyme inhibitors, such as captopril and enalapril. In a similar manner verapamil and propranolol, both of which have negative inotropic properties, can precipitate cardiac failure in a susceptible patient.

Antagonism

Opportunities for competitive antagonism abound in clinical practice. Some are obvious—for example, β agonists and blockers, adenosine and aminophylline, vitamin K and warfarin, thiazide diuretics and hypoglycaemic agents. Others are more esoteric, such as the abolition of the ulcer healing effect of carbenoxolone by spironolactone and the reduction of the sedative effects of benzodiazepines by theophylline. A classic example of antagonism results in the suppression of the bactericidal activity of penicillins (which act on dividing bacteria) by tetracycline, which reduces

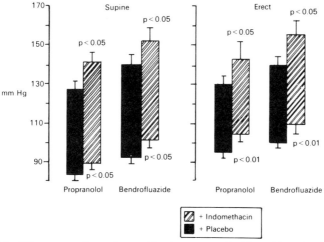

FIG 4.3—Effects on supine and erect blood pressures of adding either placebo or indomethacin to treatment with propranolol or bendrofluazide. (Taken from Watkins J, Abbott EC, Hensby CN, Webster J, Dollery CT. Attenuation of hypotensive effect of propranolol and thiazide diuretics by indomethacin. *BMJ* 1980;**281**:702–5.)

bacterial protein synthesis and hence growth. The reversal of the hypotensive effects of thiazide diuretics and β blockers by non-steroidal anti-inflammatory agents suggests a local renal mode of action mediated by prostaglandins for these antihypertensive agents (fig 4.3).

Indirect receptor effects

Drug combinations may act by an interplay of receptor effects that include physiological or biochemical control loops. Non-selective β blockers such as propranolol may prolong the duration of hypoglycaemia in a diabetic patient treated with insulin by inhibiting the compensatory breakdown of glycogen. This is mediated by β_2 receptors, and cardioselective agents such as atenolol or metoprolol are less likely to provoke such a response. This interaction is much less important than the masking of the sympathetically mediated warning signs of hypoglycaemia such as tachycardia and tremor, which occur with all these drugs.

An indirect receptor effect may also be responsible for the neurotoxicity (lethargy, confusion, and ataxia) reported in some patients treated with lithium and prescribed a neuroleptic, methyldopa, or carbamazepine. The potentiation of "first dose" hypotension with prazosin and withdrawal hypertension with clonidine by pretreatment with a β blocker are probable consequences of unopposed peripheral α adrenergic stimulation.

Cellular transport systems

Drugs that act by using physiological transport systems offer a rich source of potential interactions. The antihypertensive effect of the little used adrenergic neurone blockers (guanethidine, bethanidine, and debrisoquine) may be reversed by tricyclic antidepressants that block their uptake by neurones. Other drugs that interact with these antihypertensives include neuroleptics and indirectly acting sympathomimetics such as ephedrine, phenylpropanolamine, and phenylephrine, often found in proprietary cough and cold mixtures. Tricyclic antidepressants also antagonise the hypotensive effect of clonidine and guanfacine, probably by preventing their uptake into adrenergic nerves.

Fluid and electrolyte disturbance

A reduction in the serum concentration of potassium after treatment with diuretics, corticosteroids, or amphotericin will increase the risk of cardiotoxicity with digitalis and of ventricular arrhythmias with some antiarrhythmic drugs such as sotalol, quinidine, procainamide, and amiodarone. Loop diuretics such as frusemide may increase renal concentrations of nephrotoxic drugs like gentamicin and cephaloridine. The successful treatment of congestive cardiac failure may improve the metabolising capacity of the liver and thereby hasten the elimination of lipid soluble drugs that the patient is already receiving.

Over the counter drugs and alcohol

Drugs bought over the counter are known to be used by most patients. Interactions with sympathomimetics found in cold cures, non-steroidal anti-inflammatory drugs such as ibuprofen and aspirin, and antihistamines have already been discussed.

Alcohol has a variable effect on drug metabolism. Circulating concentrations inhibit the biotransformation of many lipid soluble agents, and chronic excess results in enzyme induction. Synergistic respiratory depression occurs with other psychoactive drugs, particularly chlormethiazole. A disulfiram-like reaction (flushing, headache, palpitations, tachycardia, nausea, and vomiting) may be produced in patients who are receiving chlorpropamide, metronidazole, or some cephalosporins. Alcohol may also have short term effect in reducing the standing blood pressure, but heavy consumption produces transient hypertension. These properties make it a dangerous drug for hypertensive patients, especially those receiving drug treatment.

Conclusions

Drug interactions are ubiquitous but only rarely result in major adverse repercussions for the patient. In assessing their probable clinical relevance three factors need to be considered: the number of reports; the quality of documentation; and (most importantly) the degree of variation in outcome among patients. Thus one patient may show little effect, whereas another may manifest a catastrophic life threatening interaction with the same combination of drugs.

An understanding of the pharmacology of the drugs concerned will make the difficult task of avoidance easier. Aides memoire in the form of charts, textbooks, and computer programs will identify well recognised interactions, but as the number of potential pitfalls with old and new agents is limitless, constant vigilance is required. Fortunately it is possible to anticipate an unwanted effect with several drugs that pose a particular risk either by measuring their circulating concentrations—for example, anticonvulsants, theophylline, digoxin, and lithium—or by monitoring their pharmacological effects—for example, anticoagulants, antihypertensives, and hypoglycaemic agents. The early clinical detection of an adverse interaction greatly reduces the risk of serious toxicity.

Thought is required before altering treatment, particularly in an ill or elderly patient receiving several powerful therapeutic agents. Constant suspicion of an iatrogenic cause for any deterioration in symptoms or signs will ensure that an adverse interaction is not overlooked.

Aarons L. Kinetics of drug-drug interactions. *Pharmacol Ther* 1981;4:321–44.
Amdisen A. Lithium and drug interactions. *Drugs* 1982;24:133–9.
Aronson JK, Grahame-Smith DG. Adverse drug interactions. *BMJ* 1981;282:288–91.

Balis FM. Pharmacokinetic drug interactions of commonly used anticancer drugs. *Clin Pharmacokinet* 1986;**11**:223–35.

Bint AJ, Burt I. Adverse antibiotic drug interactions. *Drugs* 1980;**20**:57–68.

Breckenridge AM, Back DJ, Orme ML'E. Interactions between oral contraceptives and other drugs. *Pharmacol Ther* 1979;**7**:617–26.

Brodie MJ. Drug interactions in epilepsy. *Epilepsia* 1992;**33**(suppl 1)S13–S22.

Brodie MJ. Adverse drug interactions. In: Beattie AD, Ireland J, eds. *Emergencies in medicine*. London: Pitman Medical 1984: 80–90.

Brodie MJ, Harrison PI. *Practical prescribing*. Edinburgh: Churchill Livingstone, 1986

Buckley M, Feely J. Antagonism of the antihypertensive effect of guanfacine by tricyclic antidepressants. *Lancet* 1991;**337**:1173.

Cadwallader DS. *Biopharmaceutics and drug interactions*. New York: Raven Press, 1983.

Caranasos GJ, Stewart RB. Clinically desirable drug interactions. *Annu Rev Pharmacol Toxicol* 1985;**25**:67–95.

Crook JE, Nies AS. Drug interactions with antihypertensive drugs. *Drugs* 1978;**15**:72–9.

D'Arcy PF, McElnay JC. Drug interactions involving the displacement of drugs from plasma protein and tissue binding sites. *Pharmacol Ther* 1982;**17**:210–20.

Griffin JP. D'Arcy PF. *A manual of adverse drug interactions*. Bristol: John Wright, 1979.

Grogono AW, Seltzer JL. A guide to drug interactions in anaesthetic practice. *Drugs* 1980;**19**:279–91.

Hansen JM, Christensen LK. Drug interactions with oral sulphonylurea hypoglycaemic drugs. *Drugs* 1977;**13**:24–34.

Hansten PD. *Drug interactions*. Philadelphia: Lea and Febiger, 1985.

Hayes AH. Therapeutic implications of drug interactions with acetominophen and aspirin. *Arch Intern Med* 1981;**141**:301–4.

Hoyumpa AM, Schenker S. Major drug interactions: effect of liver disease, alcohol and malnutrition. *Annu Rev Med* 1982;**33**:113–49.

Hurwitz A. Antacid therapy and drug kinetics. *Clin Pharmacokinet* 1979;**2**:269–80.

Kendall MJ, Beeley L. Beta-adrenoceptor blocking drugs: adverse reactions and drug interactions. *Pharmacol Ther* 1983;**21**:351–69.

Levy RH, Koch KM. Drug interactions with valproic acid. *Drugs* 1982;**24**:543–56.

McInnes GT, Brodie MJ. Drug interactions that matter—a critical reappraisal. *Drugs* 1988;**36**:83–110.

Park BK, Breckenridge AM. Clinical implications of enzyme induction and enzyme inhibition. *Clin Pharmacokinet* 1981;**6**:1–24.

Perucca E, Richens A. Drug interactions with phenytoin. *Drugs* 1981;**21**:120–7.

Petrie JC. *Clinically important adverse drug interactions*. Vol 1. *Cardiovascular and respiratory disease therapy*. Amsterdam: Elsevier/North Holland Biomedical Press, 1980.

Petrie JC. *Clinically important adverse drug interactions*. Vol 2. *Nervous system, endocrine system and infusion therapy*. Amsterdam: Elsevier/North Holland Biomedical Press, 1984.

Petrie JC. *Clinically important adverse drug interactions*. Vol 3. *Gastrointestinal, haematological and infectious disease therapy*. Amsterdam: Elsevier/North Holland Biomedical Press, 1985.

Ragheb M. Drug interactions in psychiatric practice. *Int Pharmacopsychiat* 1981;**16**:92–118.

Rodighiero V. Therapeutic drug monitoring of cyclosporin. *Clin Pharmacokinet* 1989;**16**:27–37.

Schou JS. Drug interactions and (pharmacodynamically active) receptor sites. *Pharmacol Ther* 1982;**17**:119–210.

Serlin MJ, Breckenridge AM. Drug interactions with warfarin. *Drugs* 1985;**25**:610–20.

Somogyi A, Muirhead M. Pharmacokinetic interactions of cimetidine. *Clin Pharmacokinet* 1987;**12**:321–66.

Stockley I. *Drug interactions and their mechanisms*. London: Pharmaceutical Press, 1981.

Tollefson GD. Monoamine oxidase inhibitors: a review. *J Clin Psychiatry* 1983;**44**:280–8.

Webster J. Interactions of NSAIDS with diuretics and β-blockers: mechanisms and clinical implications. *Drugs* 1985;**30**:32–41.

Welling PG. Interactions affecting drug absorption. *Clin Pharmacokinet* 1984;**9**:404–35.

Wettrell G, Andersson KE. Cardiovascular drugs. II. Digoxin. *Ther Drug Monit* 1986;**8**:129–39.

5 Prescribing for infants and children

GEORGE W RYLANCE

Rational drug treatment for infants and children requires an understanding of the wide variability in drug handling and response in the early years of life. Such understanding without knowledge of the many and varied practical aspects of drug administration during this period is insufficient, however, and treatment therefore depends on a comprehensive theoretical and practical approach to prescribing.

Drug handling

The main changes in drug handling with age occur in the first three or four years of life and particularly in the first few months. The table summarises these changes, which form the basis for altering the dosage for relevant groups of patients who may be affected. Often several determinants of dosage—for example, increased distribution of water soluble drugs in neonates who have diminished excretion—may be altered simultaneously. In some instances these work in opposite directions, producing no overall change in drug concentration.

ABSORPTION

Physiological changes during infancy and childhood have little effect on the rate or extent of gastrointestinal absorption. Though the rate of absorption may be increased by using liquid preparations that do not require any time for dissolution, the widespread use of such preparations in young children has little clinical importance except in the long term use of drugs that are eliminated rapidly—for example, carbamazepine and theophylline. Adverse effects relating to higher peak concentrations, and also reduced control of symptoms or signs owing to lower trough concentrations at the usual intervals between doses, may be more prevalent in the young as a result of this increased rate of absorption.[1] The rate and extent of absorption of drugs administered intramuscularly varies little with age and is far more dependent on other factors—for example, perfusion.[2]

The newborn baby born at full term has a mature skin with barrier properties similar to those of the child or adult. Infants born before 33 weeks of gestation, however, have a poorly developed epidermal barrier, but this has limited therapeutic possibilities owing to the lack of a convenient and reliable method of transdermal drug delivery, though some success has been achieved with theophylline.[3] Modifying the transdermal systems used for delivering nitroglycerine and clonidine may also be useful.

DISTRIBUTION

The total volumes of body water and extracellular fluid related to body weight are greatest during the neonatal period and infancy. These values decrease with age most appreciably during the first three months of life and thereafter more gradually. Water soluble drugs that are distributed mainly in extracellular water therefore have the largest volumes of distribution in newborn and young infants.[4] Furthermore, the blood–brain barrier may be functionally incomplete in neonates, which permits increased penetration by some drugs.

Though there are small differences in the extent of protein binding with age throughout childhood (lower values in neonates and young infants),[2] these are generally not clinically important. The displacement of bilirubin from albumin by sulphonamides and some other drugs in the newborn is well recognised,[5] and it should not be forgotten that the transfer of drugs in breast milk may be a source of inadvertent treatment to the neonate.

BIOTRANSFORMATION

Biotransformation of most drugs proceeds comparatively slowly in the first few weeks of life (table). This is particularly so in preterm infants and relates to the comparative immaturity of the hepatic microsomal enzyme systems.[6 7] Oxidation and glucuronidation are particularly slow. After a few weeks (about 2–12, the time varies according to the process of biotransformation) the rates increase rapidly and remain fairly high for most drugs during the first two or three years of life. After this they reduce gradually until adolescence. There are, however, several exceptions to these

TABLE 5.1—*Pharmacokinetics of drugs in children compared with "normal" adults (↑ = faster or enhanced, ↓ = slower or reduced, ↔ = unchanged)*

	Age of child					
	Newborn preterm	Term (0-4 weeks)	Infancy	1-4 years	5-12 years	Comments
Absorption	↓	↔	↔	↔	↔	No clinical relevance
Distribution:						
Body water	↑↑↑	↑↑	↑	↑	↑	Weight related doses produce lower blood concentrations of water soluble drugs in the neonates
Body fat	↓ ↓	↓ ↓	↓ Slight	?↔	?↔	Minimal clinical effect
Plasma albumin	↓	↓	↓ Slight	↓↔	↔	Minimal clinical effect
Biotransformation:						
Oxidation/hydrolysis	↓ ↓	↓ ↓	↑ ↑ (After some weeks)	↑	↑ Slight	Reduce dosage for neonates and young infants; increased dosage subsequently
N-demethylation	↓ ↓ ↓	↓ ↓	↑ ↑	↑ ↔	↔ ↓	Applies to theophylline, caffeine
Acetylation	↓	↓	↑	←	↔	Reduce dose in neonates—for example, sulphonamides
Conjugation-glucouronidation	↓	↓	↔	↑	↑	Reduce dose in neonates—for example, chloramphenicol
Renal excretion:						
Glomerular filtration	↓ ↓	→ →	→ Slight to 6 months	↓ ↓	↓ ↓	Reduce dose in first few months
Tubular secretion	↓	→	→			

general changes—for example, conjugation by sulphation does not seem to be altered.[8]

EXCRETION

The glomerular filtration rate increases steadily in early infancy to reach "adult" values related to surface area at 2–5 months old. Tubular secretion and reabsorption matures during a similar period.[9] Thus most drugs that are primarily excreted unchanged by the kidney are eliminated more slowly in the first few months of life. Again, this is a particular feature in preterm babies, in whom the glomerular filtration rate may be less than one sixth of that of the normal older child and adult.[10] The reported higher clearance rates of some drugs that are primarily eliminated by the kidney in young children compared with adult rates are probably due to enhanced extrarenal biotransformation (few drugs are totally eliminated by renal excretion). There are therefore considerable differences in the rates of drug biotransformation among infants and children of a similar age but less appreciable differences in the rates of elimination of those drugs that are primarily excreted unchanged by the kidney.

Receptor sensitivity

Differences in the sensitivity of receptors related to age that have been seen in animal studies may also be present in man, but to date this has not been shown. There is, however, indirect evidence of some differences as shown by the higher doses of digoxin, related to weight (or surface area), required in infancy compared with those at other ages. Infants have higher ratios of myocardium to plasma and erythrocyte to plasma concentrations of digoxin.[11]

The paradoxical effects of some drugs (for example, hyperkinesis with phenobarbitone), previously considered to be peculiar to childhood, also occur in some adults and may not represent a difference in drug sensitivity related to age.

Prescribing

The difference in drug handling and response among infants and children of different ages and among children and adults as described above needs to be considered carefully at each stage of prescribing.

59

CHOICE OF DRUG

Though drugs that have been used widely without undue untoward effects for many years may be considered to be the safest, this assumption should be regularly reviewed and questioned. The comparatively recent evidence of the relation between aspirin and some cases of Reye's syndrome supports this approach.[12]

ROUTE OF ADMINISTRATION AND DRUG FORMULATION

Most children aged 5 years or more will successfully take solid preparations. The use of liquids, with a greater chance of spillage and therefore less accurate dosage, is thus inappropriate for an older child. Some liquid preparations still contain sucrose, with no alternative sweetener available. The long term use of medicines that contain sucrose increases the incidence of tooth caries and gingivitis.[13]

Sustained release preparations that reduce fluctuations in drug concentration between doses should be particularly useful in those children who will metabolise drugs rapidly. Young children aged under 4 years, however, who might be expected to benefit most in this respect, cannot generally swallow large solid preparations. Accommodating the needs of young children by crushing or cutting the tablets usually destroys the sustained release properties.

Some liquid medicines and tablets contain dyes and colouring agents. Sensitivity to these—for example, tartrazine—is much commoner in children than in adults, though the number who react adversely is probably small.

Inhalation offers many advantages for drug administration to the respiratory tract, although much of what is known may not be applicable to children. Young children have difficulty in co-ordinating their breathing. A variety of drug delivery devices are available and the following general statements are appropriate:

● Children aged less than 2.5 years can use a metered dose inhaler (MDI) with close fitting soft mask attached to a large volume spacer device

● Children between 2.5 and 5 years can use a large volume spacer and metered dose inhaler with or without a face mask

● Metered dose inhalers without spacer devices are not generally appropriate in children less than 10 years

• A nebuliser may be appropriate for children under 1 year and of other ages.

The topical application of drugs to the skin is appropriate only for skin conditions except possibly for the limited purpose of delivering theophylline to preterm neonates.[3] Inflamed or broken skin is a poor barrier to drug absorption, and topical agents used to treat diseased areas may therefore cause systemic effects. Topical treatment, leading to drug absorption through the skin, may therefore have toxic consequences. Extensive nappy rashes, eczema, and blistered skin conditions are examples of conditions in which the risk of toxicity from the repeated use of topical agents is enhanced. Problems have been reported after the percutaneous absorption of alcohol, iodine, salicylic acid, oestrogens, steroids, hexachlorophene, antibiotics (for example, neomycin), and urea.

Intramuscular injections are often painful. Hydrocortisone, aminophylline, and paraldehyde are particularly irritating. There is generally little advantage in giving drugs by this route. When indicated, and temporary use in a vomiting child may be considered to be an appropriate indication, the quadriceps muscle is the safest site; the upper and outer quarter of the buttock should not be used (the course of the sciatic nerve is more transverse in this area in children than in adults). Babies of low gestational age have little muscle bulk, and intramuscular injection is therefore generally inappropriate in preterm babies.

DOSAGE

The larger volumes of distribution in young children, particularly in the first few months of life, mean that single doses of drugs according to weight need to be comparatively larger at this age to produce similar drug concentrations in the blood. In repeated dosing the total daily doses according to weight vary widely with age. In newborn and particularly preterm infants daily doses of drugs that are metabolised in the liver should be lower, as drug clearance is slow at this age because the microsomal enzymes are immature.[67] After a few weeks the appropriate dose changes rapidly over a fairly short period, so that daily doses according to weight in early infancy are higher than at any other time of life. Subsequently the relative daily dose decreases gradually throughout childhood until it reaches that normal in the adult. Weight related daily doses of drugs that are primarily eliminated by the kidney are similar at all ages after renal function has matured at about 6 months old. Measuring drug concentrations in plasma may provide information useful for determining the appropriate dose and dosage interval. The time taken to reach a steady state is usually shorter for most metabolised drugs after the first few weeks of life because of their shorter half life in children.

Mistakes in administered doses occur in children as in patients of other ages, and some of these relate to difficulties in measurement. Small errors in the volumes of liquids containing drugs at high concentrations particularly those designed for "adult" markets, can be important in the very young.

FREQUENCY OF DOSING

Most hepatically metabolised drugs have a shorter elimination half life in young children. At "standard" intervals between doses that are accepted for adults fluctuations in the drug concentration may be great and clinically unacceptable.[1] For example, children receiving carbamazepine at the same treatment intervals as adults may show evidence of toxicity at peak concentration times and breakthrough convulsions immediately before dosing. Increasing the frequency of dosing during the child's shorter wakeful day (about 12 h) is a compromise that has little effect on the total fluctuation over 24 h.

For drugs for which there is no relation between concentration and effect the frequency of dosing is governed by other considerations. Compliance should be improved by reducing the number of daily doses. Dosing with steroids once a day produces less toxicity than using divided doses.

COMPLIANCE

The definition of compliance used in reported studies varies widely. It is therefore difficult to compare rates of compliance in children with those in other age groups. About one half of children taking long or short term treatment, however, take drugs according to the advice of the prescriber.[14] This rate is similar to that reported in other groups. Most children are not responsible for their own treatment, and the requirement for a third party (usually a parent) and the tendency for young children to refuse to comply at the time of administration might be expected to increase the incidence of poor compliance.

Other aspects of prescribing

NEW DRUGS

The fact that children are growing and developing mentally and physically, and that late adverse effects of drugs are most likely to be seen in those who live for a considerable time after the introduction of new drugs, suggests that additional caution is necessary when treating children with new drugs. The balance between extreme and inappropriate caution and allowing children to be therapeutic orphans and therefore disadvantaged is a fine one.

The problem of restricted "availability" of drugs for children is not limited to new drugs. The regulations governing applications for product licences whereby licences are granted for age groups and indications determined by the applying institution rather than the licence granting body lead to confusion and inconsistency. Dosage guidelines indirectly representing the terms of the product licences may therefore relate to restriction in children under 6 years for some drugs, those under 4 years for others, and under 1 or 2 years for others. Demands for information by the licensing authority should have consistent and appropriate age groups for all drugs and indications submitted – for example 0–4 weeks, 4 weeks up to 1 year, 1–4 years, and 5–12 years.

Consistency in dosage guidelines relating to product licences would reduce some of the confusion and difficulty for the prescriber reading recognised information sources such as the *British National Formulary*[15] and the *Data Sheet Compendium*[16]. However, if doctors are to tell parents and children when and why they are using drugs outside the product licence[17] it is essential that the details of the drug licences are known. Although it is possible to get some idea of the restrictions by absence of recommendations on children's age, special "contraindicated" statements, or those of "not recommended" the terms are not clear. It is usual for most hospital and retail pharmacies to have no knowledge of specific product licence information. If prescribers are to follow advice[17] doctors' prescribing practice would require radical change and its effects would not be predictable—more than one third of drugs used in teaching hospitals are used outside the apparent product licence (personal communication).

INTERACTIONS

Infants and children are apparently no more likely to show the clinical effects of interactions between drugs than other age groups. Though the microsomal enzyme systems of infants and young children have a greater capacity for induction, and neonates and infants have generally less drug protein binding, the effects of interactions that are clinically relevant are few. The apparently lower rates of interaction in children probably reflect the fairly low exposure of children to many of the commonly implicated drug groups and the lower incidence of treatment with multiple drugs at this age. Anticonvulsants, theophylline, and erythromycin are the drugs most likely to be implicated in clinically relevant interactions.

ADVERSE EFFECTS

The incidence of adverse reactions to drugs in newborn infants (25%) is higher than that reported in infants and children, both in hospital and in the community (5·2–12·2%).[18–20] The nature of these adverse effects varies according to the circumstances of drug use. In "everyday" use in the community, the most commonly reported effects are drowsiness, diarrhoea, and abdominal pains.[21] These contrast with rash, drowsiness, vomiting, and suppressed bone marrow activity as the most commonly reported reactions in studies in hospitals. The types of adverse reactions due to prescribed drugs in children in the community are not appreciably different from those due to drugs obtained "over the counter."

DRUGS IN SCHOOLS

Most commonly used drug treatment does not need to be given during school hours. Even for commonly used antibiotics administration three times a day is acceptable for all conditions treatable during continued school attendance. Some drugs, however, need to be used at school, and this presents problems for the child, family, and teachers. Teachers are naturally reluctant to accept third party responsibility for the safe storage and administration of medicine, particularly when they consider the stringent regulations of the similar circumstances of medicine administration to hospital inpatients by nurses. Close liaison among parents, the child, teachers, the school nurse, and the doctor should allow a code of conduct acceptable to all parties to be formulated. Doctors clearly have a responsibility to consider this specific problem when they advise on and prescribe drugs.

1 Rylance GW, Moreland TA, Butcher GM. Carbamazepine dose frequency requirement in children. *Arch Dis Child* 1979;**54**:454–8.
2 Morselli PL, Franco-Morselli R, Bossi L. Clinical pharmacokinetics in newborns and infants. *Clin Pharmacokinet* 1980;**5**:485–527.
3 Evans NJ, Rutter N, Parr G, Hadgraft J. Percutaneous theophylline administration to the preterm neonate. *Br J Clin Pharmacol* 1985;**19**:125P.
4 Friis-Hansen B. Bodywater compartments in children: changes during growth and related changes in body composition. *Pediatrics* 1961;**28**:169–81.
5 Rylance GW. Neonatal pharmacology. In: Roberton NRC, ed. *Textbook of neonatology.* Edinburgh: Churchill Livingstone, 1986:223–38.
6 Aranda JV, MacLeod SM, Renton KW, Eade NR. Hepatic microsomal drug oxidation and electron transport in newborn infants. *J Pediatr* 1974;**85**:534–42.
7 Rane A, Tomson G. Prenatal and neonatal drug metabolism in man. *Eur J Clin Pharmacol* 1980;**18**:9–15.
8 Miller RP, Roberts RJ, Fischer LJ. Acetaminophen elimination kinetics in neonates, children and adults. *Clin Pharmacol Ther* 1976;**19**:284–6.
9 Gladtke E, Heimann G. The rate of development of elimination function in kidney and liver of young infants. In: Morselli PL, Garattini S, Sereni F, eds. *Basic and therapeutic aspects of perinatal pharmacology.* New York: Raven Press, 1975:393–403.
10 Arant B. Developmental patterns of renal function maturation compared in the human neonate. *J Pediatr* 1978;**92**:705–12.
11 Park MK, Ludden T, Arom KV, et al. Myocardial vs serum digoxin concentrations in infants and adults. *Am J Dis Child* 1982;**136**:418–22.
12 Hurwitz ES, Barrett MJ, Bregman D, et al. Public Health Service study on Reye's syndrome and medication. *N Engl J Med* 1985;**313**:849–67.
13 Roberts IF, Roberts GJ. Relation between medicines sweetened with sucrose and dental disease. *BMJ* 1979;ii:14–6.
14 Shope JT. Medication compliance. *Pediatr Clin North Am* 1981;**28**:5–21.
15 Joint Formulary Committee. *British National Formulary* No 26. London: Pharmaceutical Press and British Medical Association, 1993.
16 *Data Sheet Compendium.* Datapharm Publications, 1993.
17 Schutt PK. Some legal considerations in prescribing. *Prescribers Journal* 1991;**31**:27–32.
18 Boston Collaborative Drug Surveillance Programme. Drug surveillance: problems and challenges. *Pediatr Clin North Am* 1972;**19**:117–30.
19 Whyte J, Greenan E. Drug usage and adverse drug reactions in paediatric patients. *Acta Paediatr Scand* 1977;**66**:767–75.
20 Choonara IA, Harris F. Adverse drug reactions in medical patients. *Arch Dis Child* 1984;**59**:578–80.
21 Woods CG, Rylance ME, Cullen RE, Rylance GW. Adverse reactions to drugs in children. *BMJ* 1987;**294**:869–70.

6 Prescribing for the elderly

CAMERON G SWIFT

The growth of information about drugs and prescribing in the elderly in the past 20–25 years has been stimulated by three main factors, which in general still retain their validity.

Firstly, there are the demographic trends, particularly the continually expanding number of people aged over 75, who present a complex range of requirements for health care, including drug treatment.

Secondly, expenditure on drugs for the elderly is proportionately greater. Data from the Prescription Pricing Authority for 1989 show that the number of prescription items per person per year (16.8) for people of pensionable age in Britain was more than three times greater than for the population below that age group (5.3).[1] Furthermore, of the growth in overall annual prescription items of over 50 000 000 during the period 1977–1988, 96% was accounted for by prescriptions to the elderly.

Thirdly, there is a disturbing apparent increase with age in susceptibility to adverse drug reactions. This has been more difficult to show historically but is an undoubted fact of life, particularly with certain drug groups such as several acting on the central nervous system, those with autonomic effects, non-steroidal anti-inflammatory drugs and a variety of cardiovascular compounds. Information has been derived from anecdotal reports, expensive drug surveillance programmes in hospitals, detection systems for adverse drug reactions (such as the yellow card system of the Committee on Safety of Medicines), and reports on samples of selected patients, such as those being admitted to psychiatric units or departments of geriatric medicine.

Underreporting and exploitation

The extent to which age is perceived as conferring increased vulnerability may be positively weighted by the greater extent of prescribing but negatively weighted by a widespread failure to detect and diagnose iatrogenic disease in the elderly and by the underreporting of adverse reactions to regulatory bodies. Such underreporting is particularly likely when the adverse effect can be readily explained as an exaggeration of the drug's main action or one of its known side effects—that is, a type A or dose related effect. Many older people, particularly those who are disabled, tend to become reconciled to less than optimum health; hence neither they nor their carers complain readily, and the more subtle, if debilitating, consequences of iatrogenic disorder are readily overlooked unless prescribers remain alert.

The rapid growth in the numbers of new drugs means that special steps must be taken to protect the interests of this vulnerable and potentially exploitable section of the population, particularly as much pharmaceutical innovation is directly aimed at the relief of longstanding disorders prevalent within this age group rather than at radical short term cure. Equally it is important to ensure that older people have the access they need to effective medication.

This chapter will first, for completeness, outline the main areas of importance that have emerged from research into drugs in the elderly, though there are numerous reviews of the topic.[2-8] Secondly, the possible implications for future prescribing, drug research, and drug development will be discussed.

Defining the problem

Although the issues mentioned above emphasise drug safety, adverse reactions, and what amounts (as far as patients collectively and individually and indeed the health service as a whole are concerned) to rather poor value for money, it is the more positive objectives of rational and effective drug treatment for older people that should be uppermost. The problems are usually subdivided into two categories: "extrinsic" factors (prescribing and drug compliance) and "intrinsic" factors (pharmacokinetics and pharmacodynamics).

PRESCRIBING PATTERNS

Several prescribing difficulties have been highlighted.

Excessive amount

Several studies have identified large numbers of elderly patients each receiving far more drugs than they can reasonably be expected to cope with in a practical way. Equally, the risk of drug interactions causing unwanted effects is positively correlated with the numbers of drugs prescribed.

Inadequate clinical indication

In the context of multiple problems with symptoms, not all require a pharmacological solution, particularly as the ratio of risk to benefit is higher in old age. Treatment without drugs is often insufficiently explored. Extrapolating clinical indications from younger age groups may also be inappropriate. The particular difficulties of accurate diagnosis in the elderly have already been alluded to. In defence of the prescriber, however, reliable data from clinical trials on drug use in the elderly have been scarce.

Excessive duration of treatment

The withdrawal of drug treatment once the original indication has resolved often needs greater initiative and discipline than initial prescribing. A reliable "prompting" process is usually needed, together with the necessary time to counsel the patient to explain and reach agreement on the drug being withdrawn. Excessive repeat prescribing without review has come in for much justifiable criticism. The stockpiling of drugs is more or less universal in all households, and every geriatrician has a favourite photograph of the vast private pharmacies encountered in the homes of older people. There is good evidence that much long term drug treatment may be neither beneficial nor necessary for a proportion of recipients; examples include hypnotics and other psychotropic drugs, diuretics, digoxin, and non-steroidal anti-inflammatory compounds.

Inappropriate dose regimens

Sufficient information now exists about most drugs to enable prescribers to decide on the best regimen for the elderly. Often the dosage is reduced. The message has probably got through about digoxin, but inappropriately high doses of many compounds (for example, antiparkinsonian drugs, β blockers, hypnotics, and anti-depressants) are still commonly prescribed. Complex dose regimens are also given when a simple once or twice daily dosage would be satisfactory and far more manageable.

DRUG COMPLIANCE

Problems of drug compliance are not primarily related to age and are considered later in this book. Doctors dealing with all age groups are becoming increasingly conscious of the problems and are taking the necessary steps to reduce them. These include:

(1) prescribing the minimum number of drugs with the simplest possible regimen;

(2) improving packaging, labelling, and instructions;

(3) identifying patients at high risk: factors include social isolation, severe illness, psychiatric disorder, and long duration of treatment. There is little point in prescribing at all for a patient who has impaired cognitive function or memory unless specific steps are taken to ensure supervision by a third party; and

(4) improving communication: several studies have highlighted the discrepancy between the prescriber's perception of what patients are receiving and their actual drug intake. A simple policy measure at all ages would be to ensure that at every consultation each patient is required to bring all drug supplies along to show the doctor. Such an inspection is probably as important as the clinical examination of the patient.

Absolute compliance can never be achieved, and the benefits of "intelligent non-compliance" in some cases have rightly been defended. The goal of rational treatment, however, requires as sensible a contract of agreement as possible between the prescriber and the patient. To achieve this requires time and patience, and the roles of mechanical aids to compliance and of counselling independent of the prescriber (for example, by pharmacists or district nurses), are undoubtedly worth exploring further.

PHARMACOKINETICS

Table 6.1 summarises the principal changes in drug handling in the elderly. These broad generalisations represent the main thrust of research to date, but the scale of change, the degree of variability among patients, and the degree of clinical importance differ appreciably among compounds.

TABLE 6.1—*Main changes in drug handling in elderly patients*

Absorption of drugs	Drug absorption by passive diffusion is substantially unaltered with age, though may be marginally slower for some compounds
	Oral bioavailability of some drugs may be increased by reduced first pass metabolism in liver or gut
Distribution of drugs	Distribution volume of water soluble compounds decreases
	Distribution volume of lipid soluble compounds increases until extreme age
	Binding to albumin may decrease, especially in ill health
	Reactant phase protein binding shows little change with age in itself
Metabolism of drugs	Microsomal oxidative (phase I) metabolism exhibits variable decrease with age
	Non-microsomal, non-oxidative (phase II) metabolism may also decrease for some compounds, particularly in the frail elderly
	Physical frailty may be an additional determinant of impaired metabolism
Renal excretion of drugs	Renal elimination of drugs is slower in elderly whether by glomerular filtration or tubular secretion

Absorption and bioavailability

Clinically important changes in passive absorption have not so far been described for any compounds, despite the physiological changes (reduced gastric pH, delayed gastric emptying, reduced blood flow in the small intestine) that might be expected to influence this. These include delayed gastric emptying and reduced blood flow to the small intestine. Gastric pH has now been shown to be unchanged in the elderly. The reduction in first pass metabolism for some drugs, however, by allowing increased peak plasma concentrations to occur after oral administration, might contribute to an increased effect after a single dose. This was undoubtedly the case in the early period of levodopa treatment, when the threefold increase in oral bioavailability of the compound, owing to reduced gastric dopadecarboxylase activity, accounted for the large number of reports of severe side effects in the elderly and the widely voiced conclusion that the drug was unsuitable for use in this age group.

Drug distribution

The reported changes in drug distribution are readily explained by the reduction in lean body mass and body water, the increase in body fat, and the reduction in plasma albumin (more especially in the context of ill health) that are known to occur in the elderly. For many drugs such changes seem to be of little immediate clinical importance, save that they may have some effect on the extent and duration of response to a drug after a single dose or, in the case of plasma concentrations used in therapeutic drug monitoring (for example, with sodium valproate). When an increase in the free fraction occurs in conjunction with other complex changes in pharmacokinetics it may assume greater importance (see discussion of acetazolamide below).

Drug metabolism

Reduced blood flow to the liver and reduced liver size appear to be the main contributory factors in the reported reduction in the hepatic clearance of some oxidatively metabolised compounds. The apparent sparing of some metabolic pathways, however, remains unexplained by these mechanisms.

The interpretation of age related changes in drug metabolism has been somewhat confounded by the scale of variability among patients. Thus though in the case of many drugs studied the changes are significant, the 95% confidence interval is extremely wide, making quantitative prediction from age alone unrealistic. The influence of environmental, dietary and genetic factors is considerable, often dwarfing the effect of age.

It is often stated that age changes in drug metabolism are of little importance. This is an oversimplification. From a practical point of view what they imply is a measurable increase in the relative risk of accumulated toxic steady state drug concentrations in elderly patients. To ensure safety it is therefore prudent—almost invariably—to begin treatment with half the normal adult dosage and to increase dosage only if absolutely necessary and with particular vigilance.

Renal excretion

The parallel decline in both glomerular filtration and tubular secretion with age is in keeping with the "intact nephron" loss hypothesis of renal changes related to age. It is therefore usually possible to correlate reduced renal clearance with estimated or measured creatinine clearance in healthy elderly subjects, irrespective of whether the drug is eliminated predominantly by tubular secretion or glomerular filtration. This is found to be the case with acetazolamide, for example, but only when allowance is made for the reduction in binding of acetazolamide to albumin. The result of the reduced binding is in effect to alter the dynamic balance of distribution and elimination of the drug. The increased concentrations of free acetazolamide are available not only to the kidney for active tubular secretion (resulting in a comparative increase in the total clearance of the drug to concentrations similar to those in a young adult) but also for uptake by red cells (giving increased concentrations of acetazolamide in the red cells). Because the side effects of acetazolamide have been related to the effects of carbonic anhydrase inhibition in the red cell it has been suggested that a complex pharmacokinetic mechanism exists to explain the poor tolerance of this drug by elderly recipients.

In general terms, however, the need for a reduced dose of renally eliminated compounds in the elderly is straightforward when there is any likelihood that accumulation may give rise to clinically important toxicity.

PHARMACODYNAMICS

Table 6.2 shows some of the more important changes in specific aspects of drug sensitivity and in homoeostatic mechanisms with age. Elucidating the precise mechanisms in humans presents difficulty for ethical and methodological reasons. Accordingly, some of the data have been derived from animal experiments, whereas elsewhere the information has been derived indirectly from concurrent measurements of indexes of drug response and plasma drug concentrations. Some of the changes are of direct, clear cut clinical importance, as in the case of the benzodiazepines and anticoagulants, though the consequences of the varying changes in autonomic function are often more difficult to pinpoint because of interaction with other autonomic pathways connected with physiological adaptive mechanisms. Pharmacodynamic changes may, however, be at least as important as alterations in drug handling in modifying the response to drugs in old age; further basic research in these topics is important.

The loss of homoeostatic reserve increases the susceptibility of older people to a whole range of side effects of drugs, which feature predominantly in medical reports. These include falls due to postural imbalance and postural hypotension, hypothermia and confusional states induced by drugs, retention of urine, faecal impaction, and urinary and faecal continence problems.

TABLE 6.2—*Drug sensitivity in elderly patients*

Several β adrenergic receptor mediated responses show attenuation
α_1 Adrenergic responsiveness is unchanged
α_2 Adrenergic responsiveness is reduced
Responsiveness to benzodiazepines and warfarin is increased
Homoeostatic mechanisms may be impaired—for example, postural stability, orthostatic responses, thermoregulation, reserve of cognitive function, mechanisms of bowel and bladder function

New drugs and the elderly

The lessons of the past and the increased knowledge now available should do much to ensure better results from drug treatment for elderly patients in the future. The basic ground rules of rational prescribing include the following:

1. care in diagnosis, requiring improved detection, accuracy, and definition based on a knowledge of modified presentation of disease in the elderly and a firm clinical indication before starting any course of drug treatment;
2. use of the minimum possible number of preparations, exploring non-pharmaceutical options whenever possible;
3. appropriate dose regimens, adjusted when indicated by pharmacokinetic or pharmacodynamic changes with age; and
4. defined duration of treatment, supported by an automatic mechanism for review or withdrawal and measures to remove stockpiled and outdated drugs.

Computerised record systems offer the opportunity to monitor prescribing performance and perform simple therapeutic audit procedures. Some districts, departments, or practices operate their own drug formularies, which should among other things reflect the needs of the elderly. Informal peer review sessions to discuss prescribing can be very effective, and it is important that the therapeutics of old age is well represented in undergraduate and postgraduate teaching programmes.

The regulatory requirements for new drugs now have built in safeguards for the elderly. The Committee on Safety of Medicines requires pertinent recommendations for drug dosage in the elderly, based on hard evidence, for all new compounds that have a prospective market among older patients. Such information is particularly sought when:

- the drug has a low therapeutic ratio;
- a reduced rate of elimination is likely;
- other aspects of drug handling or response are likely to change with age or disease;
- interactions may be anticipated; or
- the drug belongs to a class of drugs that has a history of hazardous effects.

Prescribers should check the drug data sheets carefully for the dose recommendations for older patients. In general, data on pharmacokinetics in the elderly are required, and the efficacy and safety of each compound must be attested at least by a considerable participation of elderly patients in clinical trials for a reasonable period. Although these requirements clearly constitute a safeguard, some possible disadvantages include a prolonged premarketing process, with correspondingly aggressive marketing drives after a licence has been granted, and a rather mechanical flow of data emerging from regulatory studies conducted in contract houses, possibly obscuring some of the more important findings that could emerge from critical studies undertaken in academic research settings. The content of regulatory requirements for new drugs to treat the elderly accordingly requires periodic and careful review.

There are still many unanswered questions concerning the basic mechanisms that may modify drug handling or response, or both, in old age, and it is vital that continuing research in this subject continues to receive support. There is also a need for well conducted studies into the practical aspects of presenting and administering drugs to elderly patients, including possible strategies for ensuring appropriate compliance.

Innovations in drugs during the past 15 years have undoubtedly brought benefits for the elderly, both in terms of effectiveness (for example, angiotensin converting enzyme inhibition in heart failure) and in terms of safety (for example, H_2 antagonists in peptic ulcer disease). In the future a better understanding of pharmacokinetic and pharmacodynamic mechanisms in old age may well provide a basis for developing innovative compounds specifically targeted at this age group.

1 Laing W, Hall M. *The challenges of ageing.* ABPI, 1991.
2 O'Malley K, ed. *Clinical pharmacology and drug treatment in the elderly.* London: Churchill Livingstone, 1984.
3 Vestal RE, ed. *Drug treatment in the elderly.* Sydney: ADIS Health Service Press, 1984.
4 Royal College of Physicians. Medication for the elderly. *J R Coll Phys Lond* 1984;**18**:7–17.
5 O'Malley K, Waddington JL, eds. *Therapeutics in the elderly.* Amsterdam: Excerpta Medica, 1985.
6 Caird FI. *Towards rational drug therapy in old age* (The F E Williams Memorial Lecture). *J R Coll Phys Lond* 1985;**19**:235–9.
7 Moore SR, Teal TW, eds. *Geriatric drug use: clinical and social perspectives.* Oxford: Pergamon Press, 1985.
8 Swift CG, ed. *Clinical pharmacology in the elderly.* New York: Marcel Dekker, 1987.

7 Nitrates and antianginal drugs

DEREK MacLEAN, JOHN FEELY

Antianginal drugs

Considerable progress in the medical as well as the surgical management of angina has been made in the past decade. An appreciation of the pharmacokinetics of the "oldest" antianginal drugs, the nitrates, has led to the development of effective long acting preparations and new techniques of administration. On the other hand, calcium antagonists represent another approach to the treatment of angina as an alternative to the now well established β blockers, and the two are often complementary.

We now have a greater understanding of how to reduce work done by the heart (hence oxygen consumption) and thus relieve angina. This may be achieved in various ways (fig 7.1) such as by

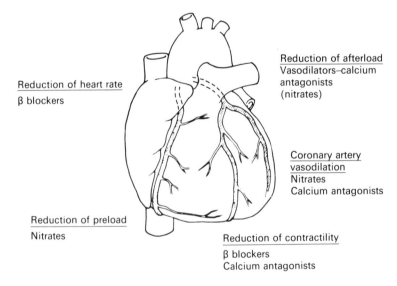

Reduction of afterload
Vasodilators–calcium antagonists
(nitrates)

Reduction of heart rate
β blockers

Coronary artery vasodilation
Nitrates
Calcium antagonists

Reduction of preload
Nitrates

Reduction of contractility
β blockers
Calcium antagonists

FIG 7.1—Site of action of antianginal drugs.

reducing venous return (preload) with nitrates or by reducing heart rate (with β blockers) or muscle contractility (with β blockers or calcium antagonists) directly. The resistance against which the heart has to pump (afterload) may be reduced by arterial dilatation (with calcium antagonists). Alternatively, the oxygen supply to the heart may be increased by reducing spasm of the coronary arteries (with calcium antagonists) or possibly redistributing blood flow to ischaemic areas (with nitrates). Clearly, drugs may act by various different mechanisms and may also be used successfully in combination with glyceryl trinitrate in angina and with long acting nitrates, β blockers, or calcium antagonists (or combinations thereof) to prevent angina.[1] The use of calcium antagonists and of β blockers in angina are considered in the next two chapters.

SILENT ISCHAEMIA

Ambulatory electrocardiographic monitoring of patients with angina shows that almost half the episodes of ST segment depression are not associated with chest pain. Nevertheless such episodes may be accompanied by unfavourable haemodynamic responses. Such episodes of "silent ischaemia", particularly in patients with unstable angina, may predict future myocardial infarction. Antianginal treatment with nitrates, calcium antagonists, or β blockers may reduce such episodes. The benefits of such treatment, however, remain to be established.[2] Many such patients are also treated with low dose aspirin.

New nitrates

Nitrates are now thought to act primarily by relaxing vascular (and particularly venous) smooth muscle, thus decreasing the return of blood to the heart. They therefore reduce the demand for myocardial oxygen by decreasing left ventricular volume, filling pressure, and also to a lesser extent afterload. They probably increase the supply of oxygen by causing redistribution of coronary blood flow (dilatation occurs only in normal vessels) and increasing collateral flow, particularly to ischaemic regions. The primary action of nitrates seems to be their conversion to nitrate ion, which generates nitric oxide.[3 4] Nitric oxide is probably the "endogenous nitrate", endothelial derived relaxant factor, which plays an important part in mediating vasodilatation. The organic nitroesters stimulate the activity of the smooth muscle enzyme guanyl cyclase. This in turn produces a cyclic nucleotide, cyclic guanosine monophosphate, which lowers intracellular free calcium concentrations and causes relaxation.

The nitrates are primarily used for angina pectoris, and several new preparations have become available. The use of nitrates in congestive heart failure, although producing a favourable haemo-dynamic response, is too limited to recommend their widespread use for this condition. In combination with hydralazine they can reduce mortality, but the efficacy and patient acceptability is probably less than with ACE inhibitors alone.

Sublingual glyceryl trinitrate (nitroglycerine, trinitrin) is rapidly absorbed and is the drug most widely used to treat angina because its rapid absorption gives almost instantaneous high serum drug concentrations.[5] The drug is also available as a metered dose aerosol that delivers glyceryl trinitrate by spray emission (Nitro-ligual spray 400 µg) on to the oral mucosa, especially under the tongue. Unlike sublingual tablets, which may lose potency rapidly (often indicated by a loss of characteristic tingling or burning sensation) if they are kept in a warm place or non-opaque bottle, this form of glyceryl trinitrate is chemically stable for at least 3 years. Its efficacy and adverse reactions (headache, flushing, and postural hypotension) are similar to those of sublingual tablets. It is, however, considerably more expensive, but it may produce even more rapid relief from angina in some patients. It may also be of use in patients affected by dry mouth. Buccal glyceryl trinitrate (Suscard) tablets are placed above the upper front teeth between the gum and lip. They undergo initial partial dissolution, which produces a rapid onset, and also have a sustained effect for 4–6 h that is quickly reversed by removing the tablet from the mouth should side effects occur. The use of these two formulations has been limited.

Glyceryl trinitrate unfortunately has only a short acting effect (usually 20–30 min). Small doses of oral long acting nitrates have proved disappointing because first pass metabolism in the liver reduces the amount of systemically available drug. Investigations by formally testing exercise capacity, ST segment depression on electrocardiography, and haemodynamic and biochemical moni-toring have shown objectively that large oral doses of nitrates—for instance, *isosorbide dinitrate* (5–20 mg two to four times a day) or sustained release glyceryl trinitrate—are effective, presumably because the doses are sufficiently large to at least partially offset first pass metabolism.[5] Isosorbide dinitrate is available in a variety of short acting tablets (e.g. Cedocard, Isordil), spray (Imtack), or modified release preparations (e.g. Isoket Retard, Sorbid SA), which may reduce the dosing frequency to twice daily. Nevertheless, isosorbide dinitrate is subject to pronounced and highly variable first pass metabolism to 2- and particularly 5-mononitrates, both of which are haemodynamically active. The *5-mononitrate of isosorbide* has become available (Elantan, Ismo, Isotrate, Monit, or Mono-Cedocard), and this drug may give higher and more consistent plasma nitrate concentrations than does an equal dose of sustained release isosorbide dinitrate. To date both seem to be equally efficacious in reducing anginal attacks and consumption of glyceryl trinitrate and increasing tolerance to exercise. Mononitrate is rapidly absorbed and excreted by the kidneys unchanged and as an inactive glucuronide metabolite, and has an elimination half life of 4–6 h. The duration of effect of a 20 mg dose is about 8 h, which correlates with its peak plasma concentration. Dosage is 20–40 mg two to three times a day. Whether this form of nitrate is more effective clinically than other nitrates has not been established. Irrespective of which is chosen the dosage for an individual patient is determined against control of angina. Nevertheless, the effectiveness of these longer acting nitrates is no longer in doubt. Sustained release formulations of isosorbide mononitrate are also available (Imdur 60 mg), which may be taken as 60 mg or 120 mg once a day. Elantan LA 50 mg provides a dual (rapid followed by sustained release) mechanism and is intended to maintain effective concentrations throughout the day but a "low nitrate" period overnight to prevent nitrate tolerance developing. High dose nitrates may, in addition to headache and nausea, produce hypotension and sometimes collapse. Caution should be exercised in giving high doses of nitrates to the elderly or patients with pronounced renal or hepatic impairment.

Nitroglycerine is also absorbed from the skin, but much more slowly than from the sublingual mucosa, again bypassing the liver. Numerous studies have shown a prophylactic antianginal effect of *glyceryl trinitrate ointment* (Percutol). The degree and duration of the benefit are directly related to the amount of ointment applied. Usually 1·2–5 cm (8–32 mg) of ointment is measured on to a special sheet (Applirule) and applied to the skin, without being rubbed in, and taped into position. The dose applied may be increased to just below that which produces troublesome nitrate induced headaches, but individual patients are best advised to find the dose and times of application most suited to them as variation between patients is considerable. The effects last 4–6 h or sometimes longer, irrespective of where on the skin the ointment is applied. For added psychological benefit it is often applied to the chest wall.

Glyceryl trinitrate ointment has proved particularly useful in those with atypical or variant angina at rest, after exercise, or causing the patient to waken during the night, when, as mentioned above, it is often associated with coronary spasm. In these cases the ointment has been shown to abolish the ST segment elevation as well as the pain. It has also helped to reduce the use of sublingual nitrate in exercise induced angina.

Many patients find the ointment somewhat messy to use, and it requires frequent application. Transdermal patches have proved more popular. A self adhesive *patch impregnated with glyceryl trinitrate* (Transiderm-Nitro, Deponit, 5 or 10 mg, Nitro-Dur, 2·5, 5, 10 and 15 mg) that is released slowly for 24 h is also available for prophylactic use. It resembles a sticking plaster, and effective plasma concentrations are usually achieved within 2 h of application and maintained for 24 h. The efficacy of these preparations, particularly during long term (more than a month) use, is in doubt.[6] This may partly be attributable to the development of tolerance (see below). Skin irritation may occasionally occur but is less likely if the site of application is varied. The patch may be applied to any area of hairless skin. Both glyceryl trinitrate (Nitrocine, Nitronal, or Tridil) and isosorbide dinitrate (Cedocard, or Isoket) are available for intravenous use when the sublingual route is ineffective in patients with ischaemic chest pain, or to treat acute left ventricular failure.

TOLERANCE

When increased dosage is necessary to obtain an effect previously obtained by a smaller dose, tolerance is considered to have developed. Mechanisms thought to mediate tolerance include the downregulation of receptors after continuous exposure to agonists (for example opiates), or increased liver metabolism with, for example, the barbiturates. Workers in munition factories quickly acquired tolerance to the vasodilator headache of nitrates only to lose it over the weekend and subsequently develop "Monday head". Tolerance to nitrates is more pronounced in arteries than in veins, which may explain why hypotension after taking nitrates is uncommon. Tolerance has been shown to the antianginal effect of nitrates.[7 8] It is particularly associated with continuous exposure to high circulating concentrations of nitrates. When concentrations are allowed to fall for part of the day tolerance is much less likely. Thus tolerance may be a greater problem with patches providing 24h therapeutic concentrations. The mechanism(s) may involve a depletion of reduced sulphydryl groups in vascular smooth muscle, as an intravenous infusion of a sulphydryl donor such as n-acetylcysteine restores sensitivity to nitrates.[8] Several strategies have been suggested to reduce the development of tolerance, including using an eccentric dosing schedule, omitting bedtime doses of isosorbide mono- or dinitrate (taking the last dose with the evening meal), or removing nitrate patches at bedtime. For patients with predominantly nocturnal pain the pattern of use should be reversed. As tolerance is a particular problem of high dosage, a lower dosage combined with a calcium antagonist or β blocker may be worth considering.

ADVERSE EFFECTS

Adverse effects common to all nitrates (throbbing headache, flushing, postural hypotension, and reflex tachycardia) are related to vasodilatation and may be minimised by removing the source of nitrate—for example, by spitting out sublingual glyceryl trinitrate after angina has been relieved or by removing patches or ointment. Although these adverse effects are too troublesome for some patients to persist with treatment, patients often become accustomed to adverse effects during prolonged treatment.

1 Packer M. Combined beta-adrenergic and calcium entry blockade in angina pectoris. *N Engl J Med* 1989;**320**:709–18.
2 Fox KM, Quyyumi AA, Levy RD. Should we treat silent ischaemia. *Drugs* 1987;**33**(suppl 4):127–30.
3 Ahlner J, Axelsson KL. Nitrates: mode of action at a cellular level. *Drugs* 1987;**33**(suppl 4):32–8.
4 Luscher TF. Endogenous and exogenous nitrates and their role in myocardial ischaemia. *Br J Clin Pharmacol* 1992;**34**(suppl 1):29–35.
5 Ekylayam U, Aronow WS. Glyceryl trinitrate (nitroglycerin ointment and isosorbide dinitrate). *Drugs* 1982;**23**:165–94.
6 Anonymous. Transdermal glyceryl trinitrate patches (Transiderm-nitro). *Drug Ther Bull* 1986;**24**:55–6.
7 Anonymous. Nitrates: the problem of tolerance. *Drug Ther Bull* 1988;**26**:57–9.
8 May DC, Popma JJ, Black WH *et al.* In vivo induction and reversal of nitroglycerin tolerance in human coronary arteries. *N Engl J Med* 1987;**317**:805–9.

8 Calcium channel blockers

JOHN FEELY, TERENCE PRINGLE,
DEREK MacLEAN

Calcium channel blocking agents or antagonists constitute an important class of drug that reduces myocardial work both directly and in many cases also indirectly by causing vasodilatation. Calcium antagonists are particularly useful in angina, and they and the nitrates are the best treatments for coronary artery spasm. Their use in hypertension is also established. One of the group, verapamil, is also highly effective in managing supraventricular and junctional tachycardias.

Action of calcium antagonists

To appreciate fully the differing profiles of activity of the members of the group an understanding of their mode of action is necessary. In the myocardium and vascular smooth muscle an essential step in the process of contraction is the entry of calcium ions into the cells.[1] In heart muscle this occurs during the "slow current" or plateau phase (2) of the action potential (fig 8.1). This entry of calcium ions into the cells causes the contractile protein to interact, thus leading to shortening fibres and increasing myocardial wall tension. The degree of this contractility (or positive inotropic state) is regulated by the amount of calcium ions that reach the contractile proteins, not only from outside the cells but also from "activator" calcium ions released from an intracellular calcium pool during the action potential. The fibres of the atrioventricular node and contraction in the arterial and venous smooth muscle cells, unlike contraction in heart muscle, rely predominantly on the entry of external calcium ions. Calcium antagonists effectively block the entry of calcium ions through the slow calcium channels ("slow channel blockers"). They thereby reduce

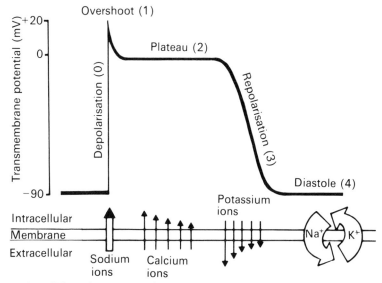

FIG 8.1—Schematic summary of the generation and different phases of an action potential in cardiac cells.

the strength of cardiac muscle contraction and slow conduction through the atrioventricular node (with a consequent increase in the PR interval on electrocardiography) and also decrease arterial and venous smooth muscle tone.[2]

Differences between calcium antagonists

Numerous calcium antagonists have been developed (table 8.1), and many are now available in the United Kingdom, nifedipine and verapamil being the most widely used. Each differs considerably from the others in terms of potency and differential effects on heart muscle contraction, atrioventricular node conduction, and arterial and venous smooth muscle tone. Some, such as verapamil, have additional modes of action. Nifedipine exerts its greatest effect on vascular smooth muscle, including that in the coronary arteries, but has much less effect on myocardial contractility and little influence on atrioventricular node conduction. Verapamil, however, exerts a much greater effect than nifedipine on myocardial contractility and atrioventricular node conduction as well as having a useful effect in reducing vascular smooth muscle tone.

TABLE 8.1—*Comparison of calcium antagonists*

Drug (proprietary name)	Negative inotropic effect	Decreased atrioventricular node conduction	Decreased smooth muscle tone	Oral dose range
Nifedipine (Adalat)	+	−	+ + +	10–20 mg three times a day
Nicardipine (Cardene)	(+)	−	+ + +	20–40 mg (usually 30 mg) three times a day
Verapamil (Cordilox)	+ +	+ +	+ +	40–120 mg three times a day
Diltiazem (Tildiem)	+ +	+	+	60–120 mg three times a day

(+) = least effect, + + + = greatest effect.

The reasons for the differential tissue specificity are not fully clear but are of considerable therapeutic importance.

NIFEDIPINE

Nifedipine is almost completely absorbed.[3] It is detectable in blood, and a hypotensive effect is seen within 5 min of buccal and 20 min of oral administration. Peak concentrations occur 1–2 h after oral use, and the drug is about 90% bound to plasma proteins. It is metabolised in the liver to inactive metabolites that are primarily excreted by the kidney. Although the plasma half life is only 4–5 h, the duration of effect may extend for 8–12 h. Nifedipine does not appear to interact with other drugs and has been safely used with β blockers, nitrates, diuretics, digoxin, anticoagulants, and other antihypertensive drugs.[3,4]

The usual starting dose is 10 mg three times a day (5 mg in the elderly). The introduction of a sustained release (10 mg, 20 mg Adalat Retard) preparation makes dosage twice a day possible in many cases. A long acting (LA) preparation is also available for once daily dosing in hypertension. Dosage is increased until symptoms are relieved (or side effects occur) to a maximum of 120 mg a day. An immediate effect may be obtained by biting the 10 mg capsule and retaining the contents in the mouth.

Adverse effects

The risk of heart failure with nifedipine is small, but some patients have experienced worsening angina or cerebral ischaemia (perhaps because of a vascular steal phenomenon).[5] Over 5% of patients develop headache and others experience nausea, flushing, and dizziness, which are occasionally severe enough to merit stopping treatment. Ankle oedema may result from the higher proximal capillary pressure consequent on dilatation of the resistance vessels and does not usually respond to diuretics. In hypertensive patients already receiving β blockade because of angina the addition of nifedipine may produce severe hypotension without improving the angina; in those circumstances the calcium antagonist should be stopped.[4,6] A similar profound hypotensive effect is sometimes seen when nifedipine is combined with β blockade in the early days after myocardial infarction.[6,7] Drug induced hypersensitivity with hepatitis may occur rarely, as may glucose intolerance. Nifedipine may possibly inhibit or prolong labour.

VERAPAMIL

Although verapamil is well absorbed after oral administration, it undergoes extensive first pass metabolism in the liver and has a bioavailability of only 10–20%.[38] This explains why, in common with other highly extracted drugs such as propranolol, to achieve comparable plasma concentrations the oral dose is 5–10 times greater than the intravenous dose. The metabolites may have some pharmacological activity and are excreted by the kidney. The elimination half life varies from 3 to 7h after a single dose, but during long term administration the first pass effect falls, the drug accumulates, and the half life is longer (up to 10h). Elimination is reduced in patients with liver disease. Verapamil is 90% bound to plasma proteins.

After intravenous administration the hypotensive effect is short lived (10–20 min) but the depressant effect on the atrioventricular node persists for up to 6h, possibly because of preferential binding of drug to this tissue.[348] The intravenous dose (5 mg by slow injection for a minute) may be repeated after 10 min while monitoring blood pressure and electrocardiogram because hypotension and asystole, especially when verapamil is combined with β blockers, have occasionally been reported in patients with myocardial damage. When given by mouth the dosage may, if necessary, be increased rapidly from 40 to 120 mg three times a day in 2–3 days. A sustained release preparation (240 mg Securon SR) may be used once a day with good antihypertensive effect.

Adverse effects

The overall tolerance to verapamil is good.[8] Many of the side effects—gastrointestinal disturbances (particularly constipation), headache and dizziness, and rashes—may be transient. Fewer patients withdraw from treatment than with nifedipine. Large doses may precipitate heart failure, but bradycardia, hypotension, and conduction disturbances are rare except when verapamil is given intravenously to patients receiving β blockers. In addition to interacting pharmacodynamically with digoxin, verapamil reduces the renal and non-renal excretion of digoxin (similarly to the interaction of digoxin and quinidine), thereby raising steady state digoxin concentrations by about 50% and increasing the likelihood of heart block.

DILTIAZEM

Diltiazem (Tildiem) is a benzothiazepine derivative similar to verapamil, which has been in use in the United States and Japan for some years. After oral administration it undergoes extensive and variable first pass metabolism in the liver.[3] In common with many drugs that undergo extensive presystemic elimination, such as verapamil and propranolol, first pass metabolism of diltiazem is saturated during long term administration and plasma concentrations increase. Metabolites, some of which are pharmacologically active, are excreted largely into bile. The pharmacokinetics of diltiazem, including its elimination half life (4–6 h), are not appreciably altered by aging but have not been studied adequately in patients who have liver disease. As expected, kidney disease does not alter the kinetics of diltiazem.

Diltiazem has similar haemodynamic and electrophysiological effects to verapamil but is less potent at producing arterial vasodilatation and has a greater tendency to slow the heart rate. Sinus bradycardia is seen occasionally and conduction through the atrioventricular node is slowed, which suggest that it should be prescribed with caution to patients who have bradycardia or sick sinus syndrome or who are receiving β blockers or digoxin. In addition to pharmacodynamic interaction with digoxin there may also be a kinetic interaction, as seen with verapamil, which reduces digoxin elimination. In common with verapamil diltiazem enhances the effect of carbamazepine.

Dosage is 180–360 mg a day, given in three or four doses, though 60 mg twice a day is often recommended initially for the elderly, as some patients show an enhanced response. A long acting (Retard) preparation allows twice daily dosing. As an antihypertensive or antianginal agent diltiazem does not seem to have any great advantage over verapamil.[4] Some evidence indicates that it may prevent early recurrence of infarction in patients who are recovering from subendocardial (non-Q wave) myocardial infarction.[9] The incidence of adverse effects (headache, dizziness, flushing, and gastrointestinal disturbance) is similar to that seen with verapamil.

NICARDIPINE

Nicardipine (Cardene), a dihydropyridine derivative, is similar to nifedipine in structure, pharmacological activity, and toxicity.[10] It is well absorbed and peak concentrations occur within an hour.

It also undergoes extensive presystemic elimination after oral administration. It is not subject to the same problem of sensitivity to light as nifedipine and may be used intravenously, although this formulation has not yet been marketed. It is rapidly eliminated (half life 1–2 h) by extensive hepatic metabolism, and inactive metabolites are excreted in bile and subsequently faeces. Elimination is not appreciably altered in patients who have renal disease or in the elderly. Patients who have liver disease clear the drug more slowly than normal. Cimetidine may also impair its metabolism, and that of other dihydropyridines.

The primary effect of nicardipine is peripheral vasodilatation.[11] This is accompanied by a reflex increase in myocardial pump activity. The heart rate may increase initially, but it returns to normal during long term treatment. Coronary vasodilatation has been shown to occur. In clinical practice no appreciable effect on conduction tissue has been seen, making nicardipine, unlike verapamil and diltiazem, safe in patients who have impaired atrioventricular conduction. In angina its efficacy is comparable to other calcium antagonists and β blockers. Although nifedipine may decrease left ventricular contraction and relaxation in patients who have coronary heart disease, nicardipine does not.[10 12] As an antihypertensive it is of similar efficacy to diuretics or β blockers.

Adverse effects

Adverse effects—namely, flushing, palpitation, headache, peripheral oedema, and hot limbs—are largely related to vasodilatation and are hence dose related and usually primarily a problem during the start of treatment. As with nifedipine, hypotension induced by exercise and, rarely, an increase in anginal symptoms, possibly due to reflex sympathetic activity, have been reported. Assessment of the quality of life according to psychological variables showed no deterioration during treatment with nicardipine. Dosage should start with 20 mg (increasing if necessary to 40 mg) three times a day. To date nicardipine seems to be almost identical to nifedipine in its effects.[13] If its lack of depressant effect on left ventricular function, particularly in patients who have compromised cardiac pumping ability, is confirmed it may prove advantageous. As with the other groups of calcium antagonists, however, we do not have sufficient comparative studies to make firm recommendations.

Four additional dihydropyridines (nimodipine, amlodipine, isradipine, and felodipine) have recently become available.

Nimodipine—Nimodipine (Nimotop) is used after subarachnoid haemorrhage to reduce or prevent cerebral vessel spasm and neurological deficits by about one third. To treat ischaemic neurological deficits it is given by intravenous infusion via central catheter, and dosage is tailored carefully to ensure that pronounced hypotension does not occur. Where oral administration is possible it should be given in tablet form for 3 weeks.

Amlodipine—Amlodipine (Istin) is a long acting agent with an elimination half life of 35–50 h. It is eliminated (like the other dihydropyridines) by the liver. A single daily dose of 5 mg (increasing to 10 mg if necessary) is effective for 24 h against angina and hypertension.

Isradipine—Isradipine (Prescal) has a shorter elimination half life (6–12 h) and 2·5 mg is commonly given twice a day. The dose should be half this in the elderly or in patients with renal or hepatic impairment. Dosage may, if necessary, be increased to 10 mg twice a day.

Felodipine—Felodipine (Plendil) has a long elimination half life (24 h) and may be used once daily (dose 5–20 mg) in hypertension. Its bioavailability is markedly increased by grapefruit, but not orange, juice.

At least another 20 new calcium antagonists are under development.[12 14] Most of these are dihydropyridone derivatives—for example, nitrendipine, and nisoldipine—that may have more selective effects on certain regional vasculature. Several phenylalkylamines (methoxyverapamil and tiapamil) similar to verapamil are also under study. Preliminary observations suggest that these drugs will not differ greatly from nifedipine and verapamil in terms of overall efficacy and toxicity.

Several older calcium antagonists such as perhexiline, prenylamine, and lidoflazine, which have complex pharmacological profiles, have been withdrawn or are used only rarely. Hepatitis associated with perhexiline was seen predominantly in patients with an inherited inability to hydroxylate several drugs.

Uses of calcium antagonists

ANGINA

Calcium antagonists may lower the oxygen requirements of the ischaemic myocardium by reducing myocardial contractility and by reducing blood pressure and therefore left ventricular pressure.[15][16] In addition, they lower myocardial wall tension as a consequence of decreasing venous tone and therefore venous return.[4] Unlike β blockers, they do not greatly reduce the heart rate. Calcium antagonists such as nifedipine, which particularly affect vascular smooth muscle and thus relieve spasm, effect dramatic relief in about 80% of patients who develop spontaneous episodes of chest pain at rest or at night that are associated with reversible ST segment elevation in the electrocardiogram (variant and Prinzmetal's angina) and are thought to be associated with coronary artery spasm (vasospastic angina). Reports suggest that if patients become asymptomatic and remain so after a few months the drug may be withdrawn cautiously. Calcium antagonists are also synergistic in combination with β blockade in many patients with classic exercise induced angina, when presumably some degree of coronary spasm accompanies structural coronary artery stenosis.[4][17] Given alone, they are generally less potent than β blockers in preventing classical angina. Nevertheless, they may be very useful when β blockers are contraindicated.

SUPRAVENTRICULAR TACHYCARDIA

Many supraventricular tachycardias, including atrial flutter and those associated with the Wolff–Parkinson–White syndrome, are maintained by a re-entry phenomenon using the atrioventricular node. Calcium antagonists that have a prominent influence on the atrioventricular node, such as verapamil,[8] slow the ventricular response to these arrhythmias and to atrial fibrillation and may also sometimes prevent or abolish them. Adenosine is increasingly supplanting verapamil in the treatment of supraventricular tachycardia (see chapter 13). Prolonged atrioventricular conduction induced by excess verapamil can best be reversed with atropine. Nifedipine does not have antiarrhythmic properties, and calcium antagonists are not helpful in managing ventricular arrhythmias.

HYPERTENSION

Calcium antagonists relax arterial muscle and so reduce raised blood pressure, though nifedipine, because of its pronounced effect in lowering smooth muscle tone, usually has a more potent antihypertensive effect than verapamil. This hypotensive effect is more striking when nifedipine is prescribed in combination with β blockade.[7] Postural hypotension and tachycardia may result from its use. Nifedipine has also been used successfully in combination with methyldopa in the long term treatment of severe hypertension. The hypotensive potency of nifedipine is similar to that of hydralazine, and that of verapamil is similar to that of thiazide diuretics. The full potential of these agents in hypertension is increasingly appreciated. At present they are recommended for first line treatment when diuretics or β blockers are contraindicated or may produce unfavourable metabolic effects, although many believe that they are first line drugs in their own right.[18] They may also be used in combination with other antihypertensive drugs, particularly when a vasodilator is indicated.

Expanding indications for calcium antagonists

The use of calcium antagonists in chronic heart failure and to preserve the myocardium after infarction is under study, although initial results are not encouraging. By causing arteriolar vasodilatation nifedipine produces symptomatic relief in patients who have Raynaud's phenomenon,[19 20] particularly the idiopathic variety rather than that secondary to collagen vascular disorders. There is less evidence to support the use of either verapamil or diltiazem in this condition.

By reducing the influx of calcium into cells calcium antagonists have a wide variety of effects, which may influence the choice of treatment in patients who have concomitant disorders. Nifedipine and verapamil have been reported to reduce the frequency of migrainous headache.[20] There is some suggestion that tolerance may occur after a few months, and effective control may be restored by changing to another calcium antagonist. Recent studies confirm that calcium antagonists have a role in reducing neurological deficits after subarachnoid haemorrhage.[20 21] Experimental data also suggest that cell death due to calcium overload—for example after cardiac arrest[22] or cyclosporin A nephrotoxicity[23]—may be reduced by calcium antagonists.

In hypertropic cardiomyopathy verapamil in particular reduces

91

cardiac symptoms and improves tolerance to exercise, even in patients who have not responded to β blockers.[24] Long term efficacy of calcium antagonists has not, however, been shown in patients who have pulmonary hypertension.

Nifedipine decreases the pressure in the lower oesophageal sphincter and has been used in patients who have diffuse oesophageal spasm and "nutcracker" oesophagus, which is a common cause of non-cardiac chest pain.[25] Biting the nifedipine capsule allows more rapid absorption for acute pain, and patients who have symptoms related to food may do this 30 min before meals. Similarly, nifedipine relaxes the internal anal sphincter and may produce some symptomatic relief in proctalgia fugax. This effect on smooth muscle may extend to other systems—for example, myometrial contraction may be reduced in patients who have dysmenorrhoea and in premature labour.[14]

To date calcium antagonists have not, in contrast with diuretics and β blockers, been associated with particular problems in managing patients who have concomitant peripheral vascular disease, gout, or asthma. Many of the above observations are preliminary, and we await detailed confirmatory studies, including an evaluation of potential additional adverse effects. Side effects may, however, be relevant when considering whether to use a calcium antagonist or drugs of similar efficacy, such as nitrates or β blockers for angina or diuretics or β blockers as the best drugs for hypertension.

1 Braunwald E. Mechanism of action of calcium-channel-blocking agents. *N Engl J Med* 1982;**302**:1618–27.
2 Anonymous. Calcium antagonists and the heart. *BMJ* 1981;**282**:89–90.
3 Echizen H, Eichelbaum M. Clinical pharmacokinetics of verapamil, nifedipine and diltiazem. *Clin Pharmacokinet* 1986;**11**:425–9.
4 Soward AL, Vanhaleweyk GLJ, Serruys PW. The haemodynamic effects of nifedipine, verapamil and diltiazem in patients with coronary artery disease. *Drugs* 1986;**32**:66–101.
5 Nobile-Orazio E, Sterzi R. Cerebral ischaemia after nifedipine treatment. *BMJ* 1981;**282**:948.
6 Sorkin EM, Clissold SP, Brogden RN. Nifedipine: a review of its pharmacodynamic and pharmacokinetic properties, and therapeutic efficacy, in ischaemic heart disease, hypertension and related cardiovascular disorders. *Drugs* 1985;**30**:181–96.
7 Dean S, Kendall MJ. Adverse interaction between nifedipine and beta-blockade. *BMJ* 1981;**282**:1322.
8 McTavish D, Sorkin EM. Verapamil: an updated review of its pharmacodynamic and pharmacokinetic properties, and therapeutic use in hypertension. *Drugs* 1989;**38**:19–76.

9 Gibson RS, Boden WE, Theroux P, *et al*. Diltiazem and reinfarction in patients with non-W-wave myocardial infarction. *N Engl J Med* 1986;**315**:423–9.

10 Turner P, Feely J, Barrett J, eds. Nicardipine: a new calcium antagonist. *Br J Clin Pharmacol* 1986;**22**(suppl 3):191–352.

11 Sorkin EM, Clissold SP. Nicardipine: a review of its pharmacodynamic and pharmacokinetic properties and therapeutic efficacy in the treatment of angina pectoris, hypertension and related cardiovascular disorders. *Drugs* 1987;**33**:296–345.

12 Freedman DD, Waters DD. Second generation dihydropyridine calcium antagonists. *Drugs* 1987;**34**:578–98.

13 Anonymous. Nicardipine: another calcium antagonist. *Drug Ther Bull* 1989;**27**:89–90.

14 Snyder SH, Reynolds IJ. Calcium-antagonist drugs: receptor interactions that clarify therapeutic effects. *N Engl J Med* 1985;**313**:995–1002.

15 Subramanian VB, Lahiri A, Paramasivan R, Raftery EB. Verapamil in chronic stable angina. *Lancet* 1980;**i**:841–4.

16 Zelis R, Flaim SF. Calcium blocking drugs for angina pectoris. *Annu Rev Med* 1982;**33**:465–78.

17 Lynch P, Dargie H, Krikler S, Krikler D. Objective assessment of anti-anginal treatment: a double-blind comparison of propranolol, nifedipine, and their combination. *BMJ* 1980;**281**:184–7.

18 Sever P, Beevers C, Bulpitt C, *et al*. Management guidelines in essential hypertension. Report of the second working party of the British Hypertension Society. *BMJ* 1993;**306**:983–7.

19 White CJ, Phillips WA, Abraham LA, Watson TD, Singleton PT. Objective benefit of nifedipine in the treatment of Raynaud's phenomenon. *Am J Med* 1986;**80**:623–5.

20 Tietze KJ, Schwartz ML, Vlasses PH. Calcium antagonists in cerebral/ peripheral vascular disorders: current status. *Drugs* 1987;**33**:531–8.

21 Pickard JD, Murray GD, Illingworth R, *et al*. Effect of oral nimodipine on cerebral infarction and outcome after subarachnoid haemorrhage: British aneurysm nimodipine trial. *BMJ* 1989;**298**:636–42.

22 Roine RO, Kaste M, Kinnunen A, Nikki P. Safety and efficacy of nimodipine in resuscitation of patients outside hospital. *BMJ* 1987;**294**:20.

23 Feehally J, Walls J, Mistry N, *et al*. Does nifedipine ameliorate cyclosporin A nephrotoxicity? *BMJ* 1987;**295**:310.

24 Fleckenstein A. The practical significance of calcium antagonists in cardiovascular therapy. In: Fleckenstein A, ed. *Calcium antagonism in heart and smooth muscle*. New York: Wiley, 1983: 286–320.

25 Anonymous. Drugs can help oesophageal motility disorders. *Drug Ther Bull* 1984;**22**:17–18.

9 β Blockers (β adrenoceptor antagonists)

ANGUS MacCONNACHIE, DEREK MacLEAN, JOHN FEELY

Currently 19 β blockers are available in the United Kingdom. These are listed in table 9.1 along with their licensed indications and routes of administration. With the development of so many agents of this type an active (and often over optimistic) marketing policy has been pursued by the pharmaceutical industry (see properties of β blockers, below), creating an element of confusion and problem of choice among prescribers.

β Adrenoceptors and β blockade

The potentially important consequences of β adrenergic blockade in relation to the role of β receptors at a variety of anatomical sites are summarised in table 9.2. For reasons that will be discussed later, the further classification of these receptors into β_1 and β_2 subtypes may have important implications when selecting a β blocker for a given indication or in the presence of coexisting disease.

Selecting a β blocker: differences between individual agents

For practical purposes the β blockers can be subdivided according to non-selectivity or (relative) cardioselectivity and to other properties such as partial agonist activity at β_1 or β_2 receptor subtypes, or both. Membrane stabilising activity, although mentioned in the text, is likely to be of no clinical consequence with the possible exception of drugs used in the treatment of hyperthyroidism (see Indications for β blockade, below).

Despite the fact that so many β blockers are now available and that particular features of molecular structure may be highlighted

94

TABLE 9.1— *The β blockers*

Drug	Licensed indications*	Route(s) of administration	Comments
Atenolol	Angina Dysrhythmias Hypertension MI, acute therapy	Intravenous Oral	Cardioselective, no PAA, no MSA, water soluble
Acebutolol	Angina Dysrhythmias Hypertension	Oral	Cardioselective (but less than atenolol), weak PAA, MSA, lipid soluble
Betaxolol	Glaucoma Hypertension	Ocular Oral	Cardioselective, no PAA, MSA equivocal, lipid soluble but long acting
Bisoprolol	Angina Hypertension	Oral	More cardioselective than atenolol, no PAA, no MSA, long acting
Carteolol	Angina Glaucoma	Oral Ocular	Non-selective, marked PAA, no MSA, long acting
Celiprolol	Hypertension	Oral	Cardioselective, selective β_2 PAA, water soluble, long acting, further vasodilator action likely
Esmolol	Dysrhythmias	Intravenous	Cardioselective, ultra short acting, no PAA
Labetalol	Hypertension with/without angina	Intravenous Oral	Non-selective, no PAA, lipid soluble, additional α blocking activity
Levobunolol	Glaucoma	Ocular	Cardioselective, no PAA, long acting
Metipranolol	Glaucoma	Ocular	Cardioselective, no PAA
Metoprolol	Angina Dysrhythmias Hypertension Migraine MI prophylaxis	Intravenous Oral	Cardioselective, relatively fat soluble, no PAA
Nadolol	Angina Dysrhythmias Hypertension Migraine	Oral	Non-selective, water soluble, long acting, no PAA
Oxprenolol	Angina Anxiety Dysrhythmias Hypertension	Oral	Non-selective, moderate PAA, some MSA, mainly fat soluble
Penbutolol	Hypertension	Oral	Non-selective, some PAA in combination with frusemide only
Pindolol	Angina Hypertension	Oral	Non-selective, marked PAA

TABLE 9.1—*contd*

Drug	Licensed indications*	Route(s) of administration	Comments
Propranolol	Angina Anxiety Dysrhythmias Hypertension Migraine MI prophylaxis Portal hypertension	Intravenous Oral	Non-selective, no PAA, possesses MSA
Sotalol	Angina Dysrhythmias Hypertension MI prophylaxis	Intravenous Oral	Non-selective, no PAA, very water soluble, class III antiarrhythmic activity
Timolol	Angina Glaucoma Hypertension Migraine MI prophylaxis	Oral	Non-selective, slight PAA
Xamoterol	Chronic mild heart failure	Oral	Cardioselective, strong β_1 PAA, use restricted to mild heart failure

MSA = membrane stabilising activity; PAA = partial agonist activity; MI = myocardial infarction

* Drugs are preferably used for their licensed indications. While it is recognised that use outwith the terms of their product licence may be justified, prescribers must be aware that no responsibility for safety can be attached to the manufacturer. The implications of this under The Consumer Protection Act should be noted.

in their promotion, relatively few important differences exist between established individual agents in practice. As a result, efficacy and tolerability has, in general, been comparable throughout the group. Newer agents are, however, appearing as a result of attempts to translate possible advantages into clinical gains.

Some pharmacokinetic differences do exist which, together with cost and individual patient preference (for whatever reason—dosage form, size and colour, et cetera), may to some extent influence choice. For practical purposes, however, prescribers are advised to familiarise themselves with one or two agents and to use these regularly. If this approach is taken as part of the management policy of a group practice, for example, the important targets of efficacy, tolerability and value for money are most likely to be achieved.

β blockers with special properties (e.g. celiprolol, esmolol and xamoterol) have recently been introduced in the United Kingdom

TABLE 9.2—*Function of β adrenoceptors and the effect of β blockade*

Anatomical site	Receptor subtype	Function	Effect of blockade
Myocardium	β_1	Increased force of contraction	Negative inotropic effect and reduced oxygen demand
Sinoatrial node	β_1	Increased rate of contraction	Negative chronotropic effect and reduced oxygen demand
Lung	β_2	Relaxation of bronchial smooth muscle	Bronchoconstriction and increased airways resistance
Peripheral vasculature	β_2	Arteriolar dilatation	Reduced perfusion, cold extremities (hands/feet), etc
Coronary arterial circulation	β_2	Dilatation	Vasoconstriction and worsening angina?
Splanchnic circulation	β_2	Dilatation	Vasoconstriction and reduction in portal pressure
Metabolic			
Atria	β_1	Reduction in atrial natriuretic peptide?	Increased atrial natriuretic peptide levels—hypotension
Blood	β_1/β_2?	Reduction in high density lipoprotein cholesterol and triglyceride	Hyperlipidaemia and increased coronary risk?
Kidney	β_1	Increased plasma renin	Hypotension
Liver	β_2	Gluconeogenesis	Hypoglycaemia
Pancreas	β_2	Insulin release	Impaired glucose tolerance in Type II diabetes mellitus
Eye (ciliary epithelium)	β_1/β_2?	Aqueous humour production?	Reduced intraocular pressure
Uterus (pregnant)	β_2	Relaxation	Increased contractility

and merit special consideration. These drugs are reviewed later in the chapter. Such drugs should be chosen after careful consideration of their potential advantages over established drugs of known efficacy and tolerability and for which relatively inexpensive brands exist.

CARDIOSELECTIVITY

This denotes the relatively greater affinity of some β blockers for β_1 (rather than β_2) receptors and is by far the most important difference ascribed to individual agents. Non-selective β blockers antagonise catecholamines equally at both β_1 and β_2 receptor sites and so have widespread effects on sympathetic autonomic and hormonal adrenergic function. This may compromise the patient to the extent that a drug is not tolerated.

For the majority of patients treated for cardiovascular conditions, however, it has been standard practice to select a β blocker that predominantly blocks β_1 receptors (so targeting the myocardium) thereby reducing the possible complications of effects at β_2 sites. In this respect atenolol has been increasingly used and remains a drug of first choice.[1] Despite this, it is stressed that the term "cardioselectivity" is only relative and limited by the nature of the drug and its dosage so that a degree of β_2 blockade can be anticipated, especially with higher doses (for example, atenolol > 100 mg daily). Therefore the use of atenolol may still pose problems in asthmatics (bronchospasm) and in patients with peripheral vascular disease (claudication).[2 3] However, it is reasonable to choose a non-cardioselective drug such as propranolol to control the widespread effects of adrenergic overstimulation, which occurs in thyrotoxicosis and anxiety.

A new generation of highly selective β_1 blockers which possess moderate but significant vasodilator activity has been developed. So far, one such agent, celiprolol, has been introduced to the British market while others, including carvedilol, have been extensively developed. These agents are discussed in more detail elsewhere.

LIPID SOLUBILITY

This largely determines the pharmacokinetic behaviour of an individual drug and may influence the choice of a β blocker in patients with limited metabolic and/or excretory capacity.[4] Thus the characteristics of a β blocker that is highly lipid soluble (such as metoprolol or propranolol) are:

1. good absorption after oral administration;
2. extensive metabolism during absorption and before reaching the systemic circulation (first pass or pre-systemic elimination);
3. relatively short half life; and
4. conversion to various metabolites which may or may not themselves be active.

The extent of the first pass metabolism may be influenced by a variety of factors including dosage (metabolic capacity is saturated with single doses of propranolol over 40 mg), genetic polymorphism, aging, the presence of food in the gut (which may reduce absorption), smoking (a recognised enzyme inducing factor), and interactions with other drugs that alter liver blood flow and/or increase or decrease liver metabolic rate (hepatic enzyme induction or inhibition). Such factors may result in a 10–20-fold difference in the plasma concentration of an essentially fat soluble drug such as propranolol and explains the wide variability in dose response seen in clinical practice.[56]

In contrast to fat soluble derivatives, β blockers that are very water soluble (for example atenolol, sotalol, and nadolol) are absorbed less from the gastrointestinal tract, are subject to little (if any) liver metabolism, and are only slowly excreted, largely unchanged, in the urine. As a result, their longer half lives make once daily dosing practical but it is important to recognise that accumulation will occur in patients with renal impairment.

As a general guide, the dose of a drug such as atenolol should be halved if the glomerular filtration rate falls below 30–35 ml/min and quartered, or administered on alternate days, if it falls to less than 15 ml/min. Note, however, that atenolol, being largely water soluble and only about 10% bound to plasma protein, is readily removed by both peritoneal dialysis and haemodialysis. The consequence of this is that immediate postdialysis dosing is recommended.

Water soluble β blockers do not interact with drugs that alter liver blood flow or influence liver metabolising capacity.

β blockers with a ratio of lipid to water solubility that approaches unity (such as acebutolol, pindolol, and timolol) are partly excreted by renal and partly by hepatic routes and are theoretically less likely to accumulate in patients with liver or kidney disease. As a result, a reduction in dosage is usually necessary only when renal function is severely impaired (for example, if the creatinine clearance is < 10 ml/min).

CENTRAL NERVOUS SYSTEM ACTIVITY AND LIPID SOLUBILITY

The incidence of side effects on the central nervous system (sleep disturbances, nightmares, mood changes, depression) may diminish as lipophilicity decreases, implying that fat soluble β blockers more readily enter the central nervous system across the blood–brain barrier. All β blockers, including very water soluble agents, are reported to produce adverse effects in the central nervous system although the incidence may be higher with a drug such as propranolol than atenolol (see Adverse effects, below).

PLASMA PROTEIN BINDING

For most drugs this is very low (10% or less in the case of atenolol, metoprolol and timolol: sotalol is virtually unbound). Propranolol is more than 90% bound to plasma protein but there is generally little or no increase in clinical response when taken with other drugs which displace it from its binding site. Its elimination half life may, however, be prolonged as a result of its high tissue binding affinity and increased volume of distribution. During chronic dosing the elimination half life of propranolol is usually 4–6 h but this is increased (for example up to 20 h) in patients with liver disease due to reduced protein binding, increased volume of distribution and impaired liver metabolism.

PARTIAL AGONIST ACTIVITY

This is also referred to as intrinsic sympathomimetic activity, a term which has been applied in the past to agents such as pindolol and oxprenolol during their promotion by the pharmaceutical industry. The implication is that β blockers with partial agonist activity are associated with fewer side effects (bradycardia, peripheral vascular insufficiency, airways resistance) because they possess a compensatory mechanism but this has largely proved of theoretical interest only and has not been demonstrated consistently in practice. However, evidence from an extensive range of postinfarction, secondary prevention trials suggests that partial agonist activity is associated with the least favourable outcome.

Xamoterol is a newer agent with considerable partial agonist activity, to the extent that it is considered a dual β agonist/β blocker. It has been actively promoted in heart failure, in which the risks from β blocker therapy are usually of sufficient importance to merit extreme caution. However, problems have been encountered with this agent. Xamoterol is discussed in more detail later in the chapter.

Epanolol is a dual β_1 selective antagonist/β_1 selective partial agonist, and is likely to be introduced soon. This agent is also discussed later in the chapter.

MEMBRANE STABILISING ACTIVITY

This property has been claimed for certain β blockers, notably alprenolol and propranolol, and implies that these drugs exert a local anaesthetic or "lignocaine-like" effect on cardiac conduction. Where it has been demonstrated, plasma concentrations considerably in excess of those which produce substantial β blockade in practice have been required and it is concluded therefore that β blockers with this activity do not have clinically useful Class I antiarrhythmic properties. It is possible, however, that membrane stabilising activity contributes to the action of propranolol in the treatment of hyperthyroidism (see Indications, below).

SLOW RELEASE (SR) FORMULATIONS

Slow release preparations of fat soluble, short acting β blockers (propranolol, metoprolol, and oxprenolol) have been introduced in an attempt to provide a smooth steady state plasma concentration profile throughout each 24 h period after once-daily dosing. However, their use automatically excludes flexibility of dose (note the earlier comments on individual variability in dose/response to fat soluble β blockers), and effective β blockade may not be achieved consistently because they produce lower peak plasma concentrations which may be delayed for several hours after dosing. As a consequence of this, some patients may require such preparations in a twice daily dosage regimen.

In the treatment of angina, continuous 24 h β blockade is desirable and may readily be achieved by frequent low doses of conventional tablets (for example propranolol 40 mg four times a day instead of 160 mg SR once daily). Dosage is more easily titrated but for some patients it is acknowledged that maximum compliance is achieved using a single daily dosage regimen. A further option is to use a very long acting drug once daily such as betaxolol, which has a half life of 20–22 h.[7] Betaxolol has been demonstrated to be of greater benefit to patients with stable angina than atenolol (half life 6–8 h) using continuous ambulatory monitoring of heart rate: patients receiving betaxolol showed reduced heart rate in the last 6 h of the dosing period than those receiving a single daily dose of atenolol. This was associated with improved treadmill exercise performance as a result of late attenuation of exercise induced reduction in left ventricular ejection fraction.

The same considerations do not apply in hypertension, where there is no correlation between plasma concentration and clinical effect. In the study mentioned above a similar hypotensive response over 24 h was achieved by both atenolol and betaxolol despite the major difference in their half lives. Therefore, it is difficult to justify the considerable increase in cost between slow release and conventional β blocker preparations in the treatment of hypertension.

Adverse effects of β adrenoceptor antagonists

HEART

Cardiac side effects,[89] which are predictable, include sinus bradycardia and precipitation or worsening of heart failure. Severe bradycardia and a high degree of heart block are absolute contraindications and, although β blockers are occasionally used in cardiac failure, this is best done under specialist supervision.

Non-selective β blockers may provoke coronary artery spasm by inhibiting β_2-mediated vasodilatation and should be used with caution in patients with unstable angina (such as those with Prinzmetal's variant angina).

LUNG

Respiratory side effects arise from blockade of β receptors (essentially β_2 although a small population of β_1 receptors also exists in bronchial smooth muscle) and include increased airways resistance and potentially severe, and even fatal, exacerbation of airways obstruction. Asthmatics are so sensitive to the effects of β blockers that bronchospasm has been precipitated by local application of timolol eye drops.

Clearly, if a β blocker is considered *essential* for a patient with obstructive airways disease a cardioselective drug is preferred, especially if combined with selective β_2 partial agonist activity (see celiprolol, below). However, it should be noted that a partial agonist will (theoretically, at least) act as an antagonist in the presence of a potent β_2 sympathomimetic drug (a pure agonist) such as salbutamol. Mild controlled asthma and chronic obstructive pulmonary disease remain relative contraindications but severe, symptomatic or "brittle" asthma is an absolute contraindication to the use of β blockade.

PERIPHERAL VASCULATURE

The fall in cardiac output produced by β blockers together with β blockade of the peripheral vasculature (predominantly β_2 sites) results in reduced perfusion—manifest as cold extremities, usually the hands and feet. This may pose particular problems for patients with existing circulatory disorders such as Raynaud's phenomenon and intermittent claudication. Absence of peripheral pulses should alert to the likelihood of intolerance to β blockade and severe or worsening claudication, ischaemic rest pain, and pregangrene are absolute contraindications. Drugs with partial agonist activity (such as pindolol) have been promoted for patients with peripheral vascular insufficiency and a case could be made for the newer, more specific vasodilator β blocker, celiprolol.

ENDOCRINE/METABOLIC[10-14]

Adverse metabolic effects of β blockers that have caused concern in the past include impaired glucose tolerance, hypoglycaemia and dyslipidaemia.

Hypoglycaemia and impaired glucose tolerance may arise as a result of β_2 blockade in the liver (impaired hepatic gluconeogenesis), and pancreas (impaired insulin release): a cardioselective drug is preferred for diabetic patients. However, hypoglycaemia has also been reported in non-diabetics and in practice it does not appear to pose a major risk in diabetes mellitus. In diabetics developing hypoglycaemia, important alerting neurohumoral symptoms (tachycardia, palpitations and tremor) may be masked and it seems reasonable to limit this to the cardiac manifestations by the use of a cardioselective drug. These agents are also less likely to delay recovery from the hypoglycaemic state.

Given the attention paid in recent years to the link between hyperlipidaemia and coronary risk and the availability of "lipid neutral" first line hypotensive drugs, the role of β blockers in hypertension has been increasingly challenged. β Blockade is associated with increased triglyceride levels and a reduction in the ratio of high density to low density lipoprotein cholesterol. Against this, however, are the known long term benefits of β blocker therapy, and in particular their cardioprotective action in patients sustaining myocardial infarction. The relative importance of hyperlipidaemia as a risk factor (compared with others such as smoking and hypertension) and the positive effect of changes in diet and lifestyle on lipid pattern must also be considered. Dyslipidaemia is less likely to be associated with a cardioselective agent than a non-selective agent, especially one with partial agonist activity, and in this respect celiprolol has been shown to *favourably* influence plasma lipid profile (by lowering low density lipoprotein cholesterol) compared with "lipid neutral" nifedipine during chronic therapy.

CENTRAL NERVOUS SYSTEM[15]

The link between lipid solubility and an increased incidence of adverse effects in the central nervous system has been discussed. Patients may report sleep disturbances, vivid dreams, hallucinations, and mood changes; psychosis and depression are extreme but rare manifestations. β Blockers, especially propranolol, should be avoided in patients with depressive illness: if they are necessary they should be used with caution, and a water soluble drug such as atenolol or sotalol is preferred.

GENITOURINARY[16]

Sexual impotence is more prevalent in male hypertensives than normotensives, probably reflecting the effect of small vessel disease on corporeal vascularisation. However, the incidence is increased further by the use of certain antihypertensive drugs, including the β blockers.

KIDNEY[17]

The renal haemodynamics in hypertensives are characterised by an increase in renal vascular resistance resulting in reduced renal blood flow. Normal glomerular filtration rate is, however, maintained by an increase in the filtration fraction but this compensatory mechanism is impaired by β blockade, causing a further reduction in renal perfusion. There is concern, therefore, over the long term safety of β blockers in patients with renal impairment, although drugs with partial agonist activity and/or cardioselective agents appear to alter renal haemodynamics only minimally, if at all. Tertatolol (discussed elsewhere) and nadolol have been shown to have no effect (or to increase) renal blood flow by a direct intrarenal mechanism which is independent of their primary β blocking action.

Drug interactions

PHARMACOKINETIC

Such interactions result in an increase or reduction in the rate of metabolism of β blockers, which are mainly lipid soluble and largely inactivated by the liver microsomal enzyme system. Enzyme *inhibitors* increase the bioavailability of drugs such as propranolol, achieving higher peak plasma concentrations, prolonging their hepatic clearance, and prolonging the β blocker's half life. Interactions of this type have been reported with cimetidine, dextropropoxyphene and the oral contraceptives but their clinical significance is unclear. Enzyme *inducers* increase the rate of liver metabolism and so reduce bioavailability and peak plasma concentration and increase hepatic clearance. Such an effect has been reported with the barbiturates and rifampicin but it is unclear whether this is of clinical importance. Hydralazine reduces liver blood flow and so reduces the rate of absorption of β blockers where hepatic extraction is flow dependent.

PHARMACODYNAMIC

Such interactions include attenuation of β blockade and loss of control of hypertension in patients treated with non-steroidal anti-inflammatory agents, particularly indomethacin. The mechanism appears to be related to inhibition of renal medullary synthesis and release of vasodilator prostaglandin, PgE, by the non-steroidal agent.

The combination of a β blocker and a calcium antagonist, although generally considered to be safe (see Angina pectoris, below), could cause an additive reduction in myocardial contractility. Caution is advised when β blockers are used with verapamil: reports of bradycardia, hypotension, heart failure, sinus arrest, and heart block associated with this combination are scattered throughout the literature. Intravenous verapamil should be avoided in the presence of β blockade.

Indications for β blockade

ANGINA PECTORIS

Myocardial oxygen demand, particularly during stress or physical exertion, is reduced as a result of the negative chronotropic and inotropic actions of the β blockers and these drugs have a major role in the prophylaxis of angina. They are widely used alone or in combination with long acting nitrates or calcium antagonists. Their antiarrhythmic action may confer additional protection on the ischaemic myocardium (see Myocardial infarction and Cardiac arrhythmias, below), and their hypotensive action makes them especially suitable when angina and hypertension coexist.

HYPERTENSION[18]

β Blockers continue to be first line drugs in the treatment of essential hypertension, despite their apparent adverse effects on the lipid profile. They are especially suitable for younger subjects who have increased sympathetic drive and those with coexisting angina pectoris, and as an alternative to the thiazide diuretics, with which they are often combined as the "next step" in the stepped care approach. Regression of left ventricular hypertrophy, an important indicator of prognosis and a target response, is reported during therapy with various antihypertensives including the β blockers.[19 20]

The mechanism by which the β blockers lower blood pressure is not clearly understood but the reduction in cardiac output that they produce is likely to be important in this respect. Other mechanisms, including a metabolic effect, probably also exist. For example, β blockade is associated, at least in the short term, with a reduction in plasma renin and aldosterone activity and an increase in atrial natriuretic peptide level, possibly producing indirect vasodilatation.[21]

Labetalol and carvedilol (see Newer β blockers, below) further reduce peripheral vascular resistance due to their combined α and β adrenoceptor blocking properties. The selective β_2 agonist action of celiprolol confers additional antihypertensive properties as a result of direct vasodilatation.

A central hypotensive role cannot be excluded.

CARDIAC ARRHYTHMIAS

All β blockers are class II antiarrhythmic drugs with the exception of sotalol, which has additional class III properties. They increase atrial refractoriness by prolonging sinus node recovery and sinus cycle length and increase the period of conduction at the atrioventricular node. Claims that some drugs (for example, propranolol) possess membrane stabilising activity, which implies lignocaine-like class I antiarrhythmic activity, are irrelevant in practice: such an effect can be demonstrated only in the laboratory using concentrations far in excess of those achieved in clinical practice.[22]

β Blockers block the response to catecholamine release and are used in the treatment of supraventricular dysrhythmias associated with sympathetic overactivity. This includes stress or exercise-induced sinus tachycardia and paroxysmal atrial tachycardia and underlies their role in situational anxiety and thyrotoxicosis (discussed below). Use of β blockers in acute myocardial infarction and for long term prophylaxis thereafter probably also reflects their ability to suppress ventricular dysrhythmias. The dextro-rotatory isomer of sotalol (D-sotalol) also has class III activity, which results in prolongation of the action potential. Sotalol has a limited role in the treatment of resistant ventricular dysrhythmias: this might be expected to make sotalol more beneficial than other β blockers when antiarrhythmic activity in addition to β blockade is required (for example following myocardial infarction) but no such advantage has been demonstrated.[23]

MYOCARDIAL INFARCTION

Intravenous β blocker therapy has been increasingly used in the acute stage (within a few hours) of myocardial infarction in order to suppress ventricular fibrillation during the period of greatest risk, to reduce infarct size and so limit early mortality and morbidity[24-26] by blocking the deleterious effects of adrenergic overstimulation on an already sensitised ischaemic myocardium. A single intravenous dose is ideally given within 4 h of an infarction but may be effective if given as late as 12 h after. Any benefits from later intervention are much less likely. If a prolonged effect is required, up to 1 week of oral therapy can be started within hours of intravenous dosing but should be discontinued gradually thereafter, unless long term prophylaxis is indicated.

The role of β adrenoceptor antagonists in preventing further infarction or sudden cardiac death and improved survival therefrom has become accepted after many large scale trials involving thousands of patients.[27-30] Given orally within the first year following myocardial infarction, they may reduce mortality by as much as 25%. Metoprolol, propranolol, and timolol have all proved to be effective but an interesting, and as yet unexplained, finding is that drugs with demonstrable partial agonist activity (such as oxprenolol and pindolol) have given the poorest, or even negative, results.

The mechanism by which β blockade reduces mortality is not clearly understood. There is little point in using the drugs for patients with good left ventricular function, but others in the age range 30–70 years in whom there are no apparent contraindications may benefit from acute intervention and/or secondary prevention.

THYROTOXICOSIS[31 32]

Propranolol has been widely used for the symptomatic treatment of Graves' disease, in which the hyperthyroid state is associated with catecholamine excess and/or increased sensitivity of peripheral target tissues to catecholamines. It also blocks the conversion of T_4 to T_3 and of rT_3 into $3,3'-T_2$ by inhibition of $5'$-deiodination, possibly via a hitherto unrecognised metabolite.[33] Possession of membrane stabilising activity appears to be a requirement for inhibition of T_3 formation.

Symptoms that respond to *non-selective* β blocker therapy (β_1 blockade alone is inadequate) include fine tremor, excessive sweating, tachycardia, palpitations, nervousness, and the characteristic "staring" appearance (which is the result of eyelid contracture). Propranolol may also be used as an adjunct to more specific therapy, for example at the outset while a decision concerning definitive treatment is awaited, to suppress symptoms pending an effective response to antithyroid drugs or radioiodine, and in preoperative management. It is of particular value in controlling supraventricular dysrhythmias caused by the thyrotoxic state, including paroxysmal atrial tachycardia and atrial fibrillation, and can be used in combination with diuretics in patients with high output cardiac failure. Atrial fibrillation and high output cardiac failure are especially common in elderly subjects.

The dose of propranolol may be difficult to establish and careful dosage titration is required. Doses higher than those used in euthyroid patients should be anticipated because the hepatic clearance of propranolol is increased in thyrotoxicosis. Because of this, nadolol, a non-selective long acting drug unaffected by liver metabolising enzymes (nadolol is excreted unchanged in the urine) is sometimes preferred to propranolol.[34] Esmolol, an ultra short acting β blocker, has been administered by continuous intravenous infusion in the perioperative management of thyrotoxicosis in a patient with cardiac decompensation in whom propranolol precipitated cardiovascular collapse.[35]

PORTAL HYPERTENSION[36]

Propranolol and other non-selective β blockers reduce portal pressure by decreasing portal–collateral blood flow and are used for prevention of recurrent bleeding from varices or gastric erosions. Their action stems mainly from blockade at β_2 sites associated with vasoconstriction in the splanchnic circulation and augmented by the fall in cardiac output produced at β_1 receptors in the myocardium. Not all patients respond, however: response rates are reported to vary from as little as 50% up to 70%, possibly due to a compensatory increase in portal–collateral vascular resistance and maintenance therefore of elevated portal pressure.

The dose of propranolol varies considerably between individuals. Most patients respond to 40–80 mg twice daily or 160 mg once daily as slow release capsules, but others require much higher doses. Heart rate is used as a guide to adequacy of β blockade, so that the dosage is titrated gradually to achieve a reduction in resting heart rate of about 25% (to a limit of 55 beats/min).

GLAUCOMA[37]

Topical β blockers are used in the treatment of chronic open angle glaucoma. They reduce intraocular pressure by reducing aqueous humour production as a result of their effects on sympathetic innervation in the ciliary epithelium. Both cardioselective (betaxolol) and non-selective (levobunolol, timolol, metipranolol, and carteolol) agents are available. Carteolol also possesses partial agonist activity, but it is not clear whether it produces fewer side effects as a result and, although betaxolol is less likely to increase airways resistance, it too must still be used with caution in patients with obstructive airways disease. Timolol and levobunolol are the most active and are used in patients who do not respond to other agents. All preparations are administered twice daily, but levobunolol is also effective in single daily dosage. Topical β blockers are all potentially irritant, and betaxolol in particular may produce local stinging on application.

MIGRAINE[38][39]

Soon after the introduction of propranolol in 1964 the serendipitous discovery in a few patients that it reduced the frequency of "vascular headache" was made. A series of trials followed, which confirmed that β blockers *without* partial agonist activity were effective in preventing migraine headaches but had less effect on the intensity or duration of headache once it had begun. A meta-analysis of the findings from studies (total 2403 patients) evaluating propranolol (modal regimen 160 mg daily) shows that the frequency of recurrent migraine headache is on average reduced by 44% using conservative criteria and by as much as 65% when assessed less objectively.

Other drugs that have proved to be effective include metoprolol, timolol, nadolol and atenolol. Typical studies have shown that propranolol (80 mg) and metoprolol (50 mg), both twice daily, compare favourably with the standard clonidine and pizotifen regimen although others suggest that high dosages (for example 240–320 mg propranolol daily) may be required. Exactly how β blockers reduce the frequency of migraine attacks is unclear, as indeed is the pathophysiology of the migraine attack itself: both vascular and neurological mechanisms have been proposed. It is possible that constriction of the extracranial vessels, which are typically dilated during an attack, is important or that platelet uptake of serotonin is favourably influenced. β Blockers also have effects on fatty acid and prostaglandin synthesis, which might have implications for the release of local inflammatory mediators. In addition, noradrenaline levels are high immediately before a migraine attack but subsequently fall during the attack; raising the possibility of modulation of central adrenergic transmission by β blockers.

ANXIETY[40]

Anxiety that is part of an acute stress reaction (situational anxiety), such as that provoked by examinations and public speaking, or that which adversely affects musical performance (violin playing is particularly vulnerable), readily responds to predosing with a β blocker. Relatively low dosage (such as 40 mg or less propranolol) is required, reflecting the high level of adrenergic overactivity associated with these stresses. Not surprisingly, therefore, the major benefit is seen as a reduction of the physical signs of stress—tachycardia, palpitations, and tremor.

In generalised anxiety disorders and phobic anxiety the β blockers are less effective than benzodiazepines or tricyclic antidepressants, except where somatic symptoms (for example, tachycardia, palpitations, tremor, paraesthesia, shortness of breath, chest pains, weakness, and blushing) predominate. A central mechanism cannot be excluded and may supervene during chronic dosing. However, peripheral effects consistently occur early and respond to other β blockers (for example nadolol) that are largely water soluble and do not readily enter the central nervous system. It is preferable, however, to use a drug that is non-selective so that a more generalised effect is obtained.

Newer β blockers

CELIPROLOL

Celiprolol[41-45] is the first of a new generation of selective β_1 adrenoceptor blockers that also possess selective β_2 partial agonist activity, reducing peripheral vascular resistance and having a minimal effect on resting heart rate or cardiac output. It is possible that a further, as yet undefined, vasodilator mechanism exists but, unlike labetalol, celiprolol has no demonstrable α blocking activity.

Celiprolol, like atenolol, is mainly water soluble, has an elimination half life of 4–7 h and can be given as a single daily dose. It also resembles pindolol in that it has partial agonist activity. It is claimed, however, that the degree of cardioselectivity and partial agonist activity is more pronounced than with these established agents. Celiprolol is currently licensed for the treatment of hypertension, in which doses of 200–400 mg once daily are comparable to the usual doses of atenolol and pindolol and other non-cardioselective β blockers. Because it is largely excreted unchanged in the urine, the dose of celiprolol should be halved in patients with moderate renal impairment (for example creatinine clearance below 40 ml/min).

Given in single daily dosage celiprolol has also proved to be as effective as twice daily regimens of propranolol in improving exercise tolerance and reducing glyceryl trinitrate consumption in patients with chronic stable angina. However, treatment with propranolol in these patients was associated with a significant reduction in resting heart rate compared with celiprolol.

Further potential advantages of a drug of this type include attenuation of the recognised adverse effects of β blockers on the lung, the peripheral circulation and on lipid profile.

Clearly a drug which possesses β_2 partial agonist activity may benefit patients with airways obstruction, although it is interesting to note that caution is advised in the product data sheet when "Celectol" is prescribed for asthmatics, particularly during acute exacerbations. In a single dose study of ten patients with stable asthma celiprolol produced a significant ($+12\%$) increase in FEV_1 and forced vital capacity, which were decreased (-9%) by single doses of propranolol. Furthermore, celiprolol appeared to inhibit the bronchoconstrictor effect of propranolol when both drugs were given concurrently. However, a worsening of airways function has also been reported after treatment with celiprolol.[46 47]

Non-selective β blockers (and to a lesser extent selective β_1 blockers) impair peripheral perfusion and so pose problems for patients with peripheral vascular insufficiency, in whom they may provoke worsening of intermittent claudication and exacerbation of Raynaud's phenomenon. Celiprolol, because of its β_2 selective agonist properties, may be better tolerated than established cardio-selective drugs in such cases but evidence from clinical trials so far is generally lacking.[48] Celiprolol may also be less likely to impair glucose tolerance or cause hypoglycaemia or dyslipidaemia and, indeed, it has been associated with a *reduction* in triglyceride levels and an *increase* in the high density lipoprotein:low density lipoprotein cholesterol ratio in non-smokers.

ESMOLOL[49]

Esmolol is a selective β_1 blocker with an ultra short duration of action because of its rapid inactivation by blood esterases: its distribution half life is about 2 min and its elimination half life about 9 min. Esmolol reduces heart rate in proportion to plasma concentration, and when it is administered by continuous intravenous infusion the extent of β blockade can be tailored to the requirements of individual patients by varying the administration (infusion) rate. Esmolol has a role in short term management—that is, when a rapid onset and termination of β blockade is desirable—such as in the treatment of supraventricular arrhythmias, to control elevated blood pressure perioperatively, and possibly after acute myocardial infarction.

XAMOTEROL[50]

Xamoterol also possesses substantial β_1 partial agonist activity (about half that of the pure agonist isoprenaline). Its use in cardiac failure is based on the concept that it will improve myocardial contractility as a result of pronounced partial agonist activity when sympathetic tone is naturally low (for example, at rest), but on exercise or during stress its β adrenoceptor antagonist action will predominate, so modulating detrimental energy demanding sympathetic overactivity. Xamoterol was introduced early in 1988 for the treatment of all grades of chronic heart failure but by August 1989 its association with a 2·5-fold increase in mortality risk compared with placebo was highlighted by the Committee on Safety of Medicines. As a result, the indications, contraindications and dosage of xamoterol have been revised so that it should now *only* be used in the treatment of chronic *mild* cardiac failure.

Beta blockers whose introduction is anticipated (table 9.3)

CARVEDILOL[51 52]

Carvedilol, a combined non-cardioselective β blocker and selective α adrenergic blocker, has been developed from labetalol, the forerunner of this group. However, carvedilol displays a lower α blocking:β blocking ratio than does labetalol and a different haemodynamic response is seen, on exercise and at rest, as a result. In view of its peripheral vasodilator action it is likely that its major

TABLE 9.3—*Newer β blockers expected soon*

Epanolol		Selective β_1 blocker/β_1 partial agonist
Carvedilol	Unlicensed at time of preparation of this text	Non-selective β blocker/selective α_1 blocker
Tertatolol		Non-selective, long acting, renal vasodilator?

use will be in the management of hypertension and that its promotion will focus on the proven secondary preventive effect of β blockers against coronary heart disease, and their potential role in primary prevention as a result of their cardioprotective action. Single daily doses of 25 mg have proved effective in the control of mild-to-moderate hypertension but it remains to be seen to what extent carvedilol will produce the postural dizziness so frequently associated with labetalol. Such an effect has been reported with higher doses, for example 50 mg daily.

EPANOLOL[53 54]

Epanolol is a β_1 selective blocker which also has β_1 selective partial agonist activity of about 20–25% that of the pure agonist, isoprenaline. It has been developed mainly as an antianginal agent. Studies to date show that a single daily dose of 200 mg is as effective as standard therapies (atenolol and nifedipine), is well tolerated, and does not induce tachyphylaxis. In particular, changes in resting heart rate, blood pressure, peripheral perfusion, and renal function occur to a lesser degree than with other cardioselective β blockers.

TERTATOLOL[55 56]

Tertatolol, a non-cardioselective, long acting β blocker, produces a fall in blood pressure after a single daily dose of 5 mg, which is comparable to that produced by 100 mg atenolol daily. Further, tertatolol, like nadolol, does not impair renal perfusion but has been shown to increase glomerular filtration rate by a modest amount, suggesting the possibility of a direct intrarenal vasodilator mechanism. Tertatolol may have a special role in hypertension associated with kidney failure when adjustment in daily dose is unnecessary even in patients with severe renal impairment.

1 Wadworth AN, Murdoch D, Brogden RN. Atenolol. A reappraisal of its pharmacological properties and therapeutic use in cardiovascular disorders. *Drugs* 1991;**42**:468–510.

2 Lipworth BJ, Irvine NA, McDevitt DG, *et al.* The effects of chronic dosing on the β_1- and β_2-adrenoceptor antagonism of betaxolol and atenolol. *Eur J Clin Pharmacol* 1991;**40**:467–71.

3 Lipworth BJ, Irvine NA, McDevitt DG, *et al.* The effects of time and dose on the relative β_1- and β_2-adrenoceptor antagonism of betaxolol and atenolol. *Br J Clin Pharmacol* 1991;**31**:154–9.

4 Johnsson G, Regardh CG. Clinical pharmacokinetics of Beta-adrenoreceptor blocking drugs. *Clin Pharmacokinet* 1976;**1**:233–63.

5 Routledge PA, Shand DG. Clinical pharmacokinetics of propranolol. *Clin Pharmacokinet* 1979;**4**:73–90.

6 Nies AS, Shand DG. Clinical pharmacology of propranolol. *Circulation* 1975;**52**:8–15.

7 McLenachan JM, Findlay IN, Wilson JT, *et al*. Twenty-four-hour beta-blockade in stable angina pectoris: a study of atenolol and betaxolol. *J Cardiovasc Pharmacol* 1992;**20**:311–15.

8 Pathy MS. Acute central chest pain in the elderly: a review of 296 consecutive hospital admissions during 1979 with particular reference to the possible role of beta-adrenergic blocking agents in inducing substernal pain. *Am Heart J* 1979;**98**:168–70.

9 Robertson RM, Wood AJJ, Vaughan WK, *et al*. Exacerbation of vasotonic angina pectoris by propranolol. *Circulation* 1982;**65**:281–5.

10 Holm G, Herlitz J, Smith U. Severe hypoglycaemia during physical exercise and treatment with beta-blockers. *BMJ* 1981;**282**:1360.

11 Belton P, Carmody M, Donohoe M, *et al*. Propranolol-associated hypoglycaemia in non-diabetics. *J Irish Med Assoc* 1980;**73**:173.

12 Barnett AH, Leslie D, Watkins PJ. Can insulin-treated diabetics be given beta-adrenergic blocking drugs? *BMJ* 1980;**280**:976–8.

13 Kristensen BO. Effect of long-term treatment with beta-blocking drugs on plasma lipids and lipoproteins. *BMJ* 1981;**283**:191–2.

14 van-Hoof R, Desager JP, Harvengt C, *et al*. Comparison of the effect of celiprolol and nifedipine on blood pressure and plasma lipids. *J Cardiovasc Pharmacol* 1992;**20**:268–73.

15 McAinsh J, Cruickshank JM. Beta-blockers and central nervous system side effects. *Pharmacol Ther* 1990;**46**:163–97.

16 Stevenson JG, Umstead GS. Sexual dysfunction due to antihypertensive agents. *Drug Intell Clin Pharm* 1984;**18**:113–21.

17 Beaufils M. Alterations in renal hemodynamics during chronic and acute beta-blockade in humans. *Am J Hypertens* 1989;**2**:233S–236S.

18 Kelly KL. Beta-blockers in hypertension. A review. *Am J Hosp Pharm* 1976;**33**:1284–90.

19 Lavie CJ, Ventura HG, Messerli FH. Regression of increased left ventricular mass by antihypertensives. *Drugs* 1991;**42**:945–61.

20 Alten JW, Kaiser PJ, Montenegro A. Effects of atenolol on left ventricular hypertrophy and early left ventricular function in essential hypertension. *Am J Cardiol* 1989;**64**:1157–61.

21 Colantonio D, Casale R, Desiati P, *et al*. Short-term effects of atenolol and nifedipine on atrial natriuretic peptide, plasma renin activity, and plasma aldosterone in patients with essential hypertension. *J Clin Pharmacol* 1991;**31**:238–42.

22 Duff HJ, Roden DM, Brorson L, *et al*. Electrophysiologic actions of high plasma concentrations of propranolol in human subjects. *J Am Coll Cardiol* 1983;**2**:1134–40.

23 Kato R, Ikeda N, Yabek SM, *et al*. Electrophysiologic effects of the levo- and dextro-rotatory isomers of sotalol in isolated cardiac muscle and their in vivo pharmacokinetics. *J Am Coll Cardiol* 1986;**7**:116–25.

24 Norris RM, Barnaby PF, Brown MA, *et al*. Prevention of ventricular fibrillation during acute myocardial infarction by intravenous propranolol. *Lancet* 1984;**2**:883–6.

25 Ryden L, Arniego R, Arnman K, *et al*. A double blind trial of metoprolol in acute myocardial infarction. Effects on ventricular tacyarrhythmias. *N Engl J Med* 1983;**308**:614–18.

26 Editorial. Intravenous β-blockade during acute myocardial infarction. *Lancet* 1986;**2**:79–80.

27 Editorial. Long-term and short-term beta-blockade after myocardial infarction. *Lancet* 1981;**1**:1159.

28 β-Blocker Heart Attack Study Group. The β-blocker heart attack trial. *JAMA* 1981;**246**:2073–4.

29 Olsson G, Rehnqvist N, Sjogren A, *et al*. Long term treatment with metoprolol after myocardial infarction. Effect on 3 year mortality and morbidity. *J Am Coll Cardiol* 1985;**5**:1428–37.

30 Yusef S, Peto R, Lewis JA, *et al*. B-blockade during and after myocardial infarction. *Prog Cardiovasc Dis* 1985;**27**:335–71.

31 Geffner DL, Hershman JM. Beta-adrenergic blockade for the treatment of hyperthyroidism. *Am J Med* 1992;**93**:61–8.

32 Utiger RD. Beta-adrenergic antagonist therapy for hyperthyroid Grave's disease. *New Engl J Med* 1984;**310**:1597–8.

33 Wiersinga WM. Propranolol and thyroid hormone metabolism. *Thyroid* 1991;**1**:273–7.

34 Gerst PH, Fildes J, Baylor P, *et al*. Long-acting beta-adrenergic antagonists as preparation for surgery in thyrotoxicosis. *Arch Surg* 1986;**121**:838–40.

35 Vijay akumar HR, Thomas WO, Ferrara JJ. Peri-operative management of severe thyrotoxicosis with esmolol. *Anaesthesia* 1989;**44**:406–8.

36 Hayes PC, Davis JM, Lewis JA, *et al*. Meta-analysis of value of propranolol in prevention of variceal haemorrhage. *Lancet* 1990;**336**:153–6.

37 Brooks AM, Gillies WE. Ocular beta-blockers in glaucoma management. Clinical pharmacological aspects. *Drugs Aging* 1992;**2**:208–21.

38 Andersson KE, Vinge E. Beta-adrenoceptor blockers and calcium antagonists in the prophylaxis and treatment of migraine. *Drugs* 1990;**39**:355–73.

39 Holroyd KA, Penzien DB, Cordingley GE. Propranolol in the management of recurrent migraine: a meta-analytic review. *Headache* 1991;**31**:333–40.

40 Tyrer P. Current status of beta-blocking drugs in the treatment of anxiety disorders. *Drugs* 1988;**36**:773–83.

41 Editorial. Celiprolol: theory and practice. *Lancet* 1991;**338**:1426–7.

42 Monopoli A, Forlani A, Bevilacqua M, *et al*. Interaction of selected vasodilating beta-blockers with adrenergic receptors in human cardiovascular tissues. *J Cardiovasc Pharmacol* 1989;**14**:114–20.

43 Milne RJ, Buckley MM. Celiprolol. An updated review of its pharmacodynamic and pharmacokinetic properties and therapeutic efficacy in cardiovascular disease. *Drugs* 1991;**41**:941–69.

44 Frishman WH, Helman M, Soberman J, *et al*. Comparison of celiprolol and propranolol in stable angina pectoris. Celiprolol International Angina Study Group. *Am J Cardiol* 1991;**67**:665–70.

45 Anonymous. Celiprolol—a better beta blocker? *Drug Ther Bull* 1992;**30**:35–6.

46 Waal-Manning HJ, Simpson FO. Safety of celiprolol in hypertensives with chronic obstructive respiratory disease. *N Z Med J* 1990;**103**:222.

47 Pujet JC, Dubrevil C, Fleury B, *et al*. Effects of celiprolol, a cardioselective beta-blocker, on respiratory function in asthmatic patients. *Eur Respir J* 1992;**5**:196–200.

48 Editorial. Celiprolol: theory and practice. *Lancet* 1991;**338**:1426–7.

49 Benfield P, Sorkin E. Esmolol: a preliminary review of its pharmacodynamic and pharmacokinetic properties, and therapeutic efficacy. *Drugs* 1988;**33**:392–412.

50 Committee on Safety of Medicines. Xamoterol (Corwin)—revised indications, contraindications, dose schedule and warnings. *Curr Probl* 1990;**28**:2.

51 Hansson L. Combined action drugs in the treatment of hypertension. *Drugs* 1988;**36**(suppl 6):26–30.

52 Rittinghausen R. Response rate with respect to the blood pressure-lowering effect of the vasodilating and beta-blocking agent carvedilol. *Drugs* 1988;**36**(suppl 6):92–101.

53 Ryden L. Efficacy of epanolol versus metoprolol in angina pectoris: a report from a Swedish multicentre study of exercise tolerance. *J Intern Med* 1992;**231**:7–11.

54 Harry JD. Clinical pharmacology of epanolol. Pharmacodynamic aspects. *Drugs* 1989;**38**(suppl 2):18–27.

55 Agnes E, Vandermercken C, Prost JF, *et al*. The Tertatolol International Multicentre Study (T.I.M.S.). Predicting factors of an efficient therapy. *Am J Hypertens* 1989;**2**:296S–302S.

56 Fallo F, Gregianin M, Bui F, *et al*. Comparison of the antihypertensive and renal effects of tertatolol and nadolol in hypertensive patients with mild renal impairment. *Eur J Clin Pharmacol* 1991;**40**:309–11.

10 Angiotensin converting enzyme inhibitors

ALASDAIR BRECKENRIDGE

The renin–angiotensin–aldosterone system (RAS) is of primary importance in the control of blood pressure, body fluid volume, and myocardial function; further it has important local functions in many organs. Most cells contain the genes and messenger RNA which encode the enzymes and polypeptides of the RAS and secrete active forms of angiotensin peptides; angiotensin converting enzyme (ACE) and angiotensin II are present in white blood cells and alveolar macrophages. Further, angiotensin II stimulates platelet aggregation, and acts as mitogen for cultured smooth muscle cells.[1] The local RAS acts not only as an endocrine system (that is, on target cells at sites distant from those secreting the peptides) but also has autocrine function (it acts on cells that produce the peptides) and a paracrine function (acting on neighbouring cells).

The development of antagonists of the RAS have proved important tools to explore the place of the various peptides of the system, as well as being valuable therapeutic agents in hypertension and heart failure. Such is the rate of advance of knowledge in this area that it is difficult for the clinician to keep abreast of all developments. This review of ACE inhibitors will thus concentrate on important recent clinical findings and will indicate probable future roles for this group of compounds.

Historical perspective

The development of ACE inhibitors is often cited as a prime example of task oriented research. The truth is far from this; as so often, chance played a large part in the development of this group of drugs. Some 25 years ago a group of Brazilian pharmacologists was searching for substances that would block the inactivation of bradykinin, a process subsequently shown to take place in humans

118

in the pulmonary vascular bed. It was shown that this was also the site for the conversion of angiotensin I to the potent vasoconstrictor angiotensin II, and that the two processes were controlled by enzymes that, if not the same, were very similar.

The importance of the RAS in the control of blood pressure has been appreciated for many years. Most early stratagems to lower blood pressure clinically, however, were based on manipulating the sympathetic nervous system, and attempts to perturb the RAS came much later. The use of effective orally active ACE inhibitors depended on translating the experiences of pharmacologists (who were interested primarily in the breakdown of bradykinin) to physiologists (who were interested in the mechanisms of controlling blood pressure) and then using the skills of medicinal chemists and clinical pharmacologists to design and test suitable compounds. A review by Ferreira, an important figure in the early development of this subject, details this interesting story.[2]

Eight orally active ACE inhibitors are currently licensed in the United Kingdom: captopril; enalapril; lisinopril; ramipril; quinapril; perindopril; cilazapril; fosinopril; and others are in various stages of development. In addition, compounds that are competitive antagonists of the angiotensin II receptor are in clinical trial. Their precise place in therapeutics remains to be defined. In this chapter studies with captopril and enalapril will be cited to illustrate the risk/benefit ratio of ACE inhibitors, because there is greatest clinical experience with these two compounds.

Mode of action

HYPERTENSION

Angiotensin converting enzyme is responsible for converting angiotensin I to angiotensin II and inactivating bradykinin. Other enzymes will also degrade bradykinin but will not cause conversion of angiotensin I. Angiotensin causes a rise in blood pressure in several ways—by causing direct vasoconstriction, hypertrophy of vascular smooth muscle, and release of aldosterone and thus sodium retention. Further, it is an important stimulus for cardiac growth. As discussed above, ACE is a ubiquitous enzyme.

The most easily understood mode of action of ACE inhibitors in hypertension is that they inhibit angiotensin conversion in vascular endothelium; resulting in vasodilatation and reversal of functional vascular changes; inhibition of bradykinin breakdown may play a minor role in lowering blood pressure. There is little evidence to support a direct central role of ACE inhibitors but there are important interactions between the RAS and sympathetic nervous system which may be perturbed by ACE inhibitors.[3]

HEART FAILURE

Among the main haemodynamic disturbances in heart failure is the angiotensin II mediated increase in systemic vascular resistance, producing increased left ventricular afterload and an increase in left ventricular filling pressure (preload), which in turn is caused by retention of sodium mediated by excess aldosterone. Decrease of angiotensin II concentrations reduces both afterload and preload both in the short and the long term.[4]

Clinical pharmacokinetics

CAPTOPRIL

Captopril is a derivative of the amino acid proline and contains a sulphydryl group. About three quarters of an oral dose is absorbed in healthy fasting volunteers, but ingestion with food reduces absorption by about 30%. Maximum plasma concentrations of captopril are reached 30–90 min after administration, when the peak ACE inhibitory and haemodynamic effects are also seen. These effects return to baseline 4–6 h after a 25 mg oral dose. Its elimination half life from plasma is 1–2 h, and it is excreted by the kidney partly unchanged and partly oxidised to form mixed disulphides (which are inactive). The elimination of captopril correlates closely with renal function, and a considerable increase in its half life is seen in patients who have creatinine clearances of less than 20 ml/min.[5]

ENALAPRIL

Enalapril is also a derivative of proline but, unlike captopril, does not contain a sulphydryl group. Some three fifths of a dose is absorbed, irrespective of food intake. Enalapril, however, is a prodrug that needs to be converted by esterase activity in the liver to the active moiety, enalaprilat. Enalapril itself achieves peak plasma concentrations 1 h after dosing and disappears from the plasma by 4 h: enalaprilat, on the other hand, reaches its peak concentration in plasma about 4 h after dosing with enalapril and has a half life of about 35 h; it is still detectable in plasma 96 h after the initial enalapril dose. The maximum inhibition of ACE activity occurs with peak plasma concentrations of enalaprilat and, unlike that of captopril, is sustained for 10 h and reverses gradually. Enalaprilat is excreted by glomerular filtration and, like captopril, will accumulate in patients who have advanced renal failure.[6]

The differences in kinetics and dynamics between captopril and enalapril mean that captopril is usually given two or three times a day whereas enalapril can be given once a day.

Clinical efficacy

HYPERTENSION

Captopril and enalapril both decrease blood pressure in patients who have different degrees of hypertension, irrespective of the underlying basis of the disease. Patients who have higher plasma renin activity (and thus higher angiotensin I concentrations) probably show greater decreases in blood pressure than those with low plasma renin activity, but hypotensive activity can be shown even in anephric patients.

The addition of a diuretic (thiazide or loop) to either ACE inhibitor will increase the hypotensive activity. This may be due to the increase in plasma renin activity that is produced by diuretics, which will therefore augment the efficacy of the ACE inhibitor as well as the additive hypotensive action of the two groups of drugs. The addition of β blockers (which suppress plasma renin activity) to ACE inhibitors is of less value than the addition of diuretics; calcium antagonists such as nifedipine have been shown to have an additive effect.[6]

The hypotensive efficacy of captopril and enalapril has been compared with that of diuretics, β blockers, and calcium antagonists. Individual studies may have claimed to show superiority of one ACE inhibitor over the others, but overall this is difficult to sustain.

The main differences in clinical efficacy between captopril and enalapril relate to doses and dosing intervals. There have been problems with both drugs in establishing initial dosing regimens and the optimum dose that should be given in hypertension and heart failure. For *captopril* it is now recommended that in patients who have mild to moderate hypertension the initial dose should be 12·5 mg twice a day and the maximum dose 50 mg twice a day. For patients taking diuretics the initial dose should be 6·25 mg twice a day. In patients who have severe hypertension 150 mg a day should not be exceeded. The dose should be kept as low as possible in the elderly and patients who have renal failure. The initial dose of *enalapril* in uncomplicated hypertension should be 5 mg daily, but if the patient is also taking diuretics a starting dose of 2·5 mg is recommended. The usual maintenance dose is 10–20 mg a day, and the maximum 40 mg. The elderly and patients with renal failure should initially receive no more than 2·5 mg daily.

Both captopril and enalapril are now recommended as first line treatment for patients who have hypertension. Captopril was formerly given to patients who had severe hypertension only when standard treatment had failed and to patients with mild to moderate hypertension as an adjunct to thiazide treatment when the response was inadequate. Similar constraints are placed on the use of enalapril, but this can now be used in all grades of hypertension.

One point should be emphasised about the use of ACE inhibitors. Patients usually feel well when taking them; whether this is a positive attribute of the drugs or because of a lack of the adverse effects that bedevil many other antihypertensive agents is an interesting debate. The phrase "quality of life" has been widely used in this discussion.[7]

HEART FAILURE

Comparison with other forms of vasodilator therapy for heart failure suggests that ACE inhibition is superior to both hydralazine and prazosin as judged by exercise performance and haemodynamic measurements in patients already given digitalis and diuretics.[8] Packer suggests that administration of either captopril or enalapril in heart failure may take several weeks to show an optimal effect, perhaps because the reversal of the slow pressor effect of angiotensin II leads to an improvement in peripheral utilisation of oxygen rather than the more immediate diuresis mediated by suppression of aldosterone secretion and the subsequent reduction in left ventricular filling pressure.[8]

Short term studies with both captopril and enalapril in patients with chronic heart failure show an increase in cardiac output, reduction in peripheral and pulmonary vasculative resistance. Further, symptoms are relieved and death rates reduced.[9]

Enalapril (40 mg once daily) was compared with captopril (50 mg three times daily) in 42 patients with chronic heart failure requiring digitalis and diuretics.[10] Both drugs caused a beneficial haemodynamic improvement but the fall in blood pressure caused by enalapril caused symptomatic hypotension. This may be the reason for the decline in creatinine and retention of potassium seen in the enalapril treated group. The authors suggest that in heart failure, shorter acting ACE inhibitors may be more advantageous.

Three recent trials of the use of ACE inhibitors in heart failure have been reported. In studies of Left Ventricular Dysfunction trial,[11] enalapril or placebo was given to patients with chronic left ventricular dysfunction but without symptomatic heart failure. No significant survival benefit for active treatment was seen over the 3 years of the trial. However, the incidence of symptomatic heart failure was lower in patients treated with enalapril.

The Save and Ventricular Enlargement trial[12] explored the clinical benefit of captopril given 3–16 days after myocardial infarction in patients with some systolic dysfunction but before the ventricle was severely dilated. A statistically significant reduction (19%) in mortality rate was seen in the actively treated patients. To explore if very early intervention with ACE inhibitors would be effective in preventing the onset of ventricular dilatation after myocardial infarction, the investigations in the Cooperative New Scandinavian Enalapril Survival Study II administered enalapril within 24 h of an acute myocardial infarction,[13] but no survival benefit was demonstrated. Reasons for this negative result are still being debated: could perfusion pressure of coronary vasculature be reduced leading to increase in infarct size? Could early administration of ACE inhibitors inhibit the early growth of myocytes and collagen that could protect against early infarct expansion?[9]

In heart failure, both captopril and enalapril therapy should be initiated in hospital under close medical supervision. The starting dose of captopril should be 6·25 or 12·5 mg to minimise any hypotensive effect and the usual maintenance dose is 25 or 50 mg three times daily. The initial dose of enalapril is 2·5 mg a day and the usual maintenance dose 10 or 20 mg per day, with a maximum of 40 mg a day.

Adverse effects

The most common adverse effect of ACE inhibitors is a *dry, non-productive cough*. All drugs in this group will cause it; its

123

mechanism is poorly understood but probably involves brady-kinin. Its frequency has varied from 1 to 14% in various studies.[5]

Large and unexpected *decreases in blood pressure* are seen with ACE inhibitors used in both hypertension and heart failure. They are most frequently seen in patients who are depleted in fluids because of excessive diuretic usage and in whom plasma concentrations of angiotensin I are raised. The higher the initial dose of ACE inhibitor, the more common is this adverse effect. It is seen earlier in the course of captopril than enalapril therapy because of the need to convert enalapril to active enalaprilat in the liver, but the effect can be more prolonged with enalapril.[10]

Renal impairment may occur as a result of the decrease in blood pressure described above, when it is usually attributed to the withdrawal of angiotensin II, which increases efferent arteriolar tone within the kidney and helps to maintain filtration pressure. It is more common in patients whose renal function is already compromised and, though it is usually reversible, cases have been reported with either drug when this is not so. A question remains whether there is a cohort of patients in whom treatment with either long term ACE inhibitor may result in an irreversible deterioration of renal function. From a regulatory standpoint this is of great concern and places a question mark over the use of this group of agents for mild hypertension that is not immediately life threatening. Monitoring renal function throughout treatment with these agents is thus mandatory.

All ACE inhibitors may cause *angioneurotic oedema*. It is unpredictable; its basis may be inhibition of bradykinin breakdown and deaths have resulted.

Loss of taste is found with captopril and may be related to the presence of the SH group. Taste may take several weeks to return.

Other effects, such as neutropenia, aphthous ulcers, and abdominal pain have been noted but are probably less common with the smaller drug doses now used.

The future

New therapeutic areas are being explored, in which ACE inhibitors may have an important role.[1] In hypertension, part of their benefit may be based not only on their ability to lower blood pressure but also on reversal of cardiac ventricular hypertrophy and alteration of regional vascular resistance by changing structural and functional changes in the arterial system and thus altering arterial compliance. The effect of ACE inhibitors on vascular biology may be of importance in coronary artery disease, especially in antagonising endothelial and smooth muscle proliferation seen, for example, after balloon angioplasty; it is now known that tissue ACE activity in the neointima is increased after this procedure, indicating a possible role for ACE inhibitors. Their role in the treatment of angina is also under investigation. The possibility that left ventricular structure may be beneficially remodelled by ACE inhibitors suggests a role in the development of left ventricular dysfunction; initial studies to explore this are described above.[11 12]

The intriguing observation that ACE inhibitors may reverse resistance to insulin, which may be causally associated with atheromatous disease and its consequences, is at present being vigorously explored. Reversal of insulin resistance is a property apparently shared with other antihypertensive agents such as α blockers, but not by diuretics, β blockers, or calcium channel antagonists which decrease insulin sensitivity.

Finally, ACE inhibitors have been shown to be beneficial in hypertensive diabetic patients in decreasing proteinuria and improving renal function. Whether this role can be extended with benefit to the non-hypertensive diabetic to preserve renal function is an intriguing possibility.

1 Erdmann E. Focus on ACE inhibition: implications for cardiovascular structure and function. *J Cardiovasc Pharmacol* 1992;**20**(suppl B):v–vi.
2 Ferreira SH. History of the development of inhibitors of angiotensin I conversion. *Drugs* 1986;**30**(suppl 1):1–5.
3 Johnston CI. Biochemistry and pharmacology of the renin–angiotensin system. *Drugs* 1990;**39**:21–31.
4 Laragh JH. Endocrine mechanisms in congestive cardiac failure: renin, aldosterone and atrial natriuretic hormone. *Drugs* 1986;**32**(suppl 5):1–12.
5 Fyhrqvist F. Clinical pharmacology of ACE inhibitors. *Drugs* 1986;**32**(suppl 5):33–9.
6 Gomez HF, Cirillo VJ, Irvine JD. Enalapril: a review of human pharmacology. *Drugs* 1985;**30**(suppl 1):13–24.
7 Croog SH, Levine S, Terta MA, *et al.* The effects of antihypertensive therapy on the quality of life. *N Engl J Med* 1986;**34**:1657–64.
8 Packer M. The role of vasodilator therapy in the treatment of severe chronic heart failure. *Drugs* 1986;**32**(suppl 5):13–26.
9 Cohn JN. The prevention of heart failure—a new agenda. *N Engl J Med* 1992;**327**:725–7.

10 Packer M, Lee WH, Yuschar M, Medina N. Comparison of captopril and enalapril in patients with severe chronic heart failure. *N Engl J Med* 1986;**315**:847–53.
11 The SOLVD Investigators. Effect of enalapril on mortality and the development of heart failure in asymptomatic patients with reduced left ventricular ejection fractions. *N Engl J Med* 1992;**327**:685–91.
12 Pfeffer MA, Braunwald E, Moya LA, *et al*. Effect of captopril on mortality and morbidity in patients with left ventricular dysfunction after myocardial infarction—results of the SAVE trial. *N Engl J Med* 1992;**327**:669–77.
13 Swedberg K, Held P, Kjekshus J, *et al*. Effects of early administration of enalapril on mortality in patients with acute myocardial infarction—results of the CONSENSUS II trial. *N Engl J Med* 1992;**327**:678–84.

11 Diuretic treatment

ANGUS MacCONNACHIE, DEREK MacLEAN

Over 40 years after their introduction, the "modern" diuretics remain one of the most widely prescribed groups of drugs for a variety of therapeutic indications.

Classification of diuretic drugs[1-3]

Diuretics are classified according to their site of action in the kidney tubule and their relative effects on sodium and potassium excretion. Three broad classes exist:

- thiazides and related drugs;
- "loop" (high ceiling) diuretics; and
- potassium sparing diuretics.

These three classes contain medium, high and low potency agents, respectively. Other diuretics, used less often and in special circumstances, include the carbonic anhydrase inhibitors and osmotically active agents (see table 11.1).

THIAZIDE AND RELATED DIURETICS[4-6]

The thiazides are medium potency natriuretic agents. They act on the cortical portion of the ascending tubule and at the beginning of the distal convoluted tubule, where less than 10% of the filtered sodium load is reabsorbed, and cause excretion of only 5–10% of the total sodium load.

Of this class of drugs 13 are in current use (table 11.1) and with few exceptions they are all equally effective at equivalent doses. Thus a single agent such as bendrofluazide is suitable in most cases: its action starts after about 2 h and lasts for 12–24 h. It may therefore be taken in a convenient single daily dose and is cheaper than most other thiazides. All thiazides taken by mouth are well absorbed and produce diuresis within 2 h of administration, but the length of action of individual drugs varies between 12 h or less and 48 h or longer. Very long acting drugs such as chlorthalidone

TABLE 11.1—*Available oral diuretic drugs: a practical classification*

Thiazides	*Thiazide related drugs*
Bendrofluazide 2·5/5 mg tablets	Chlorthalidone 50/100 mg tablets
Chlorothiazide 500 mg tablets	Mefruside 25 mg tablets
Clopamide (combination with a β blocker only)	Indapamide 2·5 mg tablets
Cyclopenthiazide 25/50 mg tablets	*Loop (high ceiling) drugs*
Hydrochlorothiazide 25/50 mg tablets	Bumetanide 1/5 mg tablets,
Hydroflumethiazide 50 mg tablets	1mg/5 ml liquid
Methyclothiazide 5 mg tablets	Ethacrynic acid 50 mg tablets
Polythiazide 1 mg tablets	Frusemide 20/40/500 mg tablets,
	1 mg/ml liquid
Potassium sparing diuretics	Piretanide 6 mg SR capsules
Amiloride 5 mg tablets	Torasemide (available soon)
Spironolactone 25/50/100 mg tablets	
Triamterene 50 mg capsules	*Mixed loop and thiazide drugs*
	Metolazone 5 mg tablets
Carbonic anhydrase inhibitors	Xipamide 20 mg tablets
Acetazolamide 250 mg tablets	
250 mg SR capsules	*Osmotically active agents*
Dichlorphenamide 50 mg tablets	Isosorbide (oral)
	Mannitol (intravenous)

and polythiazide may be taken on alternate days but may be associated with troublesome nocturia. Their length of action probably also has important consequences for potassium conservation (discussed below).

Indapamide, xipamide, metolazone, and mefruside are thiazide like diuretics that are structurally related to frusemide. As a result, their actions differ somewhat from those of the thiazide diuretics generally.

Indapamide[7]

In daily doses of 2·5 mg indapamide produces minimal diuresis but seems to lower blood pressure as effectively as a thiazide. There is evidence that it exerts a direct effect on vascular smooth muscle, possibly decreasing calcium inward currents, reducing vascular reactivity, and hence peripheral arterial resistance. Indeed, the classification of indapamide as a calcium antagonist has been proposed, but some doubt exists as to whether usual dosages cause appreciable calcium antagonism. Indapamide may have a useful role in managing hypertension in patients with prostatism or an unstable bladder, although the drug is occasionally associated with pronounced diuresis in the elderly. In contrast to the thiazides, indapamide has little or no apparent influence on concentrations of serum potassium, urate, glucose, or lipoproteins and it produces only a modest rise in plasma renin activity.

Xipamide[8]

This is chemically related to salicylic acid. At normal doses (20–40 mg once a day) it has a pronounced diuretic action similar to that of frusemide (40 mg), but its onset (about 1 h) and duration (12 h or more) of action is comparable to that of a medium acting thiazide such as hydrochlorothiazide. For practical purposes xipamide is, perhaps, best considered as having a gradual onset yet a diuretic potency similar to that of frusemide. It also exerts a potent antihypertensive effect and, given once a day, its efficacy has been compared with that of 24 h β blockade: many elderly patients, however, find the intense and prolonged diuretic action of xipamide somewhat troublesome. Increasing reports of profound hypokalaemia (possibly dose related), with serum potassium concentrations as low as 2·2 mmol/l, are also a worrying aspect of its long term use. Regular serum potassium measurement and concurrent administration of a potassium sparing diuretic are therefore often necessary during chronic therapy with xipamide.

Metolazone[9]

Metolazone is chemically a quinazolone sulphonamide. It produces pronounced diuresis within 1–2 h of oral administration and is active for up to 24 h. It is much more potent than the thiazides and, like the loop diuretics, it produces effective diuresis in patients with renal impairment. Metolazone has been used in combination with frusemide to produce diuresis when frusemide alone has been ineffective. Severe electrolyte disturbances have been reported, and metolazone should be reserved for the treatment of resistant oedema.

Mefruside[10]

This drug is a thiazide like diuretic, the action of which starts after 1–2 h and lasts for up to 24 h. Mefruside offers no advantages over thiazides generally and is not, as the name might suggest, an alternative to frusemide.

LOOP DIURETICS[11]

The loop or "high ceiling" diuretics (see table 11.1) include the carboxylic acid derivatives frusemide, bumetanide, ethacrynic acid, and most recently the benzoic acid derivative piretanide. Torasemide is likely to be added to the group in the near future. Loop diuretics are rapidly absorbed after oral administration and have a characteristically rapid onset (30–60 min) and brief duration (4–6 h) of action.

The main site of action is the thick ascending limb of the loop of Henle, where normally about 20% of the filtered sodium load is reabsorbed. Their action is brought about by irreversible binding to, and inhibition of, a carrier protein–$Na^+/2Cl^-/K^+$ cotransport system present in the luminal membrane and through which sodium reabsorption is mediated. The loop diuretics also remain effective diuretics, even if the glomerular filtration rate falls to as low as 10 ml/min, but only in large doses (up to 10-fold or more above normal). Thus the loop diuretics are potentially dangerous as the diuresis they produce is proportional to dose despite volume and electrolyte depletion.

Frusemide

This is the cheapest and by far the most widely prescribed of the current loop diuretics. Its bioavailability is, however, poor and erratic, perhaps as low as 20%, and increasing oral doses may be required in some patients who fail to respond to doses in the usual range (40–80 mg).

Bumetanide[12]

Bumetanide is 40 times more potent on a weight basis than frusemide and its bioavailability is much higher because its oral absorption is consistently good. This probably explains its apparently greater activity compared with frusemide and why it is preferred by some for those patients who fail to respond initially to oral frusemide. Bumetanide is more "potassium sparing" than frusemide (kaliuretic potency is only 20 times greater on a weight basis) and there is anecdotal evidence that it is less likely to impair glucose tolerance or cause urate retention.

Ethacrynic acid

This is a loop diuretic which also possesses uricosuric activity, but it is now little used. It has been associated with a relatively high incidence of gastrointestinal upsets including nausea, diarrhoea and abdominal pain; gastrointestinal haemorrhage and liver impairment have also been reported. Unlike other loop diuretics, however, ethacrynic acid is not a sulphonamide derivative, and it is a useful alternative in patients who develop hypersensitivity to other diuretics in which cross reactivity is a feature.

Piretanide[13]

This agent is chemically different from other loop diuretics but its actions seem to be similar. It is about six times more potent than frusemide. Piretanide is reported to exert a less variable natriuretic effect than frusemide, and its kaliuretic action is of much shorter duration. Thus it may be more "potassium sparing" than the thiazides and other loop diuretics. Piretanide, which is available only in slow release form, is licensed for use in treating mild to moderate hypertension, but low dose thiazides are most often used for this condition.

Torasemide[14]

Torasemide is likely to be marketed in the near future. It is about twice as potent as frusemide, produces an equal diuresis and natriuresis and has a longer duration of action, allowing once daily dosage without the paradoxical antidiuresis occasionally seen with frusemide. It also has a less pronounced effect on potassium and calcium excretion. In trials, so far, torasemide has proved as effective as indapamide and thiazide diuretics in lowering blood pressure in mild to moderate essential hypertension and is effective in single daily dosage in the control of oedema associated with congestive heart failure, liver cirrhosis and renal disease.

POTASSIUM SPARING DIURETICS[15–18]

Amiloride, spironolactone and *triamterene* are only weak natriuretics but they potentiate the action of the thiazides and loop diuretics, with which they are commonly used. Their most important role in such combinations, however, is the retention of potassium which, in the case of amiloride and triamterene, is promoted by their action in the distal renal tubule, as follows.

In the segment from the late distal tubule to the collecting duct, active sodium reabsorption, at the expense of potassium, takes place via specific sodium channels. These channels are blocked by amiloride and, to a lesser extent, by triamterene. Spironolactone inhibits the increase in numbers of sodium channels and the activity of the Na^+/K^+ pump, which drives the exchange process under the influence of aldosterone. Spironolactone and canrenoate (a derivative of spironolactone's active metabolite canrenone) are specifically competitive antagonists of the mineralocorticoid aldosterone.

Spironolactone or canrenoate are particularly useful in primary (Conn's syndrome) or secondary hyperaldosteronism (such as occurs in liver cirrhosis, nephrotic syndrome, or oedema associated with resistant cardiac failure). When a loop diuretic in high dosage (for example frusemide 80–160 mg) fails to adequately control heart failure, the addition of spironolactone may be indicated. This is especially the case when the 24 h ratio of urinary sodium to potassium is less than 1·0, as increasing the dose of diuretic merely promotes further loss of urinary potassium rather than sodium. As aldosterone causes a parallel increase in the excretion of magnesium and potassium, treatment with spironolactone also causes magnesium retention.

All potassium sparing diuretics (and particularly spironolactone) are more expensive than potassium supplementation, but maintain serum potassium concentrations much more reliably. Amiloride and triamterene have a rapid onset of action, but concentrations of canrenone accumulate slowly over a period of several days. The peak effect of all three agents continues for several days after treatment is discontinued, and spironolactone may remain active for up to 1 week.

Potassium sparing diuretics are mainly used to conserve potassium rather than for their diuretic and antihypertensive actions, and so are often prescribed in combination preparations containing thiazide diuretics.

OTHER DIURETICS

Acetazolamide and *dichlorphenamide* are inhibitors of the enzyme carbonic anhydrase. In the kidney they produce limited alkaline diuresis by promoting the excretion of bicarbonate and of sodium and potassium cations in the proximal tubule. Continuous administration, however, results in metabolic acidosis and the diuretic action is therefore self-limiting. Inhibition of carbonic anhydrase in the eye is associated with reduced production of aqueous humour and, consequently, lowered intraocular pressure. This has led to the more common use of acetazolamide to treat glaucoma. Finally, acetazolamide has been used to treat mountain sickness because it increases ventilation at altitude.

Mannitol is an osmotic diuretic that is used to force diuresis in patients with cerebral oedema, or occasionally after acute poisoning with drugs that are predominantly excreted unchanged in the urine. Infusion of a 20% solution of mannitol may produce useful diuresis in patients with oedema that is resistant to other diuretics; it has also been used to prevent renal failure in jaundiced patients undergoing surgery. Osmotic diuretics are contraindicated in hepatic or renal failure and in patients who have sustained recent cerebral haemorrhage.

Isosorbide is a well tolerated, orally active, osmotic diuretic that has been used occasionally to lower raised intracranial and intraocular pressures as well as to clear hepatic ascites resistant to other measures.

Adverse effects

THIAZIDE AND LOOP DIURETICS

Hyponatraemia

Hyponatraemia may result from over zealous use of diuretics. It is particularly likely to occur in the elderly and the inappropriate use of diuretics for supposed fluid retention in patients with venous stasis due to varicose veins should be discouraged. Excessive diuretic treatment is a common cause of postural hypotension and falls in the elderly, who may also experience hyponatraemia associated with the combination of a thiazide and amiloride, for example Moduretic.

Hypokalaemia

This may be intermittent, especially in hypertensive subjects, and occurs during prolonged treatment in 30–50% of patients treated with thiazides and 25–30% of those treated with loop diuretics. Its incidence, which seems to be related to the length of action of a particular diuretic, is highest after treatment with the very long acting thiazides chlorthalidone and polythiazide. The fall in serum potassium concentration, however, does not usually progress to a level at which total body stores of potassium are appreciably affected (it is essentially an intracellular ion). Occasional monitoring of serum potassium is therefore sufficient to identify the few patients who may develop clinically appreciable hypokalaemia. Hypokalaemia associated with loop diuretics is dose related and most likely to occur with prolonged diuresis (when taken twice daily).

Hypokalaemia is nearly always asymptomatic unless the serum potassium concentration falls below 2·5 mmol/l. Serum potassium therefore requires active investigation, particularly in patients treated with digoxin and other cardiac glycosides in whom the risk of serious cardiac arrhythmias is increased. Hypokalaemia may also precipitate hepatic encephalopathy and coma in patients with liver cell failure. Evidence also exists that, when acute cardiac infarction supervenes in patients who are already hypokalaemic, the risk of serious ventricular arrhythmias is doubled and that of fatal ventricular fibrillation increased almost fivefold. Adrenaline mediated augmentation of hypokalaemia may play an important part in this risk.

Hypomagnesaemia

This problem may be associated with long term thiazide and loop diuretic therapy and seems to carry a risk of cardiac arrhythmias. It is less pronounced with bumetanide than it is with frusemide. Magnesium, as well as potassium, conservation is promoted by spironolactone when added to diuretic therapy. Magnesium supplementation may be necessary in patients at particular risk, and oral and parenteral forms of magnesium are available for this purpose.

Hyperuricaemia

Hyperuricaemia, probably caused by enhanced tubular reabsorption of urate, occurs in about 40% of men receiving long term thiazide diuretic treatment and much less commonly in women. It is also associated with the loop diuretics but there is anecdotal evidence that bumetanide is less likely than frusemide to cause urate retention. Hyperuricaemia, which may be persistent throughout thiazide treatment, may precipitate gout but is usually harmless and can safely be ignored.

Impaired glucose tolerance

This may develop slowly during long term diuretic treatment but is only occasionally of clinical importance, even in diabetics whose requirements for insulin, dietary change, or altered dosage of oral hypoglycaemic drugs are not generally affected. If necessary, a combination of a thiazide diuretic and a potassium sparing diuretic, which is less likely to alter diabetic control, can be used.

Cholesterol and triglycerides

Raised serum total cholesterol and triglyceride concentration and unfavourable reduction in the ratio of high to low density lipoprotein cholesterol in patients treated with thiazide diuretics have given rise to concern that this treatment might be associated with an increase in coronary risk. However, in treating hypertension, at least, the benefit of diuretic treatment in terms of reduced incidence of stroke alone far outweighs any coronary risk.

Impotence

Impotence is reported in about one third of hypertensive men treated with various hypotensive agents, of which thiazide diuretics figure prominently. Thiazides may produce impotence in 20% of patients and, although the mechanism is unknown, the effect is usually reversible within a few weeks of discontinuing treatment. It is possible, though not yet confirmed, that the low dose regimen now advised in hypertension is associated with a reduction in the incidence of impotence.

Gastrointestinal upsets

Gastrointestinal problems (nausea, indigestion, and constipation) are reported in up to 20% of patients treated with thiazides or loop diuretics, particularly ethacrynic acid. Pancreatitis has been reported occasionally.

Skin reactions

Skin reactions, such as bullous and lichenoid eruptions and photosensitivity are relatively rare side effects.

Hearing problems

Temporary deafness and tinnitus may follow the use of loop diuretics in patients with renal failure.

Urinary problems

Acute urinary retention may be precipitated in patients with prostatism who take loop diuretics as these, by the brisk nature of their action, cause rapid filling of the bladder.

Thrombocytopenia

Mild or asymptomatic thrombocytopenia is occasionally noted in patients receiving frusemide. Regular reports of thiazide induced thrombocytopenia have also appeared in the literature but, given the extent to which these drugs are prescribed, its occurrence would appear to be relatively rare.

POTASSIUM SPARING DIURETICS

Hyperkalaemia

Sometimes fatal hyperkalaemia may result from the indiscriminate use of potassium sparing diuretics, especially in the treatment of hypertension when only low doses of thiazides are generally required. Despite this, their use in hypertension in combination with other diuretics (such as Dyazide, Moduretic) is extremely common. The risk of hyperkalaemia is greatest in patients with renal impairment, which is often the case in elderly hypertensives. See also the interaction with ACE inhibitors.

Hyponatraemia

Hyponatraemia, which is occasionally severe, especially in the elderly, has been reported with the combination of amiloride and a thiazide diuretic (for example, Moduretic) and is related to the marked effect which amiloride has on sodium flux in the distal renal tubule.

Antiandrogenic effects

Spironolactone has antiandrogenic effects, which are responsible for the tender nipples and painful gynaecomastia with which it is often associated. This reflects the steroidal structure of the spironolactone molecule, which in men also causes sexual impotence and in women menstrual irregularities and hirsutism.

Gastrointestinal upsets

These include nausea and vomiting and are associated more often with spironolactone than with other diuretics, but are less marked if doses are taken with meals. Nausea, vomiting and diarrhoea are reported in about 5% of patients treated with triamterene.

Renal problems

Renal calculi formation and deposition of crystals and casts have been attributed to triamterene but the occurrence is rare. Stones appear to be composed of triamterene metabolites and calcium oxalate.

Drug interactions

THIAZIDE AND LOOP DIURETICS

Drug interactions of possible clinical importance associated with diuretic treatment are as follows.

1. *Non-steroidal anti-inflammatory drugs* are generally more nephrotoxic in patients also treated with diuretics. These drugs, notably indomethacin but others too, inhibit the action of loop diuretics which appears to be mediated by renal prostaglandin release and may interfere with the control of heart failure. There is evidence that the active metabolites of the prodrugs sulindac and nabumetone are not concentrated in renal tissues and therefore have no inhibitory effect on renal prostaglandins.

2. *Aminoglycoside antibiotics* (gentamicin, tobramycin, amikacin, et cetera) and vancomycin enhance nephrotoxicity when combined with loop diuretics.

3. *ACE inhibitors* are generally more likely to be associated with first dose profound hypotension in patients receiving long term diuretic treatment, probably because they are salt depleted.

4. *Digoxin* toxicity is more likely to occur in patients who develop hypokalaemia while receiving diuretic treatment.

5. *Lithium* toxicity is reported in patients also receiving thiazide diuretics in whom increased lithium reabsorption at the proximal kidney tubule occurs.

POTASSIUM SPARING DIURETICS

1. *ACE inhibitors* promote potassium retention by inhibiting the release of aldosterone which is primarily stimulated by angiotensin. Therefore there is a major risk of hyperkalaemia when ACE inhibitors are used together with potassium sparing diuretics.

2. *Non-steroidal anti-inflammatory drugs*, in combination with potassium sparing diuretics may precipitate acute renal failure. Indomethacin/triamterene combinations appear to carry the

greatest risk and several reports of reversible non-oliguric renal failure have appeared.

3. *Digoxin* plasma concentrations are reported to be markedly raised by spironolactone as a result of its reduced clearance, but its positive inotropic action may also be attenuated. The clinical significance of this observation is, however, unclear.

Indications for diuretic treatment

OEDEMA

Thiazide diuretics form the mainstay of treatment for numerous conditions that are characterised by oedema, notably *congestive cardiac failure*, in which the glomerular filtration rate is reduced, aldosterone production increased, and sodium reabsorption from the kidney tubules enhanced. Mild symptoms usually respond to treatment with a thiazide diuretic introduced at low dosage (for example, bendrofluazide 2·5–5 mg daily) in addition to dietary salt restriction. An intermittent diuretic regimen (for example, on 3 days in each week) is occasionally sufficient and allows normal homoeostatic compensatory mechanisms to operate on diuretic-free days. Chronic heart failure no longer responsive to thiazides often responds dramatically to a loop diuretic, which should be substituted in a progressively increasing dosage. Oedema that is otherwise resistant may respond to a combination of a loop diuretic and a thiazide or thiazide like drug, especially metolazone, with or without an aldosterone antagonist. The combined diuretic action at different sites in the kidney tubule produces an additive inhibition of sodium reabsorption.

In the treatment of *acute pulmonary oedema* associated with left ventricular failure, loop diuretics rapidly reduce the pulmonary capillary pressure and produce prompt relief of symptoms. This occurs as a result of venodilatation and seems to be related to the secondary release of the vasodilator prostaglandin (prostaglandin E_2) and prostacyclin. Spironolactone in increasing dosage (up to 400 mg a day if the ratio of urinary sodium to potassium is less than 1·0) is the best drug for liver cirrhosis complicated by ascites, and a thiazide or loop diuretic may then be cautiously introduced. Spironolactone is similarly used in combination with other diuretics to treat *nephrotic syndrome*, another condition invariably associated with secondary hyperaldosteronism.

138

Thiazides and spironolactone have been prescribed to treat recurrent *idiopathic cyclical oedema*, particularly that affecting the ankles, which is associated with fluid retention. In this disorder, which is most often seen in premenopausal women and especially at menstruation, diuretics may have an initial cosmetic effect but long term benefit has not been established: they may, however, produce untoward metabolic side effects.

Hormone replacement therapy, now widely used to retard osteoporosis after the menopause, is, in many women, associated with *fluid retention*. Diuretics have been used to counter this but their effects on lipid balance may, to some extent, offset the favourable influence of the hormone replacement on the lipid profile.

Thiazide diuretics have often been used inappropriately to manage chronic *lymphoedema* and *ankle oedema* associated with varicose veins and poor venous return. Only rarely does this warrant treatment with diuretics, and adequate elastic support is generally more appropriate. Diuretics may also be abused as a means of achieving rapid weight loss in association with dietary restriction.

The requirement for diuretic treatment in managing oedema should be regularly reassessed so that control is achieved using the least potent agent at the minimum effective dose. When clinical judgement alone is insufficient, salt and water loss can be assessed by noting the rate and extent of weight loss. Provided that the serum sodium concentration remains normal, 1 kg of water loss corresponds to 140–150 mmol of associated sodium loss. Another useful indicator is the 24 h urinary sodium excretion: if this is less than 10–20 mmol then diuretic treatment should be considered inadequate; if it is more than 100 mmol and body weight is not decreasing then sodium excretion is satisfactory but sodium intake should be reduced. However, some patients are at risk of developing saline depletion (loss of tissue turgor, postural hypotension, and a rising serum urea concentration), which results from loss of interstitial fluid, a corresponding fall in plasma volume, and poor renal perfusion. The dose of diuretic in such patients may best be adjusted to permit mild ankle oedema in the evening, which clears overnight in bed. Excessive diuresis otherwise produces undue shrinkage of the plasma volume and results in secondary hyperaldosteronism and hypokalaemia. Excessively rapid clearance of oedema also causes malaise.

HYPERTENSION

Thiazide diuretics continue to be first line drugs for the management of hypertension in patients with normal renal function but their role has diminished somewhat in recent years as concern about their long term metabolic consequences has increased. Loop diuretics also lower blood pressure but are generally considered only for thiazide resistant hypertension or hypertension associated with renal impairment. Small doses of thiazides (for example, bendrofluazide 2·5 mg daily) lower blood pressure in both the erect and supine positions and only rarely cause postural hypotension or metabolic upset, but higher doses are likely to produce adverse biochemical changes and do not increase the hypotensive effect (the dose–response curve is characteristically flat). Thiazides may be used alone or in combination with other first line drugs: when combined with vasodilators, they often reduce the fluid retention with which vasodilators may be associated. Thiazides are particularly effective in patients with low renin hypertension, such as the elderly, for whom they remain drugs of choice.

The precise mechanism by which diuretics lower blood pressure is unclear. The initial fall in plasma volume that they produce is associated with a fall in cardiac output, but thereafter a sustained reduction in peripheral vascular resistance, unrelated to the natriuretic effect, is achieved—though only in patients with normally functioning kidneys. This is probably because of a direct action on the vessel wall or stimulation of an autoregulatory mechanism, perhaps associated with the release of vasoactive prostaglandin. The maximum hypotensive effect develops only slowly, therefore, and may not be reached for 2–3 weeks. It must be stressed that the antihypertensive effect of the thiazide diuretics is not increased by increasing the dose (that is, they have a relatively flat dose to blood pressure response curve) though the likelihood of serious electrolyte and metabolic disturbances increases with higher doses.

RENAL DISEASE

The effectiveness of thiazide diuretics depends on renal function and diminishes as glomerular filtration rate falls. However, high ceiling loop diuretics and metolazone, alone or in combination, are effective at glomerular filtration rates of less than 15 ml/min and have been used to manage acute and chronic renal failure. In acute renal failure, high dose intravenous frusemide and bumetanide will produce an effective diuresis in about one third of patients, thereby reducing the need for dialysis. Evidence exists to support the use of continuous intravenous infusions, rather than high dose bolus injections, of drugs such as frusemide. Intravenous infusions may be effective in patients who are apparently resistant to bolus intravenous doses.

CALCIUM EXCRETION

High dose intravenous frusemide (80–100 mg or more) has been used to supplement intensive hydration treatment as a short term method of increasing calcium excretion in *hypercalcaemia* of malignancy. Its effectiveness usually diminishes within a few days, however, and drugs such as pamidronate are preferred for long term control (see chapter 21).

Thiazide diuretics increase calcium retention and have been used to manage *hypercalciuria*, in which they reduce stone formation and the frequency of attacks of renal colic. This calcium sparing effect is unlikely to be of benefit in preventing osteoporosis, particularly in postmenopausal women.

CYSTIC FIBROSIS

The use of amiloride to treat the pulmonary component of cystic fibrosis is a recent development. In patients with this disease the sodium concentration of pulmonary secretions is lower than normal and as a result the water content is also reduced. Because amiloride inhibits transluminal sodium transport in the distal renal tubule, it follows that it might similarly block sodium (and water) reabsorption across epithelial surfaces elsewhere. In lung disease associated with cystic fibrosis, amiloride, administered by inhalation (for example 1 mg in 3 ml saline nebulised over 5 min four times daily), appears to improve sputum rheology and so increase mucociliary function.

Potassium supplements

Potassium supplements generally, and slow release potassium chloride tablets (Slow K) in particular, are grossly overprescribed. They are often unnecessary for patients taking only small diuretic doses and for most young ambulant hypertensive patients. In any event, compliance is often suspect, as evidenced by the vast numbers of such tablets returned to pharmacies during "dump" campaigns.

Hypertensive patients treated with a combination of diuretic and β blocker rarely, if ever, require measures to conserve potassium. The need for potassium conservation can be reduced by using the lowest possible dose of diuretic necessary to control oedema, using diuretics intermittently when possible, and restricting salt intake.

Careful appraisal of the need to conserve serum potassium is required in a few selected patients. These include:

● elderly subjects receiving long term diuretic treatment, as dietary intake of potassium is often suspect in this group;

● those taking digoxin or other cardiac glycosides who are at increased risk of developing arrhythmias;

● those with evidence of cardiac arrhythmias, recent myocardial infarction, or severe angina, also because of the risk of serious ventricular arrhythmias;

● those receiving drugs that produce hypokalaemia, such as corticosteroids or amphotericin; and

● diabetics.

In the above cases, the addition of a potassium sparing diuretic is preferable to the high dose—for example, 64 mmol a day (equivalent to eight Slow K tablets)—of potassium supplement that is invariably required but is certainly not adequately provided by the "usual" regimen of one Slow K tablet taken three times daily.

Potassium sparing diuretics should also be considered when thiazides are administered to patients concurrently receiving drugs that interfere with ventricular repolarisation. These include the neuroleptics (chlorpromazine and related phenothiazines) and tricyclic antidepressants, and appropriate intervention is warranted if the serum potassium concentration falls below 3·5 mmol/l.

Potassium supplements are at best a preventive measure rather than a treatment for established hypokalaemia and the widespread use of combinations containing a diuretic with low dose potassium is difficult to justify: most contain far too little potassium to meet the needs of hypokalaemic patients and, in any event, the administration of potassium during diuresis is merely offset by a corresponding increase in renal potassium excretion. The excessive use of such preparations therefore seems futile and wasteful. If potassium supplements are chosen it may be preferable to give the diuretic in the morning and the supplement in a sufficiently high dose later in the day, though compliance with such a regimen may be difficult to obtain. In hypertension the addition of a β blocker or ACE inhibitor to thiazide treatment usually obviates the need for potassium supplements or a potassium sparing diuretic.

1 Anonymous. Symposium on diuretics in the 1980s: issues and insights. *Drugs* 1986;**31**(suppl 4):1–211.
2 Lant A. Diuretics: clinical pharmacology and therapeutic use, part I. *Drugs* 1985;**29**:57–87.
3 Orme M. Thiazides in the 1990s. *BMJ* 1990;**300**:1668–9.
4 Costanzo LS. Mechanism of action of thiazide diuretics. *Semin Nephrol* 1988;**8**:234–41.
5 Thompson WB. An assault on old friends: thiazide diuretics under siege. *Am J Med Sci* 1990;**300**:152–8.
6 Ramsay LE, Yeo WW, Jackson PR. Thiazide diuretics: first line therapy for hypertension. *J Hypertens* 1992;**10**(suppl):S29–S32.
7 Chaffman M, Heel RC, Brogden TM, *et al*. Indapamide: a review of its pharmacodynamic properties and therapeutic efficacy in hypertension. *Drugs* 1984;**28**:189–235.
8 Prichard BN, Brogden RN. Xipamide. A review of its pharmacodynamic and pharmacokinetic properties and therapeutic efficacy. *Drugs* 1985;**30**:313–32.
9 Brater DC. Resistance to loop diuretics. Why it happens and what to do about it. *Drugs* 1985;**30**:427–43.
10 Brogden RN, Speight TM, Avery GS. Mefruside: a preliminary report of its pharmacological properties and therapeutic efficacy in oedema and hypertension. *Drugs* 1974;**7**:419–25.
11 Wittner M, Di-Stefano A, Wangemann P, *et al*. How do loop diuretics act? *Drugs* 1991;**41**(suppl 3):1–13.
12 Brater DC. Disposition and response to bumatanide and furosemide. *Am J Cardiol* 1986;**57**:20A–25A.
13 Clissold SP, Brogden RN. Piretanide: a preliminary review of its pharmacodynamic and pharmacokinetic properties and therapeutic efficacy. *Drugs* 1985;**29**:489–530.
14 Friedel HA, Buckley MM. Torasemide. A review of its pharmacological properties and therapeutic potential. *Drugs* 1990;**41**:81–103.
15 Horisberger JD, Giebisch G. Potassium-sparing diuretics. *Renal Physiol* 1987;**10**:198–220.
16 Kleyman TR, Cragoe EJ. The mechanism of action of amiloride. *Semin Nephrol* 1988;**8**:242–8.
17 Krishna GG, Shulman MD, Narins RG. Clinical use of the potassium-sparing diuretics. *Semin Nephrol* 1988;**8**:354–64.
18 Skluth HA, Gums JG. Spironolactone: a re-examination. *Drug Intell Clin Pharm* 1990;**24**:52–9.

12 Thrombolytic treatment

TERENCE PRINGLE, DEREK MacLEAN,
JOHN FEELY

Injury to a blood vessel results in the formation of a haemostatic plug of platelets, and fibrin is laid down to reinforce it to form a thrombus. Once the repair process is established the fibrinolytic system is activated to remove fibrin, and tissue plasminogen activators produced at the site of the injury convert plasminogen to active plasmin, which lyses fibrin. The plasmin produced is active only within the thrombus, and any leakage is destroyed by circulating antiplasmins in the plasma. Thus the fibrinolytic system plays an important part in maintaining the patency of the vascular tree.

Two thrombolytic agents—streptokinase and urokinase—have been available for clinical use for several years.[1] Unlike urokinase (which is isolated from human urine), streptokinase, the metabolic product of β haemolytic streptococci, is antigenic in humans. Streptokinase combines with plasminogen to form an activator complex, which converts plasminogen directly. The generalised lytic state caused by both of these drugs results in the dissolution of thrombi, but it also produces a haemostatic defect throughout the entire vascular system. For this reason these drugs should not be given to patients who are actively bleeding or who have had recent surgery, stroke, or cardiopulmonary resuscitation. Uncontrolled hypertension and active peptic ulceration are also contraindications to treatment.

In recent years other drugs have been developed that act locally at the site of thrombus formation and have a lesser systemic effect. Recombinant tissue plasminogen activator (rt-PA, alteplase), produced by recombinant DNA technology from human tissue cultures, specifically activates plasminogen already bound to fibrin, and its action on circulating plasminogen is limited. A second drug, anisoylated plasminogen streptokinase activator complex (APSAC, anistreplase), is inactive in plasma. When it attaches to

144

fibrin deacylation occurs, plasminogen activator complex is formed, and plasmin production is localised to the thrombus.

Myocardial infarction

Coronary angiography performed in patients within hours of the onset of pain has confirmed that coronary artery occlusion is the cause of myocardial infarction in most patients.[2] This supports the view of pathologists that rupture of an atheromatous plaque with subsequent thrombosis of the coronary artery is the precipitating event. Consequently there has been a resurgence of interest in thrombolysis for acute myocardial infarction despite the inconclusive results of earlier trials.

Streptokinase infused directly into the occluded coronary artery lyses the thrombus in up to four fifths of patients.[3] In addition to the angiographic evidence of clot lysis and return of flow in the coronary artery, other less exact variables—for example, pain relief, resolution of ST segment elevation on the electrocardiogram, emergence of predominantly benign arrhythmias, and early release of creatine kinase[4]—suggest that myocardial perfusion is effective. The re-establishment of coronary artery patency is not consistently accompanied by an improvement in left ventricular function or a reduction in death rate.[5] Although one placebo controlled randomised study of intracoronary streptokinase[6] showed a decrease in death rate at 30 days after streptokinase treatment, this benefit was not evident at 1 year.

The inherent delays in intracoronary thrombolytic therapy and lack of universal access to specialised facilities for its administration led to the investigation of intravenous thrombolytic therapy. Angiographic studies have shown that high dose streptokinase lyses coronary thrombi in 50–60% of patients. Although this is not as often as the intracoronary route, the ease of intravenous administration means that it can be given very early after patients present with myocardial infarction. Streptokinase given by this route reduces the size of the infarction and improves left ventricular contraction in the region of the infarction.

Two large placebo controlled studies have confirmed that streptokinase reduces mortality by up to 21% in patients with myocardial infarction.[7 8] The most impressive results were in those patients who were treated within 4 h from the onset of pain but patients benefited even when the delay to treatment was up to 24 h.[8] Aspirin reduced mortality when administered alone for 1 month and had an additive effect in decreasing death rates when given with streptokinase.[8] In addition to haemorrhage and allergic reactions streptokinase may cause chills, back and abdominal pain, nausea and vomiting in a small percentage of patients.

Alteplase has theoretical advantages over streptokinase:

- it is not antigenic as it is produced from tissue culture of human cells. Systemic hypotensive reactions, sometimes encountered when streptokinase is given too rapidly, do not occur;
- it has a short half life, about 10 min, and is administered as an infusion after an initial bolus injection;
- intravenous alteplase lyses more coronary arteries than streptokinase acutely but this early advantage is lost after 24 h unless intravenous heparin is given directly after alteplase;[9]
- alteplase produces a less systemic fibrinolysis than streptokinase, but this is not reflected in a lower prevalence of haemorrhagic complications at puncture sites. When given intravenously, it is effective in reducing the mortality from myocardial infarction by 26% compared with placebo.[10]

Anistreplase has a fairly long half life of 1–2 h and may be given as a single intravenous bolus injection. It is also highly effective in reopening coronary arteries.[11] In the doses required, however, it produces as much systemic fibrinolysis as non-anisoylated streptokinase, and the side effects are similar. In myocardial infarction, intravenous anistreplase results in a death rate 47% lower than placebo; elderly patients gain most from this treatment.[12] The ease of administration of anistreplase means that out of hospital thrombolysis by general practitioners in rural areas on first contact with the patient is feasible, and results in an improvement in mortality and left ventricular function.[13]

Recent large studies comparing these two newer thrombolytic drugs with streptokinase have shown no differences in mortality rates between treatments. Streptokinase and anistreplase cause more allergic and hypotensive reactions than alteplase but the incidence of stroke, albeit low, was greater after alteplase and anistreplase than streptokinase.[14][15]

After successful thrombolysis high grade stenoses remain in 70% of infarct related arteries. Reocclusion of the coronary artery occurs in 20% of patients[16] and may be more common with alteplase unless treatment is followed by intravenous heparin.[9] Reinfarction is clinically apparent in only 8%,[16] which may reflect the lack of myocardial salvage despite successful thrombolysis. Nevertheless, various strategies have been evaluated to maintain the blood supply to the myocardium, including anticoagulation, coronary angioplasty, and coronary artery bypass surgery. Studies have revealed that surgical intervention should be reserved for those patients who have postinfarction angina or ischaemia induced by exercise.[17]

Although it is expensive (£80–£1000), thrombolysis is now established as initial treatment for myocardial infarction. (Alteplase and anistreplase are six and ten times, respectively, more expensive than streptokinase.) It is most effective when given as soon as possible after the onset of the infarction, and benefit is greatest in those with ST segment elevation and in those with anterior infarction. The ease and effectiveness of intravenous administration means that thrombolytic drugs may be given on first contact with the patient. It is important that the public are educated to seek help quickly when they experience chest pain. Rapid transport to hospital and speedy treatment in casualty departments will reduce delays. The training of paramedics, general practitioners and hospital based teams to administer thrombolytic treatment in the community will also help to provide maximum benefit from this form of therapy.

Pulmonary embolism and deep vein thrombosis

Sequential pulmonary angiography and lung scans have shown that thrombolytic agents are highly effective in lysing large pulmonary emboli. In the first 24 h after treatment urokinase and streptokinase both produce greater lung reperfusion and reduction in pulmonary artery pressure than prophylactic anticoagulation with heparin.[18] By 7 days the advantage from thrombolysis is lost and no difference is apparent between the lung scans of patients treated with thrombolytic agents followed by anticoagulation and those treated with anticoagulants alone: tests of lung function, however, suggest that benefit continues for up to 1 year after thrombolysis.[19] Presumably this reflects the lysis of small clots within the peripheral pulmonary microcirculation that are beyond the resolution of pulmonary angiography or scanning. One study suggests that alteplase is more effective than urokinase in treatment of pulmonary embolism but its effects on mortality could not be evaluated.[20] Although the choice of treatment for pulmonary embolism will also determine the treatment for the source of the clot within the deep veins, anticoagulation remains the most popular treatment for isolated deep vein thrombosis. Thrombolysis is successful in dissolving thrombi in up to 70% of patients, which is more than three times more effective than heparin.[21] This has resulted in improved venous valve function and in a lower late complication rate of post phlebitic syndrome.

Thrombolysis is indicated in life threatening pulmonary embolism and may have advantages over anticoagulation in treating less severe episodes. Patients with proximal deep vein thrombosis of less than 1 week's duration should be selected for thrombolytic therapy.[21] No large studies have as yet evaluated the use of alteplase or anistreplase in thromboembolic disease: the results of such trials are awaited before any alteration to standard therapeutic policies is considered.

Peripheral arterial occlusion

Many studies have reported the effects of systemic thrombolysis on peripheral arterial occlusions and emboli.[1] Only up to two fifths of arteries are revascularised with high dose intravenous infusions. Success seems to depend on the duration of symptoms, and arterial occlusions that have occurred less than 72 h before treatment are most likely to be reopened. In recent years a low dose infusion of streptokinase has been delivered into the occluded artery close to the thrombus and has been reported to recanalise the artery in 70% of patients, including those who have had symptoms for 2 years.[22] Thrombolytic treatment is a useful alternative to surgery when it is contraindicated or in treatment of lesions not amenable to surgery. It may also be successful in lysing a thrombotic arterial occlusion that complicates peripheral arterial angioplasty.

1 Brogden RN, Speight TM, Avery GS. Streptokinase: a review of its clinical pharmacology, mechanism of action and therapeutic uses. *Drugs* 1973;5:357–445.

2 DeWood MA, Spores J, Notske R, *et al.* Prevalence of total coronary occlusion during the early hours of transmural myocardial infarction. *N Engl J Med* 1980;**303**:897–902.

3 Rutsch W, Schmutzler H. Intracoronary thrombolysis: organizational prerequisites, technique, and results. *Cardiovasc Intervent Radiol* 1986;**9**:245–52.

4 Anderson JL, Marshall HW, Askins JC, *et al.* A randomized trial of intravenous and intracoronary streptokinase in patients with acute myocardial infarction. *Circulation* 1984;**70**:606–18.

5 Yusuf S, Collins R, Peto R, *et al.* Intravenous and intracoronary fibrinolytic therapy in acute myocardial infarction: overview of results on mortality, reinfarction and side effects from 33 randomized trials. *Eur Heart J* 1985;**6**:556–85.

6 Kennedy JW, Ritchie JL, Davis KB, Fritz JK. Western Washington randomized trial of intracoronary streptokinase in acute myocardial infarction. *N Engl J Med* 1983;**309**:1447–82.

7 Gruppo Italiano per lo Studio della Streptochinasi nell'Infarcto Miocardico (GISSI). Effectiveness of intravenous thrombolytic treatment in acute myocardial infarction. *Lancet* 1986;**i**:397–401.

8 ISIS-2 (Second International Study of Infarct Survival) Collaborative Group. Randomised trial of intravenous streptokinase, oral aspirin, both, or neither among 17 187 cases of suspected acute myocardial infarction: ISIS-2. *Lancet* 1988;**ii**:349–60.

9 White HD. GISSI-2 and the heparin controversy. *Lancet* 1990;**336**:297–8.

10 Wilcox RG, Olsson CG, Skene AM, *et al.* Trial of tissue plasminogen activator for mortality reduction in acute myocardial infarction. Anglo–Scandinavian Study of Early Thrombolysis (ASSET). *Lancet* 1988;**ii**:525–30.

11 Hillis WS, Hornung RS. The use of BRL26921 (APSAC) as fibrinolytic therapy in acute myocardial infarction. *Eur Heart J* 1985;**6**:909–12.

12 AIMS Trial Study Group. Effect of intravenous APSAC on mortality after acute myocardial infarction: preliminary report of a placebo-controlled clinical trial. *Lancet* 1988;**i**:545–9.

13 GREAT Group. Feasibility, safety, and efficacy of domiciliary thrombolysis by general practitioners: Grampian region early anistreplase trial. *BMJ* 1992;**305**:548–53.

14 The International Study Group. In-hospital mortality and clinical course of 20 891 patients with suspected acute myocardial infarction randomised between alteplase and streptokinase with or without heparin. *Lancet* 1990;**336**:71–5.

15 ISIS-3 (Third International Study of Infarct Survival Collaborative Group). A randomised comparison of streptokinase vs tissue plasminogen activator vs anistreplase and of aspirin plus heparin vs aspirin alone among 41 299 cases of suspected acute myocardial infarction. *Lancet* 1992;**339**:753–70.

16 Schaer DH, Ross AM, Wasserman AG. Reinfarction, recurrent angina and reocclusion after thrombolytic therapy. *Circulation* 1987;**47**(suppl II):57–62.

17 Rogers WJ, Baim DS, Gore JM, *et al.* Comparison of immediate invasive, delayed invasive, and conservative strategies after tissue-type plasminogen activator. Results of the thrombolysis in myocardial infarction (TIMI) phase II-A trial. *Circulation* 1990;**81**:1457–76.

18 Sasahara AA, Hyers TM, Cole CM, *et al.* The urokinase pulmonary embolism trial: a national cooperative study. *Circulation* 1973;**47**(suppl II):1–108.

19 Sharma GVRK, Burleson VA, Sasahara AA. Effect of thrombolytic therapy on pulmonary–capillary blood volume in patients with pulmonary embolism. *N Engl J Med* 1980;**303**:842–5.

20 Meyer G, Sors H, Charbonnier B, *et al*. Effects of intravenous urokinase versus alteplase on total pulmonary resistance in acute massive pulmonary embolism: a European multicenter double-blind trial. *J Am Coll Cardiol* 1992;**19**:239–45.
21 Rogers LQ, Lutcher CL. Streptokinase therapy for deep vein thrombosis: a comprehensive review of the English literature. *Am J Med* 1990;**88**:389–95.
22 Hess H, Ingrisch H, Mietaschk A, Rath H. Local low-dose thrombolytic therapy of peripheral arterial occlusions. *N Engl J Med* 1982;**307**:1627–30.

13 Antiarrhythmic drugs

W S HILLIS, B WHITING

Antiarrhythmic drugs remain the mainstay of the treatment of patients with cardiac arrhythmias, although there is an increasing role for other manoeuvres, including catheter ablation of atrioventricular accessory connections, the use of automatic implantable defibrillators and antiarrhythmic operations for medically refractory patients. The major aims in drug treatment are:

1. to afford symptomatic relief to patients with troublesome, but not life threatening arrhythmias;
2. to prevent the onset of arrhythmias producing major haemodynamic sequelae;
3. to prevent recurrent life threatening arrhythmias.

The ideal antiarrhythmic compound should have a wide range of therapeutic activity against atrial, junctional and ventricular arrhythmias and should be available in parenteral and oral formulations to allow rapid activity and sustained prophylactic use with simple dosage schedules. It should have pharmacokinetic properties to allow predictable long term plasma levels and should have no proarrhythmic action, depressant haemodynamic effects or significant non-cardiac side effects. Non-invasive and invasive investigations of patients using serial assessment may help guide the choice of antiarrhythmic drugs. These methods have included ambulatory monitoring, exercise testing, electrocardiogram signal averaging and invasive electrophysiological testing.

Original observations, particularly in patients with acute myocardial infarction, suggested that suppression of so called warning arrhythmias (not life threatening or haemodynamically significant in themselves) might prevent the onset of serious life threatening arrhythmias such as ventricular tachycardia and ventricular fibrillation.[1] Suppression of ventricular extrasystoles has been regarded as a surrogate for potential antiarrhythmic efficacy in clinical trials, particularly of Class I antiarrhythmic drugs. The Cardiac Arrhythmia Suppression Trial (CAST) study has caused confusion and controversy, as drugs which were given to patients who showed successful suppression of ventricular ectopic activity caused an increased mortality rate compared to placebo. This has enhanced interest in the study of proarrhythmic effects, and has questioned the viability of the suppression hypothesis and thus the endpoints of antiarrhythmic trials. Interest has focused on β blockers and class III antiarrhythmic agents in an attempt to prevent sudden death, with a potentially diminishing role for the standard class I agents.

Invasive electrophysiological testing can determine the mechanisms of arrhythmias and can be used to locate arrhythmic foci using mapping techniques. Electropharmacological testing assumes that drug efficacy can be inferred from suppression of an arrhythmia previously inducible in the baseline state. Studies have shown, however, considerable spontaneous temporal variation in the inducibility of ventricular tachycardia in the drug free state, and the results of suppression using intravenous drugs may be different from those obtained when the drug is given orally. In hypertrophic cardiomyopathy, positive suppression evidenced by electrophysiological testing has not necessarily been predictive of a reduced incidence of sudden death. Despite these observations and reservations, tailoring of a drug regimen to a patient's responses remains the best clinical option. Continued critical observations of the use and limitations of the investigation methods are required. Drugs are therefore often chosen on an empirical basis by trial and error, either alone or in combination.

Following selection of a drug, therapeutic drug monitoring may play an important role in this difficult therapeutic area. Rapid analytical methods are available to measure concentrations of many antiarrhythmic drugs. Patients with arrhythmias may have other conditions that lead to considerable pharmacokinetic variability in the individual subject and between patients. This variability in absorption, distribution, and clearance may lead to pronounced differences in relation to doses and plasma concentrations of drugs. The plasma concentrations associated with safe and effective antiarrhythmic treatment are usually confined to a narrow range, and this necessitates careful tailoring of the dose. Efficacy remains difficult to assess if the arrhythmia, although potentially serious, occurs infrequently. Inappropriate changes in treatment may occur if adequate guidelines are not followed in assessing the time of sample collection. Moreover, several drugs (for example, verapamil, procainamide, and amiodarone) have active

TABLE 13.1—*Vaughan Williams' classification of antiarrhythmic drugs*

Class I		Class II	Class III	Class IV
A	Quinidine Procainamide Disopyramide	β Adrenoreceptor blocking compounds Bretylium	Amiodarone Sotalol Bretylium	Verapamil Diltiazem Adenosine
B	Lignocaine Mexiletine Aprinidine Phenytoin Tocainide			
C	Flecainide Encainide Propafenone Lorcainide			

metabolites, and the plasma concentration of the parent drug only may not be helpful. The degree of protein binding should also be known so that the active free fraction may be assessed. Rational antiarrhythmic treatment should entail the achievement of target plasma concentrations that are known to be associated with successful suppression of arrhythmias through appropriate dosage adjustments dictated by monitoring plasma concentrations and by clinical observation.

Classification of antiarrhythmic agents

Compounds with antiarrhythmic activity show great variation in their chemical structure, and may be classified according to:

1. their anatomical site of action (for example, sinus node, atrium, atrioventricular node, anomalous pathway, or ventricle);
2. their clinical range of activity; and
3. their electrophysiological action on isolated cardiac fibres

(Vaughan Williams' classification, see table 13.1).

Vaughan Williams' classification, although it follows observations on electrophysiological effects of drugs on isolated tissues, allows drugs to be characterised at the preclinical phase of development. It is of limited clinical value and excludes some agents with antiarrhythmic activity, such as the cardiac glycosides. Four principal modes of basic activity are recognised, although future developmental agents may require further classes to be recognised. In addition, some drugs may have more than one action, though therapeutic success is usually associated with one dominant action.

Class I contains agents that interfere with the rapid sodium current, with the slowing of conduction or an increase in the refractory period, or both. These agents usually have local anaesthetic properties and membrane stabilising activity. The electrophysiological effects tend to reduce spontaneous automaticity, and these agents may be further subdivided according to the influence on duration of the action potential, which may lengthen (group IA) shorten (group IB), or be unaffected (group IC).

Class II agents reduce the potential for arrhythmias to develop in response to catecholamines. Bretylium blocks the release of sympathetic transmitters. The β adrenoreceptor blocking compounds act as competitive antagonists and also block the possible arrhythmogenic effect of cyclic adenosine-5-monophosphate.

Class III agents prolong the duration of the action potential, with resulting prolongation of the effective refractory period, without influencing the inward sodium current.

Class IV agents inhibit the slow inward calcium mediated current and depress phases 2 and 3 of the action potential. These actions have an important influence on the upper and middle parts of the atrioventricular node, and these effects may have particular value in blocking one limb of a re-entry circuit.

Class I antiarrhythmic agents

QUINIDINE

Quinidine is the parent compound of the class I antiarrhythmic drugs. All class I agents interfere with sodium channel activity and have a potentially negative inotropic effect. Group 1A drugs have more negative inotropic activity than group 1B drugs.

Mechanism of action

Quinidine reduces the maximum rate of depolarisation, depresses spontaneous phase 4 diastolic depolarisation in automatic cells, and in general slows conduction through atrial, ventricular, and Purkinje fibres. Its antivagal action may accelerate atrioventricular nodal conduction.

Clinical use

Quinidine is now of limited clinical use. The lack of an adequate parenteral formulation restricts its use to prophylaxis after cardioversion or after short term administration of lignocaine. It is active against atrial and ventricular arrhythmias.

Pharmacokinetics

About 70% of an oral dose is absorbed from the gut, peak concentrations occur in 1–3 h, and the half life is relatively short (6–7 h). Slow release preparations are now available, but their bioavailability may be lower than that of standard release products. Antiarrhythmic effects on atrial and ventricular arrhythmias occur at drug concentrations of 2–5 mg/l. Quinidine is highly protein bound (80–90%) and is metabolised by hydroxylation. In liver disease the clearance is reduced, half life increased, and protein binding reduced. Lower total plasma concentrations may be effective. In congestive heart failure the half life is not affected. Quinidine interacts with digoxin and may precipitate digoxin toxicity; the dose of digoxin may require reduction.

Adverse effects

Cardiac—Myocardial depression occurs at high plasma concentrations and is associated with vasodilatation and hypotension. Sinus arrest, sinoatrial block, atrioventricular dissociation, and progressive QRS and QT interval prolongation may occur. QT interval prolongation may facilitate the development of re-entry arrhythmias.

Other effects—Gastrointestinal effects (nausea, vomiting, and diarrhoea) may occur. Cinchonism and hypersensitivity reactions such as fever, purpura, thrombocytopenia, and hepatic dysfunction may also occur.

PROCAINAMIDE

Procainamide shows electrophysiological properties similar to those described for quinidine.

Clinical use

Procainamide is available for parenteral and oral use and may be effective in the treatment of atrial, junctional, and ventricular arrhythmias. The standard intravenous dose is 100 mg given over

2 min, repeated to a total of 1000 mg in the first hour. Oral treatment may be given prophylactically.

Pharmacokinetics

The bioavailability of oral procainamide is about 85%. Absorption is rapid, peak plasma concentrations occurring about 1 h after administration. It is metabolised to an active metabolite, N-acetyl procainamide. The rate at which metabolism occurs is determined genetically, patients being classified as fast or slow acetylators. Subjects who are slow acetylators require smaller doses during long term treatment. High plasma concentrations of procainamide and N-acetyl procainamide may be obtained in renal impairment and cardiac failure. The therapeutic range of the parent compound is 4–10 mg/l; toxic effects are related to the concentration and may start at 8–10 mg/l. Toxicity is pronounced at concentrations of about 16 mg/l. The half life is about 3–5 h, which necessitates frequent dosage; slow release preparations are available.

Adverse effects

Cardiac—Rapid intravenous administration may lead to reduced cardiac output with hypotension and vasodilatation. PR segment prolongation may proceed to increased degrees of heart block, and QRS and QT segment prolongation may also occur, particularly in slow acetylators.

Other—Long term oral use may be associated with a drug induced lupus erythematosus syndrome if antinuclear factor is present. The kidneys are rarely affected, and the effects are usually reversible.

DISOPYRAMIDE

The electrophysiological properties of disopyramide are similar to those of quinidine.

Clinical use

Parenteral and oral preparations are available. The range of activity includes action against atrial and ventricular arrhythmias, including supraventricular tachycardia and ventricular extrasystoles.

Pharmacokinetics

Disopyramide is commercially available as the base compound and as the phosphate salt. Bioavailability is about 70–80%. The half life in normal subjects is 6–8 h. The main metabolite is the N-dealkylated form of disopyramide. This is excreted by the kidneys, as is most of the parent compound. The dose should be reduced in severe renal failure. The therapeutic range is 2–5 mg/l.

Adverse effects

Cardiac—Myocardial depression may be clinically important and is related both to the plasma concentration and to the rate of administration of the compound. Use of the drug is therefore contraindicated in heart failure or severe left ventricular dysfunction. QT interval prolongation related to concentrations of the drug may also occur, and this may predispose to ventricular arrhythmia with a re-entry mechanism. Sinus node depression may also occur.

Other—Disopyramide has anticholinergic activity, and urinary retention, dry mouth, and blurred vision often occur. Glaucoma may also be precipitated.

LIGNOCAINE

Lignocaine has typical class I electrophysiological effects.

Clinical use

Lignocaine remains the first line drug for treating ventricular arrhythmias after acute myocardial infarction and cardiac operations.[1] After intravenous administration, long term treatment may be continued by giving an alternative class I antiarrhythmic drug orally. After intramuscular injection absorption is erratic, and blood concentrations achieved vary widely according to the haemodynamic state of the patient. The most appropriate strategy for administering lignocaine remains controversial. Prophylactic treatment has been suggested, even in the absence of warning arrhythmias but this does not appear to have a great advantage over a selective strategy and administering lignocaine on the appearance of specific warning arrhythmias only.

Pharmacokinetics

Lignocaine is hydrolysed in the gastrointestinal tract and is subjected to extensive first pass metabolism in the liver: adequate blood concentrations are therefore not obtained after oral administration. After intravenous administration the elimination half life is about 2 h. Clearance is related to hepatic blood flow, and hepatic function and clearance is prolonged in the elderly, in cardiac failure, and in hepatic disease. Infusion rates require appropriate adjustment in these circumstances. Therapeutic efficacy is associated with blood concentrations in the range 1·5–5·0 mg/l. Toxicity may occur at a wide range of total blood concentrations and may show considerable overlap with the therapeutic range. The rate of injection may be important in precipitating toxic reactions. The degree of toxicity, however, relates better to the free drug concentration than to the total plasma concentration. Protein binding may be important in many clinical conditions. The free fraction may vary from 20% to 40% and is determined largely by the concentration of acute phase proteins, notably α_1 acid glycoprotein. After myocardial infarction, long term infusion leads to progressively increasing plasma concentrations, and a true steady state may not be achieved. Although this may be related to diminished clearance, it may also reflect increasing concentrations of α_1 acid glycoprotein. In these patients, although total lignocaine concentrations are raised, the free fraction may remain fairly constant. However, the precise relation between total and free concentrations of lignocaine and antiarrhythmic activity remains to be clarified.

Adverse effects

Cardiac—In therapeutic doses lignocaine has little haemodynamic effect. High concentrations may cause bradycardia, hypotension, and even asystole.

Other—Gastrointestinal upset with nausea and vomiting may occur. At concentrations above 5 mg/l central nervous system side effects, including paraesthesiae, twitching, and grand mal seizures, may occur.

MEXILETINE

Mexiletine is a primary amine with electrophysiological actions similar to those of lignocaine.

Clinical use

Mexiletine is effective after intravenous or oral administration to treat ventricular arrhythmias.

Pharmacokinetics

Peak plasma concentrations are obtained 2–4 h after oral administration. Mexiletine is extensively metabolised. The half life is 9–12 h in normal volunteers but may be prolonged for up to 26 h in patients with cardiac disease, particularly those who have sustained an acute myocardial infarction. Administration of narcotic analgesics may be associated with reduced absorption. About 10–20% of an administered dose is excreted unchanged in the urine at normal urinary pH, but renal clearance depends on urinary pH and may be reduced if the urine is alkalinised. Effective plasma concentrations are in the range of 0·75–2·0 mg/l.

Adverse effects

Cardiac—Adverse effects include hypotension, bradycardia, and transient atrioventricular block.

Other—Neurological side effects are common and include tremor, nystagmus, diplopia, dizziness, dysarthria, paraesthesiae, ataxia, and confusion.

TOCAINIDE

Tocainide is a primary amine with electrophysiological and antiarrhythmic properties similar to those of lignocaine.

Clinical use

Tocainide is active after intravenous or oral administration and may be used to treat acute or chronic ventricular arrhythmias.

Pharmacokinetics

The bioavailability of tocainide is almost 100%, and peak plasma concentrations are achieved within 60–90 min. The elimination half life is about 11–15 h. Plasma protein binding is about 50%. At least 40% of the drug is excreted unchanged in the urine, and the remainder is excreted by hepatic metabolism. About 25% is excreted as N-carboxy tocainide; other metabolites include glucuronide and lactoxylidide salts, which are inactive. Hepatic clearance is low. Antiarrhythmic activity occurs in the plasma concentration range of 6–12 mg/l.

Adverse effects

Cardiac—No appreciable adverse haemodynamic effects occur at plasma concentrations within the therapeutic range.

Other—Gastrointestinal side effects include anorexia, nausea, vomiting, constipation, and abdominal pain. Effects in the central nervous system are similar to those associated with mexiletine and seem to be related to peak plasma drug concentrations. Rashes and interstitial pulmonary alveolitis have occasionally necessitated withdrawal of the drug. Haematological side effects, including agranulocytosis, aplastic anaemia, and thrombocytopenia occurring during the first 12 weeks of treatment have restricted its long term use, except for life threatening arrhythmias.[2]

Class IC agents

FLECAINIDE

Mechanism of action

Flecainide acetate is a sodium channel blocker that slows conduction in the atria, the His–Purkinje conduction system, accessory pathways, and ventricles. Its use is associated with PR and QRS segment prolongation. It has a negative inotropic action, although no evidence exists of reduction in cardiac output or rise in pulmonary capillary wedge pressure.

Clinical use

Flecainide has been shown to be useful for a wide range of arrhythmias, including recurrent ventricular arrhythmias and the Wolff–Parkinson–White syndrome. Up to 2 mg/kg can be given intravenously over 30 min. It has broad range efficacy against atrial arrhythmias, tachycardias utilising accessory pathways, and ventricular arrhythmias. It is as successful as amiodarone in converting atrial fibrillation to sinus rhythm, particularly in patients with a short history.

Pharmacokinetics

Flecainide is well absorbed orally; it is not extensively protein bound, and 27% is excreted unchanged in the urine. Active metabolites are formed. The elimination half life in normal subjects is 14h; this is prolonged to 20h in cardiac and renal failure.

Adverse effects

Flecainide may exacerbate pre-existing conduction disorders. Caution is required in patients with sinoatrial or atrioventricular node disease or bundle branch block. The threshold in patients with implanted pacemakers may be increased, with failure to capture. An appreciable proarrhythmic effect is seen after the use of flecainide. Preliminary results from the cardiac arrhythmia suppression trial show that patients treated with encainide or flecainide had a 2·5-fold greater death rate and a fourfold greater rate of sudden death or non-fatal cardiac arrests.[3] Flecainide is now used only for atrioventricular nodal reciprocating tachycardia (such as Wolff–Parkinson–White syndrome with accessory pathways and anterograde or retrograde conduction), symptomatic sustained ventricular tachycardia, or ventricular extrasystoles or non-sustained ventricular tachycardia), which cause disabling symptoms when these conditions are resistant to other treatment or when patients cannot tolerate other agents. In the treatment of supraventricular arrhythmias, no increased mortality has been shown in patients treated with flecainide compared to groups treated with alternative agents.

PROPAFENONE

Electrophysiological effects are similar to those of other class IC agents, but propafenone has β adrenoreceptor blocking effects with, in addition, minor calcium channel blocking activity.

Clinical use

Propafenone has been shown to be effective in treating ventricular arrhythmias, in SVT, and in atrial fibrillation.

Pharmacokinetics

Propafenone is metabolised in the liver; conjugation leads to variable concentrations of the parent compound and the active metabolite, 5-hydroxy propafenone. The elimination half life may be fairly long, up to 32h in slow metabolisers. This is determined by genetic variation in the presence of the hepatic cytochrome *P*-450.

Adverse effects

Propafenone may induce conduction defects and may also have proarrhythmic activity and a moderate negative inotropic action.

ENCAINIDE

Electrophysiological effects are similar to those of flecainide, but with relatively little inotropic activity.

Pharmacokinetics

This drug is well absorbed, and is metabolised to O-demethyl-encainide and 3-methoxy-O-demethyl-encainide. Both metabolites have antiarrhythmic activity. In poor metabolisers the half life of the parent compound encainide is increased.

Proarrhythmias

The observations from the cardiac arrhythmia suppression trial have stimulated interest in the well recognised problem of inducing arrhythmias by antiarrhythmic compounds. These may be dose related (as with procainamide), and features suggesting a proarrhythmic mechanism include:

1. initiation of sustained ventricular tachycardia in patients in whom only non-sustained ventricular tachycardia is inducible on electrophysiological testing;

2. conversion of sustained ventricular tachycardia that could, by prolonged electrical stimulation at base line, be converted to one that required cardioversion for termination during drug treatment;

3. initiation of ventricular tachycardia by a less aggressive mode of stimulation than that required at base line; and

4. development of spontaneous or incessant ventricular tachycardia.[4]

Proarrhythmias may include torsade de pointes seen with class IA drugs and amiodarone, incessant tachycardia seen with class IA and IC agents, and wide sine wave type ventricular tachycardia seen after class IC drugs.

Class II agents

β ADRENORECEPTOR BLOCKING COMPOUNDS

New β adrenoreceptor blocking compounds continue to be developed in large numbers. Some agents, such as esmolol and flestolol, have very short half lives, which may limit their side effects as they are rapidly reversible. The antiarrhythmic properties of all β blockers seems to be identical, despite different properties regarding cardioselectivity, partial agonist activity, and potency of membrane stabilising activity.

Mechanism of action

Catecholamine augmented phase 4 depolarisation is blocked. The action potential is shortened, and the functional refractory period of the atrioventricular node is prolonged.

Clinical use

β Adrenoreceptor blocking drugs may be used when arrhythmias are associated with high levels of catecholamine production, including arrhythmias induced during anaesthesia.

The long term use of β blockers after myocardial infarction has been extensively reviewed, and beneficial effects have been shown with timolol, propranolol, atenolol, and metoprolol in secondary prevention trials. Although propranolol remains the reference compound, in clinical practice intravenous administration of atenolol or metoprolol is most widely used. These agents may be used as first line or adjunctive treatment to reduce the ventricular rate in atrial flutter and atrial fibrillation or to cardiovert paroxysmal atrial tachycardia. Atenolol and metoprolol afford long term oral treatment. There has been increasing use of sotalol, which has additional mild class III activity and may therefore show a wider range of activity. Additional clinical conditions that may benefit from β blockers include mitral valve prolapse, hypertrophic cardiomyopathy, and the hereditary prolonged QT interval syndromes.

Adverse effects

Cardiac—Myocardial depression and hypotension or cardiac failure may occur in patients with little cardiac reserve. Agents with partial agonist activity may give fewer haemodynamic effects.

Other—Increased airways obstruction and reduction of peripheral arterial blood flow may occur secondarily to blockading β_2 receptors by non-selective agents. β Blocking agents are therefore contraindicated in patients with obstructive airways disease.

BRETYLIUM

Bretylium has adrenergic neurone blocking activity and may have some class III activity in Purkinje fibres; it is therefore effective in ventricular arrhythmias.

Clinical use

Bretylium is used particularly for ventricular fibrillation that is refractory to lignocaine or procainamide or to repeated electrical defibrillation.

Bretylium is eliminated by the kidney and has a half life of 7–12 h. Adverse effects include hypotension. It is administered cautiously by the intravenous route (5–10 mg/kg) or intramuscularly (5 mg/kg).

Class III agents

AMIODARONE

Amiodarone prolongs the duration of the action potential and the effective refractory period in all cardiac tissues. It is also a non-competitive α and β adrenoreceptor antagonist, and may have additional class I activity.

Clinical use

Amiodarone is effective in a wide range of supraventricular and ventricular arrhythmias, particularly those associated with the Wolff–Parkinson–White syndrome, and in resistant ventricular arrhythmias. Although it has a minor negative inotropic effect, efficacy has been shown in ventricular arrhythmias associated with severe left ventricular impairment. Loading dose schedules have been varied from 600–1200 mg a day for 7–14 days; doses are then reduced to 400 mg a day. Full therapeutic action may take several weeks to develop. Amiodarone may be given intravenously and may be very effective in short term conversion or control of supraventricular and ventricular arrhythmias, particularly recent onset atrial flutter and fibrillation. The dosage schedule is 300 mg intravenously over 30 min, followed by 1200 mg over 24 h. Local chemical irritation may lead to pronounced phlebitis, and the drug is therefore usually infused into a central vein.

Pharmacokinetics

After oral administration considerable accumulation occurs in tissue. Amiodarone is metabolised to an active metabolite. Therapeutic plasma concentrations are 1–2 mg/l. An initial relatively rapid distribution half life of 1–2 days is followed by an extremely slow terminal half life of more than 30 days. The amiodarone molecule is diiodinated and blocks peripheral conversion of thyroxine to triiodythyronine.

Adverse effects

Cardiac—Haemodynamic effects after intravenous amiodarone are usually unimportant, as amiodarone has little negative inotropic action. Occasional vasodilatation may cause hypotension. Sinus node function and intracardiac conduction may be depressed, and amiodarone should be used cautiously with sinoatrial or atrioventricular nodal disease. Proarrhythmic effects, including torsade de pointes, may occur.

Other—Non-cardiac side effects are common and are potentially serious. Cutaneous manifestations of photosensitivity are extremely common, and direct exposure to sunlight should be avoided; hyperthyroidism or hypothyroidism may occur, and neurological side effects may include tremor and ataxia. More potentially serious are hepatitis and pulmonary infiltration, and routine screening of patients receiving long term treatment is essential.[5] Corneal microdeposits of yellow–brown granules warrant serial eye examinations.

SOTALOL

Sotalol is a non-selective β blocker without intrinsic sympathomimetic activity, but which possesses class III activity that prolongs the atrioventricular action potential duration and the refractory period.

Clinical use

Sotalol is effective in supraventricular tachycardias involving accessory pathways and ventricular arrhythmias. Therapeutic control can be obtained with a dose of 80–320 mg twice a day.

Side effects

Side effects of sotalol are similar to those of other β blockers, although proarrhythmic effects associated with its class III activity may occur.

Class IV agents

VERAPAMIL

Mechanism of action

Verapamil inhibits slow inward calcium mediated current.

Clinical use

The main action of verapamil is exerted on conduction through the atrioventricular node. Ventricular response in atrial fibrillation and flutter is controlled, and cardioversion of paroxysmal re-entrant atrioventricular nodal tachycardia is often achieved. Verapamil is the best drug for paroxysmal supraventricular tachycardia. Intravenous verapamil is administered by infusion or rapid injection of 5–10 mg. Oral dosage is established at 40 mg three times a day and, if there are no side effects, is quickly escalated to 80 or 120 mg three times a day. Use of slow release preparations limit differences between peaks and troughs and results in sustained activity.

Pharmacokinetics

Verapamil is active when given intravenously or by mouth. Bioavailability is only 10–20% because of a pronounced hepatic first pass effect. Its elimination half life is normally 3–7h but is prolonged in patients with liver disease, when the volume of distribution is increased and the clearance is diminished. Renal excretion accounts for 70% of the oral dose. Norverapamil, an active metabolite, is formed by hepatic metabolism.

Adverse effects

Myocardial depression may occur in patients with cardiac failure. Drug interactions may occur with digoxin, with which it has a pharmacodynamic interaction on the atrioventricular node and a pharmacokinetic interaction leading to an increase in plasma digoxin concentrations. Concomitant intravenous treatment with β blockers should be avoided in view of the pharmacodynamic interaction, which may lead to profound bradycardia and hypotension. Verapamil should be avoided in patients with the sick sinus syndrome or atrioventricular node disease.

DILTIAZEM

Diltiazem shows effects on the atrioventricular node similar to those of verapamil, but the effects are less pronounced.

Clinical use

Although not yet available for clinical use, intravenous diltiazem has been shown to be effective in atrioventricular node re-entrant tachycardia, and oral diltiazem was found to be effective in controlling ventricular response at rest and during exercise in patients with chronic atrial fibrillation.[6]

ADENOSINE

Adenosine is an endogenous purine nucleoside which has effects including potassium channel opening and has an inhibitory effect on the sinus and atrioventricular nodal conduction in humans.

Mechanism of action

Adenosine is a potent atrioventricular nodal blocking agent. In patients in sinus rhythm, sinus bradycardia develops 10–20 s after an injection and has associated progressive AH prolongation and atrioventricular block, which lasts for less than 10 s and is followed by a sympathetically mediated sinus tachycardia.

Clinical use

Adenosine is used as a therapeutic agent for the treatment of supraventricular tachycardia, but may also be used as a diagnostic agent in broad or narrow complex regular tachycardia, where the origin is uncertain. In patients with supraventricular tachycardia involving the atrioventricular node (atrioventricular nodal re-entrant or atrioventricular re-entrant tachycardia) cardioversion is successful in over 90%.[8]

Pharmacokinetics

In physiological concentration adenosine has a very short half life of 0·6–1·5 s. In therapeutic dosing, its effects last 20–30 s. Its effects are antagonised by aminophylline and potentiated by dipyridamole. The suggested dosage schedule is 3 mg by rapid intravenous bolus over 2 s and if no effect is seen within 1–2 min, then a further dose of 6 mg over 2 s, and followed 1–2 min later by a dose of 12 mg given rapidly.

Adverse effects

Excess sinus or nodal inhibition may occur, and transient new arrhythmias may recur after chemical cardioversion. Dyspnoea, flushing and chest pain are common, but are short lived (2–20 s). Bronchoconstriction may occur and may persist for up to 30 min. Hypotension, even in the absence of cardioversion, is generally not troublesome.

1 McMahon S, Collins R, Peto R, Coster RW, Yusuf S. Effects of prophylactic lignocaine in suspected acute myocardial infarction. An overview of results from randomised control trials. *JAMA* 1988;**260**:1910–16.
2 Oliphant LD, Goddard M. Tocainide associated neutropenia and lupus-like syndrome. *Chest* 1888;**94**:427–8.
3 Cardiac arrhythmia suppression trial (CAST) investigators. Preliminary report: effect of encainide and flecainide on mortality in a randomised trial of arrhythmia suppression after myocardial infarction. *N Engl J Med* 1989;**321**:406–12.
4 Rae AP, Kay HR, Horowitz LN, Spielman SR, Grenspan AM. Proarrhythmic effects of antiarrhythmic drugs in patients with malignant ventricular arrhythmias evaluated by electrophysiological testing. *J Am Coll Cardiol* 1988;**12**:131–9.
5 Magro SA, Lawrence EC, Wheeler SH, Krafchek J, Lin H, Wyndham CRT. Amiodarone pulmonary toxicity prospective evaluation of serial pulmonary function tests. *J Am Coll Cardiol* 1988;**12**:781–8.
6 Maragno I, Saniostasi G, Gaion RM, *et al.* Low and medium dose diltiazem in chronic atrial fibrillation. Comparison with digoxin and correlation with drug plasma levels. *Am Heart J* 1988;**116**:385–92.
7 Woosley RL. Role of plasma concentration monitoring in the evaluation of response to anti-arrhythmic drugs. *Am J Cardiol* 1988;**62**:9H–17H.
8 Camm AJ, Garratt CJ. Adenosine in supraventricular tachycardia. *N Engl J Med* 1991;**325**:1621–9.

14 Drugs in cerebral and peripheral arterial disease

GORDON D O LOWE

Stroke, intermittent claudication, foot ischaemia, and Raynaud's phenomenon are common and disabling diseases. Compared with other cardiovascular disorders, however, their treatment has been relatively neglected by doctors and clinical pharmacologists, partly because of a lack of facilities. It is paradoxical that young patients with critical strokes are "abandoned" in the corners of general wards, often with little medical treatment, whereas patients 30 years older (and often less ill) are rushed to coronary care units for intensive monitoring and treatments that require such specialised units to show their efficacy. It is equally strange that patients with peripheral arterial disease are routinely referred to surgeons, who operate on only a minority. The United Kingdom and United States, traditionally performers of randomised controlled trials, lack stroke units and angiologists who receive unselected referrals. The paucity of large randomised studies is therefore not surprising.

Few "new" drugs have been approved in recent years for treating cerebral or peripheral arterial disease in the United Kingdom, although several are under clinical trial and some may soon receive product licences. Several "old" drugs, however, have recently been evaluated further in randomised controlled trials of reasonable size, which will be reviewed, though few trials are large enough to give definite conclusions about whether treatments are beneficial, harmful, or of no value. Overviews and meta-analyses may help clinicians to make provisional assessments in the meantime.

Potential sites of action

ARTERIES

Most drugs traditionally promoted for cerebral or peripheral arterial disease are vasodilators. There is little theoretical rationale

169

for dilating larger vessels, except in Raynaud's phenomenon and in subarachnoid haemorrhage, in which large vessel spasm has been found. Furthermore, doses that produce systemic vasodilatation may "steal" blood from ischaemic areas and also produce systemic adverse effects (table 14.1). However, ischaemia of the brain or limbs is not a simple plumbing problem of large vessel diameter (table 14.2). Large vessel occlusion arises not only from spasm and atherosclerotic stenoses but also from thromboemboli of platelets and fibrin. Potential roles therefore exist for platelet inhibitors, anticoagulants, thrombolytic agents, and drugs that enhance endogenous fibrinolysis.

MICROCIRCULATION

Ischaemia depends ultimately on disturbance of nutritive microvascular flow rather than macrovascular obstruction. Vasoactive drugs may prevent or reduce the microcirculatory flow disturbance that succeeds large vessel occlusion—for instance, by direct action on small vessels. Many vasoactive drugs affect not only vessels but also the flow or interaction with vessel walls, or both, of circulating blood cells (table 14.2). This is not surprising considering that vessels and cells share a common mesenchymal origin and several common chemical mediators (such as serotonin and prostacyclin). The intrinsic flow resistance of blood (its rheological behaviour) deteriorates in ischaemia and is predictive of adverse prognosis: several drugs have potentially beneficial rheological effects that may increase microvascular flow. Such effects include increased red cell deformability (in capillaries) and decreased red cell aggregation (in venules) under ischaemic conditions; reduction

TABLE 14.1—*Adverse effects of vasodilators and cautions in their use*

Adverse effects	Cautions
Hypotensive dizziness and faints, especially postural and exercise induced	Angina, recent myocardial infarction
Tachycardia, palpitations	Bradycardia, heart block
Flushing, headache	Recent haemorrhage
Nausea, vomiting	Other hypotensive drugs

TABLE 14.2—*Potential sites of action for drugs to treat ischaemia*

Sites	Conditions	Drugs
Arteries	Atherosclerosis	Lipid reducers Blood pressure reducers
	Platelet or fibrin thrombus	Antiplatelet agents Anticoagulants Thrombolytic agents Stimulators of endogenous fibrinolysis
	Arterial and collateral vessel smooth muscle	Vasodilators
Arterioles	Arteriolar smooth muscle	Vasodilators
	Platelet aggregates	Antiplatelet agents
Capillaries	Platelet aggregates	Antiplatelet agents
	White cell plugging	White cell antiactivators
	Red cell deformation	Haemorheological agents
Venules	Red cell aggregation	Haemorheological agents
	White cell adhesion	White cell antiactivators
Tissue cells	Calcium influx	Calcium channel blockers
	Oxygen radical damage	Free radical scavengers
	Metabolic derangement	Metabolic regulators
	Oedema	Hyperoncotic solutions

in platelet microaggregates, which can block arterioles and capillaries; and decreased activation of white cells, which may obstruct capillary or venular flow, adhere to endothelium, and damage cells by producing lysosomal enzymes, leukotrienes, or toxic oxygen derivatives.

TISSUE CELLS

Finally, drugs may act by protecting brain or limb cells from ischaemic damage rather than by increasing microvascular flow. Possible mechanisms for such "cytoprotection" include protection against toxic products of ischaemia (for example, by scavengers of toxic oxygen products), reduction of calcium influx (for example, by calcium channel blockers), increased oxidative metabolism with reduction of lactic acidosis (for example, by naftidrofuryl), and decreased oedema (for example, by hyperoncotic solutions of mannitol, sorbitol, or glycerol).

171

Cerebral arterial disease

ACUTE ISCHAEMIC (OR UNSELECTED) STROKE[1 2]

As with myocardial infarction, specific treatment of acute cerebral infarction is most likely to benefit the patient when given in the first few hours, before infarction of the whole ischaemic area: one should not wait an arbitrary 24h to let a "transient ischaemic attack" become a "completed stroke." An accurate diagnosis should be made, by computed tomographic scanning as well as clinical evaluation, to identify the sizable minority of patients with intracranial haemorrhages, tumours, or lacunar infarctions, and make them secondary exclusions from studies of major cerebral infarction. The most relevant end points to the patients are death and long term (several months) or short term (one month) disability. Unfortunately, most reported studies have been too small, have not included routinely performed computed tomography, and have reported the outcomes as neurological scores (which interest neurologists) rather than activities of daily living (which interest patients).[1 2]

Isovolaemic haemodilution with dextran 40[3]

Several small studies have suggested that dextran infusions may be beneficial in acute cerebral infarction, possibly by lowering the packed cell volume and thus blood viscosity. Two recently reported large, multicentre, randomised, controlled trials from Italy (1267 patients) and Scandinavia (373 patients) assessed the value of isovolaemic haemodilution (by venesection and dextran 40 infusion) in acute cerebral infarction that had been confirmed by computed tomography in almost all patients. Mean packed cell volume was reduced from 43–44% to 37–38%. As no benefit was observed in either study, we can be confident that the routine application of this regimen is not useful for treating acute cerebral infarction. Possible explanations include the facts that more patients with stroke die only if they have high (over 48–50%) packed cell volumes; that dextran increases plasma viscosity; and that cardiac output in elderly patients with stroke fails to increase sufficiently to compensate for the reduction in haemoglobin concentration and thus in oxygen transport. Future studies of haemodilution should evaluate patients with high packed cell volumes; plasma expanders such as hetastarch, which do not increase plasma viscosity; and haemodynamic monitoring.[3]

Glycerol

Glycerol may be beneficial in acute infarction by reducing cerebral oedema. Analysis of the eight published randomised controlled trials showed that treatment reduced the risk of short term (within 6 weeks) death by about 36% (95% confidence interval −4% to −58%).[1] Analysis of the four trials that reported longer follow up showed a non-significant reduction in death rates of 21% (95% confidence interval −51% to +28%).[1] Further studies of larger numbers, diagnosed by computed tomography and followed up for long term disability as well as death, are required.

Naftidrofuryl

This drug has several actions, including increased oxidative metabolism by ischaemic cells and reduction of lactic acidosis. An analysis of the two published studies of acute stroke (in 100 and 89 patients) found a 29% reduction in death rates within three months, but with wide confidence intervals.[1] The second, more recent study used computed tomography to establish the diagnosis of infarction. Further larger studies are required.

Nimodipine

This calcium channel blocker has a greater antivasoconstrictive effect on cerebral than on limb arteries, crosses the blood–brain barrier, and may reduce ischaemic brain cell damage. A controlled trial of 186 patients with acute ischaemic stroke, confirmed by computed tomography, observed a 70% lower death rate within 4 weeks (95% confidence interval −12% to −90%), and the death rate difference was maintained at 6 months.[1] All patients in this study also received dextran and heparin. Larger studies of nimodipine are in progress. Nicardipine is another calcium channel blocker also under evaluation for treating cerebral ischaemia.

β Adrenergic blockers

A study of 302 conscious patients with clinically diagnosed hemisphere strokes (few underwent computed tomography) randomised to receive atenolol (50 mg daily), slow release propranolol (80 mg daily), or placebo, all starting within 48 h, showed no significant differences in death or disability at 6 months' follow up,

173

but again the 95% confidence intervals were wide.[4] Larger studies with computed tomography are therefore required.

Corticosteroids

Corticosteroids may reduce cerebral oedema and were assessed in several small studies between 1956 and 1976. Two more recent randomised trials of over 100 patients showed no benefit in death or disability. The first trial did not use computed tomography and had a 1 year follow up; the second did and had a 3 week follow up.[5]

Epoprostenol (prostacyclin) and its analogues

Intravenous infusion of prostacyclin causes systemic vasodilatation (especially in the skin) and inhibits platelet aggregation. After several small studies, a randomised controlled trial of 86 patients with ischaemic stroke confirmed by computed tomography showed no benefit.[5] Stable analogues of prostacyclin are currently under evaluation.

Full dose anticoagulants

Full therapeutic doses of heparin and oral anticoagulants have been used to treat acute stroke for many years, with continuing controversy about the balance of benefits (preventing thromboembolic extension or recurrence) and risks (bleeding, even when computed tomography is used to exclude non-ischaemic stroke). Recent controlled studies have not shown overall benefit in patients with or without potential cardiac sources of embolism.[2] Pending results of larger trials, the use of full dose anticoagulants is not recommended. The defibrinating enzyme, ancrod, reduces plasma fibrinogen concentrations and thus reduces plasma and blood viscosity as well as producing anticoagulation, but only one small study has been reported.[5]

Low dose heparin and heparinoids

Deep venous thrombosis is common in patients with acute hemiparetic stroke, and pulmonary thromboembolism is an important cause of death. Dextran 40 was ineffective in preventing deep vein thrombosis in a subgroup of patients in the Scandinavian haemodilution study.[2] Recent studies have shown that low dose subcutaneous standard heparin or the heparinoid ORG 10172 are effective in reducing the incidence of deep vein thrombosis in patients with acute stroke and do not cause appreciable bleeding.

Although one large study that did not use routine computed tomography also reported reductions in pulmonary embolism and in total deaths,[6] use of computed tomography is advisable to exclude intracranial haemorrhage before using even low dose anticoagulants. Further large trials of low dose heparin, heparin fractions, and heparinoids are certainly required.

Thrombolytics

Treatment with thrombolytics risks causing cerebral bleeding and cerebral oedema, and their use is still experimental.[7]

INTRACRANIAL HAEMORRHAGE

No medical treatment has been proved to be beneficial against intracerebral haemorrhage; a study of dexamethasone showed no benefit.[2] Two studies of subarachnoid haemorrhage showed that the fibrinolytic inhibitor tranexamic acid reduced the incidence of rebleeding but increased the incidence of delayed cerebral ischaemia and did not reduce death rates.[8] Controlled trials of nimodipine, however, showed significantly lower incidence of neurological deficits after cerebral vasospasm.[8] Nicardipine is also under evaluation. It may be logical to combine calcium entry blockade with fibrinolytic inhibition in future studies.

PRIMARY PREVENTION OF STROKE

A recent community based study of first ever stroke caused by cerebral infarction confirmed that hypertension preceded over half the strokes. The most efficient drug treatment to prevent stroke is probably to give older hypertensive patients (with diastolic blood pressure persistently over 100 mmHg) a thiazide diuretic.[9] According to the trial of the European working party on high blood pressure in the elderly, treating 100 older hypertensive patients for 2 years can prevent two fatal and two non-fatal cardiovascular events, especially stroke. Treating younger patients with similar blood pressure levels is less efficient, though the Medical Research Council working party on treating mild hypertension suggested guidelines for treating younger hypertensive people who may benefit more—for example, using bendrofluazide for men aged 55–64 who smoke or propranolol for non-smoking men.[10]

The lack of suitable screening tests to indicate increased platelet reactivity, which would be analogous to measuring blood pressure, hinders the use of aspirin or other antiplatelet agents. Despite this disadvantage, two studies of aspirin treatment as primary prevention of cardiovascular events showed that fewer treated people experienced cardiovascular events, including strokes.[11] However, long term aspirin treatment possibly increases the incidence of haemorrhagic or disabling stroke, as well as having the proven side effect of gastrointestinal bleeding.[11]

Recent evidence suggests that oestrogen replacement treatment may reduce the incidence of stroke in postmenopausal women.[12]

SECONDARY PREVENTION OF STROKE

About one third of patients admitted to hospital die soon after their stroke, and another third have major disability. The remaining third make a complete or good recovery, however, and it is important to establish whether drugs can reduce the risk of subsequent cardiovascular events. Although only about 15% of strokes are preceded by a transient ischaemic attack, such events are worrying for patients and doctors, and the value of drugs to prevent the completion of a stroke should also be considered. An overview of trials of antiplatelet treatment in patients with transient ischaemic attacks or minor ischaemic strokes (as in patients with unstable angina or myocardial infarction) showed that 15% fewer treated patients died and 30% fewer had non-fatal strokes or myocardial infarctions.[13]

Aspirin (150–300 mg a day) appears to be as effective as any other antiplatelet treatment. Lower doses of aspirin (50–150 mg a day) might have a higher ratio of benefit to risk. Doctors who do not (or cannot) institute computed tomography for patients with stroke to exclude the 10–15% with intracranial haemorrhage should appreciate that aspirin may cause further bleeding in these patients.[14]

As for other antiplatelet drugs, little evidence exists that sulphinpyrazone or dipyridamole are effective in preventing secondary stroke when used without aspirin, but dipyridamole is being compared with low dose aspirin in a current large study. Ticlopidine, a newer antiplatelet agent, has been assessed in two trials of prevention after a stroke or transient ischaemic attack (CATS and TASS), whose results were positive. The high percentage of patients who cannot tolerate aspirin makes it necessary to evaluate other antiplatelet agents.

Another review suggested that treating hypertension in patients with transient ischaemic attacks or minor strokes may also reduce subsequent strokes by up to half.[8] Treatment with antihypertensives as well as aspirin should therefore be considered.

VASCULAR (MULTI-INFARCT) DEMENTIA

This continues to be a controversial subject. Vascular dementia is less common than Alzheimer's (senile) dementia, their differential diagnosis can be difficult, and assessing drugs to treat them is difficult. There is no convincing evidence that vascular drugs make an important contribution to the care of patients with dementia.

Peripheral arterial disease

INTERMITTENT CLAUDICATION

In this common condition of older people, the prognosis for the legs is relatively benign and fewer than 10% progress to critical ischaemia (rest pain or gangrene). The general prognosis gives cause for concern, however, because the associated coronary and cerebral arterial diseases carry a high risk of fatal or non-fatal myocardial infarction or stroke. Intervention to prevent vascular events and death should therefore be as important as treating the cramping pain. Yet studies of preventing secondary cardiovascular disease in patients with claudication are surprisingly rare. No large studies have been undertaken to assess the clinical benefit of lowering either blood pressure or serum lipid concentrations in patients with claudication. When treating hypertension it may be preferable to avoid β adrenergic blocking drugs because some studies showed them to have adverse effects on walking distance and circulation in the legs. No large studies of the clinical benefit of aspirin in patients with claudication have been undertaken, although a reduction in the progression of femoral atherosclerosis was observed in one study of low dose aspirin. A study of oral anticoagulants in recipients of limb grafts showed significantly improved survival of the patients (if not the grafts), which, if this result is confirmed, may lead to a renaissance in anticoagulant treatment for patients with claudication.

The prevention of atherosclerotic complications with ketanserin (PACK) study was a large placebo controlled trial of this serotonin antagonist to prevent cardiovascular events in patients with intermittent claudication.[15] Ketanserin has antihypertensive, antiplatelet, and rheological actions. Patients using potassium losing diuretics, however, experienced drug interactions associated with a higher death rate, which counteracted a beneficial trend in the other patients. The study has, however, provided a useful basis for planning trials of other interventions that might reduce the risk of vascular events in patients with claudication. Smaller studies of ticlopidine in preventing vascular events in patients with claudication, are also promising.[16]

The placebo group in the large PACK study underwent serial treadmill walking distance studies in several centres, and the results confirm the findings of previous studies that walking distance tends to improve spontaneously, noticeably, and for several months, especially if patients are encouraged to "stop smoking and keep walking." Evaluating drugs in relieving the symptoms of claudication is therefore difficult: strict selection and large numbers of patients are required. Despite the statement in the current *British National Formulary* that "no controlled studies have shown any improvement in walking distance," large controlled studies have shown positive results for isoxsuprine, naftidrofuryl,[17] oxpentifylline,[18] and ticlopidine.[16] Although the mean increase in walking distance compared with that in patients receiving placebo is often small, some patients do show impressive responses. While the anticipated benefits of time, regular exercise, and stopping smoking are awaited, therefore, one or more of these agents may be worth trying in patients whose daily activities are severely curtailed. Little evidence exists that vasodilatation in itself increases blood flow to ischaemic leg muscles, but several other mechanisms (such as rheological or metabolic actions) have a sound rationale. Furthermore, it seems inappropriate to have a double standard for claudication and angina pectoris, whose placebo response is also well documented. Patients are as frustrated if they cannot walk because of a sore lower half as because of a sore upper half, and doctors who discriminate at the umbilicus may hit below the belt.

The theoretical importance of blood viscosity in intermittent claudication has been substantiated by a recent controlled trial of haemodilution in selected patients with claudication who have haemodynamically appropriate lesions (long stenoses) that might be expected to result in low shear stresses, under which the increased viscosity of blood may become a limiting factor in muscle blood flow. Haemodilution is not "user friendly" but should be considered in severely disabled patients with claudication who do not respond to simpler measures and have no contraindications (such as severe ischaemic heart disease).

The most obvious way to relieve claudication is to relieve haemodynamically important obstructions in major arteries. Bypass grafting carries a risk of death of 0·5–3%, and grafts fail progressively in time, especially in smokers. Recent alternatives in selected cases include angioplasty (balloon or laser) and treatment with thrombolytic drugs. Recent acute onset or worsening of claudication suggests thrombosis of a stenosed artery, and angiography may give evidence of thrombosis that has been confirmed in some cases by reperfusion after thrombolytic treatment. The current popularity of thrombolytics for treating acute myocardial infarction has promoted a renaissance of interest in applying thrombolytic treatment to subacute as well as acute limb ischaemia.[19] The main adverse effect is bleeding, the most serious manifestation of which is the death of about 1% from intracranial haemorrhage (for example, from an unsuspected intracranial aneurysm). This death rate, however, is comparable to that risked by surgery and may be reduced by modifications currently being investigated. The modifications include local infusion of the thrombolytic agent proximal to or into the thrombus via the catheter used to show the lesion by angiography and combining thrombolytic treatment with aspirating thrombus fragments to shorten the duration of treatment.

CRITICAL ISCHAEMIA

This may arise acutely (because of major thromboembolism) or subacutely (caused by progressive occlusion at a critical stenosis, for example, by overlying thrombus formation). Although embolectomy, angioplasty, or bypass grafting are used as appropriate, there is also increasing interest in treatment with thrombolytics, including local infusions proximal to or into the thrombus.[19]

Some evidence exists that infusions of vasodilators such as inositol nicotinate, naftidrofuryl, and prostanoids (prostaglandin E_1, epoprostenol (prostacyclin, prostaglandin I_2), or stable prostacyclin analogues) may relieve subacute rest pain, promote ulcer healing, or both;[20] however, the results of large controlled studies are awaited before treatment with vasodilators can be recommended with confidence. As with intermittent claudication, several mechanisms exist by which vasodilatation may act (table 14.1), which can be helpful in "buying time" while patients are evaluated for operation, angioplasty, or thrombolytic treatment. As with claudication, the main problem in trials is the response of rest pain and ulceration to placebo treatment and the passage of time.

RAYNAUD'S DISEASE

The mainstays of treatment of Raynaud's disease are general measures such as keeping warm, wearing gloves (including heated gloves), and excluding causes such as drugs, vibrating tools, and diseases of the cervical ribs or connective tissue. Drug treatment should be considered for severe cases, and placebo controlled trials of nifedipine, inositol nicotinate, and prostanoids suggest that they are helpful.[21] The benefit of these vasodilators is, however, often tempered by their systemic side effects (table 14.1).[21]

1 Sandercock P. Important new treatments for acute ischaemic stroke? *BMJ* 1987;**295**:1224–5. (Editorial overview of published trials of glycerol, naftidrofuryl, and nimodipine in acute stroke. The pessimistic view: read in conjunction with next reference.)

2 Steiner TJ. Medical care of the early stroke patient. *Clin Rehab* 1988;**2**:151–60. (Useful review, with references for most clinical trials up to 1987, including recent trials of anticoagulants. The optimistic view.)

3 Heros RC, Korosue K. Hemodilution for cerebral ischemia. *Stroke* 1989;**20**:423–7.

4 Barer DH, Cruickshank JM, Ebrahim SB, Mitchell JRA. Low dose β blockade in acute stroke ("BEST" trial): an evaluation. *BMJ* 1988;**296**:737–41. (Large study using the "pragmatic" approach (no confirmation of cerebral infarction by routine computed tomography) argues for this minority approach.)

5 Rose FC, ed. *Stroke: epidemiological, therapeutic and socio-economic aspects.* London: Royal Society of Medicine, 1986: 1–169. (Useful conference proceedings covering epidemiology, assessment, and socioeconomic aspects of stroke, as well as update on trials of steroids, prostacyclin, and naftidrofuryl in acute stroke.)

6 McCarthy ST, Turner J. Low-dose subcutaneous heparin in the prevention of deep-vein thrombosis and pulmonary emboli following acute stroke. *Age Ageing* 1986;**15**:84–8. (Low dose standard heparin reduced total deaths, pulmonary embolism at necropsy, and deep vein thrombosis in this large, if enigmatically reported, study.)

7 Del Zoppo GJ, Ferbert A, Otis S, *et al.* Local intra-arterial fibrinolytic treatment in acute carotid territory stroke. A pilot study. *Stroke* 1988;**19**:307–13. (Of 20 patients treated with intra-arterial urokinase or streptokinase, 15 showed recanalisation, 10 improved clinically, and four showed haemorrhagic transformation.)

8 Pickard JD, Murray GD, Illingworth R, *et al.* Effect of oral nimodipine on cerebral infarction and outcome after subarachnoid haemorrhage: British aneurysm nimodipine trial. *BMJ* 1989;**298**:636–42. (Nimodipine reduced the incidence of cerebral infarction by 33% and the incidence of poor outcomes by 40%.)

9 McMahon S, Culter JA, Furberg CD, Payne GH. The effects of drug treatment for hypertension on morbidity and mortality from cardiovascular disease: a review of the randomised controlled trials. *Prog Cardiovasc Dis* 1986;**29**(suppl 1):99–118.

10 Medical Research Council Working Party. Stroke and coronary disease in mild hypertension: risk factors and the value of treatment. *BMJ* 1988;**296**:1565–70. (How to choose, through the retrospectoscope, which patients to give which antihypertensive agents to prevent most strokes, bearing in mind the adverse effects of treatment.)

11 Hennekens CH, Peto R, Hutchison GB, Doll R. An overview of the British and American aspirin studies. *N Engl J Med* 1988;**318**:923–4.

12 Paganini-Hill A, Ross RK, Henderson BE. Postmenopausal oestrogen treatment and stroke: a prospective study. *BMJ* 1988;**297**:519–22. (Interesting spin off of oestrogen replacement treatment: deaths from stroke roughly halved.)

13 Antiplatelet Trialists' Collaboration. Secondary prevention of vascular disease by prolonged antiplatelet treatment. *BMJ* 1988;**296**:320–1.

14 Sandercock P. Aspirin for strokes and transient ischaemic attacks. No panacea. *BMJ* 1988;**297**:995–6. (Counsels appropriate caution before reflex prescription of aspirin for all strokes.)

15 Prevention of Atherosclerotic Complications with Ketanserin Trial Group. Prevention of atherosclerotic complications: controlled trial of ketanserin. *BMJ* 1989;**298**:424–30. (Largest study of patients with claudication (3899 patients) and their clinical course.)

16 Boissel JP, Peyrieux JC, Destors JM. Is it possible to reduce the risk of cardiovascular events in subjects suffering from intermittent claudication of the lower limbs? *Thromb Haemost* 1989; **62**: 681–5.

17 Trubestein G, Böhme H, Heidrich H, *et al*. Naftidrofuryl in chronic arterial disease. Results of a controlled multicentre study. *Angiology* 1984;**35**:701–8. (In 104 patients treated for 12 weeks placebo and active treatment gave similar increases in total walking distance, but active treatment was associated with a greater increase in pain free walking distance.)

18 Rössner M, Müller R. On the assessment of the efficacy of pentoxifylline (Trental). *J Med* 1987;**18**:1–15. (In-house meta-analysis of the efficacy of oxpentifylline in increasing walking distance in claudication in 14 double blind randomised studies. In total, 35% of patients receiving active treatment doubled their walking distance, compared with 8% of control patients.)

19 Graor RA, Risius B, Denny KM, *et al*. Local thrombolysis in the treatment of thrombosed arteries, bypass grafts and arteriovenous fistulas. *J Vasc Surg* 1985;**2**:406–14. (Large series of patients treated with low dose intra-arterial streptokinase; discusses efficacy, coagulation changes, complications, and choice of patients.)

20 Negus D, Irving JD, Fiedgood A. Intra-arterial prostacyclin compared to Praxilene in the management of severe lower limb ischaemia: a double-blind trial. *J Cardiovasc Surg (Torino)* 1987;**28**:196–9. (After either treatment about half the patients had symptomatic relief and avoided amputation. Discusses previous studies of both epoprostenol and naftidrofuryl in critical ischaemia.)

21 Corbin DOC, Wood DA, Macintyre CCA, Housley E. A randomised double-blind cross-over trial of nifedipine in the treatment of primary Raynaud's phenomenon. *Eur Heart J* 1986;**7**:165–70. (Treatment reduced number of attacks in most patients; 61% had side effects (especially flushing and acroparaesthesiae).)

15 Asthma and allergic rhinitis

K FAN CHUNG, PETER J BARNES

This chapter highlights some of the important advances in therapeutic aspects of respiratory medicine that have emerged recently. Although only a few drugs have been introduced for treating respiratory disease since this subject was last reviewed,[1][2] many drugs with potential are now being developed and may represent useful advances in the next few years. This has been made possible by our increasing understanding of the pathophysiology of many respiratory conditions. We review new drugs for asthma and allergic rhinitis.

Asthma

During the past 10 years there has been an increase in disability and death from asthma.[3-6] Despite the fact that the current trend in deaths from asthma coincides with increasing sales of all classes of drugs for treating asthma,[7] it has been suggested that those who die of asthma have not received optimum treatment.[8] Too much reliance may have been placed on β adrenoceptor agonists, resulting in the development of tachyphylaxis to such drugs and of possible dangerous arrhythmias,[9][10] but there is no convincing evidence to support this view. Use of regular inhaled β_2 agonists, rather than intermittent on demand usage may worsen asthma control.[11] Although this area remains controversial, emphasis has been placed on the use of inhaled short acting β_2 agonists on demand only and on the early use of regular anti-inflammatory treatment.[12]

It is important to realise that inflammatory changes in the airways of asthmatic patients may underlie the bronchial hyperreactivity and clinical symptoms of asthma.[13] Drugs that prevent or suppress inflammation of the airways have been advocated as a prophylaxis against attacks of asthma.[14] In two reports the bronchial hyperresponsiveness of mild asthma in children and adults was reduced by regular treatment with inhaled steroids but was worsened, if anything, by regular treatment with inhaled β_2 agonists.[15 16] These studies support the view that the strategy for antiasthma treatment should consist of regular prophylactic treatment, with β_2 agonists being used only for short term relief of wheezing and dyspnoea.

An important development in the past decade has been improved delivery of antiasthma drugs, such as spacer devices to increase deposition of inhaled aerosols and the development of controlled release theophylline preparations. Nedocromil sodium, a mast cell "stabiliser" and anti-inflammatory agent, has been introduced as an asthma prophylactic. A long acting inhaled β_2 adrenergic agonist, salmeterol, has recently been introduced, together with a new topical corticosteroid, fluticasone propionate.

DRUG DELIVERY

Slow release bronchodilators

The introduction of slow release preparations of theophylline has given a new impetus to the use of these methylxanthines in treating asthma. Increased rational use of these preparations has been made possible by the availability of reliable and convenient theophylline assays and subsequently by a greater understanding of their pharmacokinetics. Sustained release preparations have been particularly useful in treating nocturnal asthma, as therapeutic plasma concentrations of theophylline may be maintained overnight by giving a single dose in the evening.[17] The dose of slow release aminophylline needed to abolish completely the nocturnal decrease in peak expiratory flow is about 10 mg/kg body weight, taken once before bedtime.[17]

Several slow release theophylline preparations are now available for prescription in the United Kingdom.[18] Although it is possible to tailor the doses of these preparations to achieve therapeutic concentrations throughout 24 h, it is most important to prevent bronchoconstriction at night, as asthmatics can resort to inhaled β_2 adrenergic agonists during the day. The temporal variations in plasma theophylline concentrations, with reduced plasma concentrations at night in adults,[19] may be due to posture, as higher theophylline concentrations in the blood are found on standing than when lying down, possibly because of reduced gastric absorption when lying down.[20]

Sustained release theophylline preparations may be given twice a day and provide greater efficacy, fewer side effects, and greater compliance than immediate release theophylline preparations.[21][22] This difference has been attributed to the reduced fluctuations in plasma concentrations of theophylline seen with the sustained release preparations. More recently an ultrasustained release theophylline, Uniphyllin, suitable for administration once a day, has become available. A single dose of slow release Uniphyllin (800 mg) in the evening was found to prevent nocturnal wheeze more effectively than theophylline 370 mg twice a day.[23][24] Dosing with Uniphyllin in the evening rather than in the morning is better at controlling the early morning dip in pulmonary function.[25] When Uniphyllin was given in a dosage of 10 mg/kg to asthmatic patients, peak concentrations within the therapeutic range 10–20 mg/kg were achieved within 8 h.[26] To ensure that the peak concentrations coincide with the occurrence of early morning wheeze it is probably best to take ultraslow release theophylline at around 20.00.

The side effects of various theophylline preparations (including nervousness, nausea, vomiting, anorexia, abdominal discomfort, and headache) do not always seem to be related to the concentration of theophylline in the blood; patients may experience substantial side effects even at subtherapeutic concentrations.[27] The gradual introduction of theophylline has been recommended so that these side effects are minimised.[28] The risk of serious toxic effects such as seizures and cardiac arrhythmias increases when the plasma concentrations exceed 30 mg/l.[29] More recently it has been appreciated that theophylline is associated with learning difficulties and sleep disturbance in children.[30] This questions the value of regular oral theophylline for children.

In view of the considerable variation in the absorption and clearance of theophylline in and between patients, the dose of slow release preparations should be adjusted according to the clinical response and to blood concentrations of theophylline. The clearance of theophylline may be affected by various factors, including cigarette smoking, age, diet, and drugs such as erythromycin, cimetidine, allopurinol, ciprofloxacin, and propranolol. As different slow release preparations differ in their characteristics of release it is unwise to change from one preparation to another without careful monitoring.

Oral slow release β_2 adrenergic agonists are effective at controlling the morning dip in pulmonary function in some patients.[31] Slow release terbutaline and a new controlled release salbutamol preparation using an osmotically controlled delivery system may both be effective. A recent study showed that infusion of subcutaneous terbutaline (14 µg/kg/day) may alleviate the severe morning dip in patients who are not helped by oral treatment.[32] This may have been achieved through higher blood concentrations of terbutaline than would have been provided by conventional oral doses.[33] Bambuterol is an inactive compound but is converted to terbutaline when absorbed (that is, it is a prodrug). It can be administered once a day and produces effects similar to terbutaline given twice a day.[34]

Inhalation devices

Many patients, particularly elderly patients and young children, cannot master the use of the metered dose inhaler, which requires proper coordination between actuating the inhaler and inhaling, followed by holding the breath. Important advances have been the introduction of the spacer or reservoir devices for use with the metered dose inhaler (for example, Nebuhaler or Volumatic), of dry powder inhalers (for example, Rotahaler with Rotacaps), and of self-actuating metered dose inhalers on inspiration. A metered dose powder inhaler, Turbohaler, will deliver small quantities of active compound (less than 1 mg/activation) without any carrier compound. At present the Turbohaler can be prescribed to deliver terbutaline or budesonide. In a recent study terbutaline inhaled via the Turbohaler gave a more rapid onset of action, greater maximum brochodilatation, and a longer duration of action without side effects when inhaled at doses (up to 4 mg) above the recommended dose of 0·5 mg.[35] These devices circumvent the necessity for coordination between actuating the metered dose inhaler and inhaling. The spacer devices also increase the amount of aerosol that is actually deposited in the lungs: with the metered dose inhaler attached to a Nebuhaler about 2·5 times more aerosol is deposited in the lungs of patients who have obstructive airways disease than with the metered dose inhaler alone (21% versus 9%) during the inhalation of a single puff of aerosol.[36] After four puffs from the metered dose inhaler into a Nebuhaler followed by two

185

inhalations with breath holding, 15% deposition was obtained in the lungs.[37] Another advantage of using a spacer device is the decreased deposition of aerosol in the oropharynx, with most of the aerosol particles remaining in the spacer reservoir itself.[37] This is achieved by slowing down the aerosol in the chamber and by the subsequent evaporation of the fluorocarbon propellant, thus producing a finer and more slow moving aerosol cloud to be inhaled into the lungs.

The airway response to a β agonist is greater in normal and asthmatic subjects who use a metered dose inhaler with a Nebuhaler than in those who use a metered dose inhaler alone or even a Mini-neb nebuliser.[36] A Nebuhaler is as effective as a nebuliser in chronic stable asthma[38] or in acute severe asthma.[39] The smaller proportion of oropharyngeal deposition occurring means that less of the inhaled drug is absorbed, which results in reduced systemic and local side effects. High dose inhaled steroid treatment, such as budesonide 400–1600 µg/day, when used with a Nebuhaler is associated with a reduced risk of oropharyngeal candidiasis and with an appreciable increase in antiasthmatic effect.[40] The spacer reservoir can be particularly useful for children receiving inhaled corticosteroids, as a reduction in the systemic absorption of steroids may decrease any potential adverse effects on growth. In addition, the use of a reservoir device makes it possible to administer more potent inhaled corticosteroids and β agonists.

Home nebulisers

Nebulisers driven by compressed air for use at home have increased in popularity and are used to administer bronchodilator aerosols. Many patients, particularly those who have moderately severe obstruction, find greater subjective relief from bronchodilators delivered from such nebulisers than from those delivered from their metered dose inhaler. There is little evidence, however, that these nebulisers used at home provide more bronchodilatation or that they are more clinically effective than the metered dose inhaler, particularly when the metered dose inhaler is used with a spacer device.[36 41 42] Home nebulisers are of undoubted benefit in treating small children and patients who have acute asthma, permitting larger doses of bronchodilators to be administered,[43] but they should be prescribed with caution for adults with asthma, as increasing dependence solely on β agonists for relief of symptoms may mask the need for corticosteroid treatment.[44]

LONG ACTING β_2 AGONISTS

Two new β agonists with long durations of bronchodilator action, salmeterol and formoterol, have been developed for inhaled use, and salmeterol is available in the United Kingdom for use in asthmatic adults and children over 4 years. Salmeterol has been shown to be a potent selective β_2 agonist with a duration of action of more than 10 h, and its mode of action appears to be due to exoreceptor binding. A portion of the salmeterol molecule presumably occupies a site adjacent to the receptor in the cell membrane, which allows the molecule to anchor and then interact freely with the β receptor.[45] In adults with asthma, salmeterol in single dose studies, with doses of up to 100 mg, has been shown to have a duration of action of up to 12 h and has similar side effects to salbutamol[46] with little evidence of tachyphylaxis. Inhaled formoterol, in cumulative dosing studies of patients with asthma, has been shown to be about ten times more potent than salbutamol.[47] Formoterol at 12 and 24 µg was seen to have a duration of action of about 11 h, compared with only 4 h for salbutamol 200 µg.[48] It also protects against histamine induced bronchoconstriction for at least 5 h in adults and for 12 h in children.[49] The onset of bronchodilatation with formoterol seems to be more rapid than with salmeterol.

Long acting β_2 agonists are useful in controlling asthma symptoms, particularly those at night, but because they possess no anti-inflammatory properties, they should not replace the use of prophylactic antiasthma drugs such as inhaled corticosteroids. It is recommended that patients who need to use long acting β_2 agonists should be established on inhaled corticosteroid therapy first, usually after a minimum dose of 800 µg/day. Although studies have not shown tachyphylaxis to the bronchodilator effect of salmeterol or formoterol, there is a rapid loss of the protective effect of salmeterol against bronchoconstrictor challenges.[50] A recent multicentre trial in the United States of mild-to-moderate asthma showed that salmeterol given twice daily is superior to salbutamol given either four times daily or as needed.[51]

NEDOCROMIL SODIUM

Nedocromil sodium is a pyranoquinoline dicarboxylic acid that has recently been developed and marketed for prophylactic use in adults who have asthma. It is chemically remote from sodium cromoglycate, but it retains similar antiallergic properties with increased anti-inflammatory effects. In the classic models of immediate hypersensitivity in the rat nedocromil sodium is as effective as sodium cromoglycate;[52] however, in contrast to sodium chromoglycate, it considerably inhibits the release of inflammatory mediators from mast cells that have been obtained by bronchoalveolar lavage from sensitised monkeys and people and challenged with antigen or antibody to IgE.[53 54] Nedocromil sodium also inhibits bronchoconstriction induced by antigens in vivo in monkeys[55] and humans.[56] The activation of human eosinophils and neutrophils,[57] human macrophages,[58] and rat platelets[59] is also inhibited.

Studies of patients with asthma have shown that nedocromil sodium has a similar range of activity, usually with greater potency, against several triggers of bronchoconstriction. Thus nedocromil sodium in single therapeutic doses can inhibit the early and late phase responses after antigen challenge,[60] asthma induced by exercise,[61 62] and bronchoconstriction induced by inhaling cold air,[63] sulphur dioxide,[64 65] or fog.[66] Small but appreciable improvements in bronchial hyperreactivity have been seen during the pollen season in patients with asthma who are sensitive to pollen.[67]

In several clinical trials nedocromil sodium, taken for 4 or 12 weeks, was better than placebo at controlling symptoms of asthma in patients with atopic or non-atopic asthma who received bronchodilator treatment only.[68] The concurrent use of nedocromil sodium with inhaled steroids has been shown to confer additional therapeutic benefit, but it has been unable to control the deterioration in asthma that occurs after the withdrawal of inhaled steroids.[68] In a more recent study, however, some beneficial effect was shown.[69] Nedocromil sodium was not found to be effective in replacing oral corticosteroids for asthma.[70]

Nedocromil sodium (Tilade) is formulated as a pressurised aerosol, and the recommended dose is two puffs (2 mg/puff) twice a day; the dose may be increased to four times a day. It has been well tolerated by patients with asthma who have taken it for up to 1 year.[71] No serious side effects have been reported, but some patients complain of an unpleasant taste and occasional nausea. When inhaled by normal subjects nedocromil sodium is rapidly absorbed and is excreted totally unchanged in the bile and urine. There is no accumulation of the drug on multiple dosing.

Although nedocromil sodium has been shown to be effective in treating asthma, its exact place in managing asthma remains to be assessed. The initial studies suggest that nedocromil sodium is more active in a wider range of patients with asthma, including adult and non-atopic patients, than sodium cromoglycate, but does not seem to be as potent as inhaled corticosteroid treatment.

ENPROFYLLINE

Slow release preparations of theophylline are used to manage nocturnal and early morning wheeze and chronic asthma not adequately controlled by β agonist and steroid aerosols. Although there is now a better understanding of the pharmacokinetics of theophylline, and plasma concentrations of theophylline can be monitored, the wide variation in the rate of hepatic metabolism may make it difficult to achieve adequate therapeutic concentrations in individual patients. The toxicity and side effects of theophylline also remain a great problem.

Of great interest is the recently developed xanthine derivative enprofylline, which is five times more potent than theophylline in causing bronchodilatation and does not have the stimulating effects on the central nervous system such as anxiety, tremor, seizures, and respiratory stimulation.[72] In contrast with theophylline, enprofylline does not increase gastric secretion or cause diuresis or the release of free fatty acids into the circulation. Both drugs, however, cause a similar degree of nausea (which is the most troublesome side effect of theophylline), relaxation of the lower oesophageal sphincter, and headache, which is presumably due to vasodilatation of cerebral arteries.[72]

The mechanism of action of enprofylline as a bronchodilator is uncertain.[73] In contrast with theophylline, enprofylline is not an adenosine antagonist, which probably explains its lack of side effects on the central nervous and cardiac systems. Theophylline antagonises the effect of infused adenosine in humans, but enprofylline has no such effect,[74] indicating that theophylline probably exerts its antiasthma effect by another mechanism. Methylxanthines may have effects other than relaxation of the smooth muscle in airways, such as inhibition of microvascular leakage and thus inhibition of oedema in airways. Enprofylline and theophylline both inhibit the late phase response to antigen challenge,[75] an effect that may be related to the inflammation of airways.

Enprofylline is well absorbed throughout the gastrointestinal tract, is metabolised only minimally, and is eliminated unchanged

189

by the kidneys.[76] Thus, in contrast with theophylline, enprofylline blood concentrations do not depend on a variable rate of hepatic metabolism. The renal clearance of enprofylline is linearly related to renal function in patients who have varying types of renal dysfunction.[77] A sustained release preparation given twice a day will maintain therapeutic plasma concentrations for 24 h.

Oral enprofylline in a single dose (4 mg/kg) caused a similar degree of bronchodilatation to a standard oral dose of terbutaline in patients with stable asthma.[78] Enprofylline has been shown to be more potent than theophylline in treating acute asthma.[79] Patients with asthma treated with enprofylline for 2 weeks had a lower score for asthmatic symptoms, but a greater prevalence of headaches, than when they were receiving theophylline.[80] Further development of enprofylline has now been abandoned.

NEW INHALED CORTICOSTEROIDS

Recent studies have demonstrated that topical corticosteroids, in addition to restoring the integrity of the airway epithelium, markedly suppress the inflammatory influx in the airway submucosa of patients with mild asthma.[81 82] Inhaled corticosteroids also improve bronchial hyperresponsiveness and symptoms associated with a reduced usage of inhaled β_2 agonist therapy.[83] With the wide range of dosages available (for example 100–2000 µg daily for beclomethasone dipropionate or 100–1600 µg daily for budesonide), the dose may be adjusted to the minimum required to control asthma symptoms. There is a strong argument for instituting inhaled steroid therapy as early as possible in asthma.

Currently available topical steroids possess a combination of high topical anti-inflammatory effect in the airways and effective metabolic inactivation in the liver after uptake into the systemic circulation. The systemic contribution of the large swallowed function of inhaled steroids is rather small because of the low oral bioavailability of inhaled steroids. There is little evidence that low doses of topical steroids (up to 800 µg daily) cause systemic side effects, but at higher doses systemic adverse effects may occur with changes in biochemical markers such as plasma corticols or serum osteocalcin levels. It is currrently not clear how much risk there is of developing osteoporosis while on long term high dose inhaled steroid therapy, particularly in patients at risk such as postmenopausal women.

New topical glucocorticoids are under development with the

main aim of enhancing topical anti-inflammatory activity while reducing oral bioavailability and increasing hepatic metabolism. Fluticasone propionate for inhalation through the Diskhaler has recently been marketed and is also available as a nasal spray for the treatment of rhinitis. In animal studies and in skin vasoconstrictor tests in humans, it has been reported to be more active than beclomethasone dipropionate. Low systemic oral bioavailability with extensive first pass hepatic metabolism has also been shown. Fluticasone propionate has twice the potency of beclomethasone dipropionate (as shown in clinical trials). Other topical steroids under clinical development include tipredane and mometasone furoate.

The introduction of these new corticosteroids may mean that the early use of inhaled steroids may be more justified with compounds possessing the potential for lower risk of systemic side effects. A substantial proportion of more severely asthmatic patients may not have to resort to chronic oral corticosteroid therapy with its attendant side effects.

STEROID SPARING AGENTS

Some patients with asthma may need maintenance treatment with oral corticosteroids in addition to high dose inhaled cortico-steroids to remain symptom free. Preventive measures against the development of steroid induced osteoporosis should be con-sidered. Drugs such as gold salts and methotrexate have been advocated as steroid sparing agents and may be introduced with the aim of reducing steroid maintenance dosage, thus reducing side effects of oral steroid treatment. Two recent studies have shown the efficacy of low dose methotrexate (15 mg a week), but patients should be monitored carefully and have regular blood counts and liver function tests.[84 85] Gold salts have also been shown to be effective.[86] Cyclosporin may improve lung function in steroid dependent asthmatics.[87] However, all of these agents could cause serious side effects and patients needing steroid sparing drugs should be treated in specialised asthma centres.

A minority of asthmatic patients do not appear to respond (in terms of their airways obstruction) to very high doses of systemic steroid therapy. Although in some of them part of the underlying reason may be fixed irreversible airways obstruction, in others the cause of steroid resistance is still unclear.

Acute asthma

The treatment of acute asthma has for a long time been empirical, and only recently have objective data been obtained about the effectiveness and possible toxic effects of various bronchodilator treatments. No new drugs (apart from enprofylline) have been developed to treat acute asthma, and recent studies have evaluated β agonists, aminophylline, and anticholinergic drugs.

Corticosteroids are undoubtedly beneficial in treating acute asthma.[88–91] A recent study has shown that intravenous hydrocortisone confers no additional advantages when used with oral prednisolone and bronchodilators to treat acute severe asthma without ventilatory failure.[92] Nebulised β₂ agonists, rather than intravenous aminophylline or parenteral β₂ agonists, remain the best bronchodilator treatment for acute asthma, as they produce prompt relief of wheezing and dyspnoea with few side effects.[93 94] The combination of aminophylline and β agonists does not seem to offer any advantage and could increase any side effects.[95] In addition, theophylline toxicity may be a problem in patients who are already taking slow release methylxanthines.

The α agonist activity of adrenaline could reduce oedema and thus be useful in treating acute asthma, but when compared with an inhaled β agonist nebulised adrenaline was no better at relieving airways obstruction in acute asthma.[96] Similarly, subcutaneous adrenaline was no more effective than subcutaneous terbutaline in treating acute asthma.[97]

The anticholinergic drug atropine sulphate is less effective as a bronchodilator than as a β agonist in acute severe asthma.[98] The use of nebulised salbutamol followed by another anticholinergic agent, ipratropium bromide, however, produces considerably more bronchodilatation in acute severe asthma than sequential treatments with salbutamol alone.[99] A mixture of a β₂ agonist and an anticholinergic may be more effective than a β₂ agonist alone.

FUTURE DIRECTIONS IN TREATING ASTHMA

Few new drugs are under development that are likely to have a great impact. Improving the topical potency of inhaled steroids may be useful, as this will permit greater control of inflammation and may be helpful to patients with asthma who still need oral corticosteroid treatment despite maximum doses of the inhaled steroids currently available. Steroids that have topical potency but that are metabolised locally with reduced systemic absorption would be useful. An increase in the understanding of the mechanism of action of corticosteroids may make it possible to develop drugs that retain the beneficial anti-inflammatory effects (such as the anti-eosinophil action) without the harmful effects. The development of a once daily inhaled steroid would improve patient compliance.

Glucocorticosteroids may act by inducing the synthesis of a new protein, lipocortin, which inhibits phospholipase A2 and thus the generation by inflammatory cells of prostaglandins, leukotrienes, and platelet activating factor.[100] Lipocortin may represent the forerunner of a new generation of anti-inflammatory drugs for treating several diseases, including asthma. Drugs such as oxatomide and lodoxamide, which stabilise mast cells, have not been of clinical benefit in asthma.

Antagonists of putative mediators of asthma are now available. Potent antihistamines such as terfenadine (see below) have considerable effects in antagonising bronchoconstriction induced by histamine[101] but are unlikely to be useful in asthma.[102] Antagonists of leukotrienes are currently being tested for their effectiveness in asthma, but the initial compounds have shown weak inhibitory effects in the airways and appreciable side effects.[103] More recently, leukotriene receptor antagonists have been shown to improve symptoms and to reduce the need for inhaled β agonists in patients with mild asthma.[104] There has also been interest in platelet activating factor as a mediator of asthma, as it is able to induce sustained bronchial hyperresponsiveness in humans.[105] Platelet activating factor antagonists have been tested clinically,[106] but results have been disappointing. Because symptoms of asthma may result from an interaction among these mediators, a combination of these antagonists would presumably be necessary. Inhibitors of specific phosphodiesterase isozymes such as Type IV are currently being tested, and may afford protective effects against bronchoconstrictor challenges in addition to being effective in inhibiting inflammatory cell activation (for example, of eosinophils and lymphocytes). However, they could induce headaches and vomiting.

The development of new bronchodilators is probably unnecessary, as inhaled β_2 agonists are effective and do not have appreciable side effects. Other bronchodilators, such as prostaglandin E, vasoactive intestinal peptide, and forskolin (which directly activates adenylate cyclase), have not proved to be clinically useful.[107] Similarly, calcium antagonists such as nifedipine and verapamil have been disappointing, as they show no bronchodilator response and only a weak protective effect against induced bronchoconstriction.[108] Potassium channel activators such as cromokalim are now being developed, which seem to be effective as bronchodilators and have the advantage of having a long duration of action when given orally.[109] They have recently been shown to be effective against nocturnal asthma,[110] but may cause headaches and hypotension.

Allergic rhinitis

The introduction of non-sedating H1 antihistamines has improved the treatment of several allergic conditions, including allergic rhinitis, urticaria, and allergic conjunctivitis. The use of previously available antihistamines such as chlorpheniramine was severely limited because of their sedative side effects.

Two new antihistamines, terfenadine and astemizole, do not possess the central sedative and anticholinergic side effects of other preparations.[111][112] These drugs differ appreciably in their pharmacokinetics. Astemizole has a slow onset of action, with a long half life up to 19 days. It is released slowly from hepatic lysozymes, binds almost irreversibly to H1 receptors, and has some affinity for serotonin receptors.[113] Astemizole is therefore better used for maintenance treatment, and its once daily dosage may help long term compliance. Terfenadine has a rapid onset and end of action, which makes it ideal for intermittent use.[114] Nevertheless, a prophylactic effect may be obtained by taking 60 mg twice a day. Terfenadine may also help in an acute attack of urticaria.

One study showed that after 8 weeks of treatment astemizole was more effective than placebo or terfenadine at controlling itchy eyes, sneezing, and runny but not blocked nose, but there was a high failure rate for both drugs.[115] In a double blind study, terfenadine was found to be as effective as chlorpheniramine at improving all symptoms of allergic rhinitis and conjunctivitis.[116] Astemizole and terfenadine were both found to be more effective than placebo at controlling symptoms of hay fever.[117] Patients taking terfenadine noticed alleviation of their symptoms within hours, whereas those taking astemizole noticed it within days. Astemizole reached a similar degree of efficacy to terfenadine before the fourth day of treatment. The efficacy of H1 antihistamines in chronic perennial rhinitis remains less clear. Terfenadine provides only a modest benefit in the treatment of perennial rhinitis, and its effect is no different from that of chlorpheniramine (8 mg twice a day) or placebo.[118] Other antihistamines that have been introduced in recent years include loratidine and cetirizine, which may be given once daily with relatively few side effects.

The treatment of allergic rhinitis has also improved considerably since the introduction of topically acting corticosteroids such as beclomethasone, flunisolide, and budesonide.[119] These corticosteroids are extremely effective at controlling allergic rhinitis, particularly when used in combination with histamine H1 antagonists. Fluticasone propionate is a newly introduced topical steroid for the nose, and may be used once daily. Topical steroids cause no systemic side effects, and local adverse reactions, such as dryness and bleeding, occur only occasionally. Finally, patients with severe seasonal rhinitis may benefit from specific immunotherapy.[120]

1 Flenley DC. New drugs in respiratory disease. *BMJ* 1983;**286**:871–5.

2 Flenley DC. New drugs in respiratory disease. *BMJ* 1983;**286**:955–9.

3 Burney PGJ. Asthma mortality in England and Wales: evidence for a further increase. *Lancet* 1986;**ii**:323–6.

4 Fleming DM, Crombie DL. Prevalence of asthma and hay fever in England and Wales. *BMJ* 1987;**294**:279–83.

5 Stewart CJ, Nunn AJ. Are asthma mortality rates changing? *Br J Dis Chest* 1985;**79**:229–34.

6 Sly RM. Increases in death from asthma. *Ann Allergy* 1984;**53**:20–5.

7 Keating G, Mitchell EA, Jackson R, Beaglehole R, Rea H. Trends in sales of drugs for asthma in New Zealand, Australia, and the United Kingdom 1975–81. *BMJ* 1984;**289**:348–51.

8 Rea HH, Scragg R, Jackson R, Beaglehole R, Fenwick J, Sutherland DC. A case-control study of deaths from asthma. *Thorax* 1986;**41**:833–9.

9 Stolley PD, Schinnar R. Association between asthma mortality and isoproterenol aerosols: a review. *Prev Med* 1978;**7**:519–38.

10 Wilson JD, Sutherland DC, Thomas AC. Has the change to beta agonists combined with oral theophylline increased cases of fatal asthma? *Lancet* 1981;**i**:1235–7.

11 Sears MR, Taylor RD, Print CG, *et al.* Regular inhaled beta-agonist treatment in bronchial asthma. *Lancet* 1990;**336**:1391–6.

12 British Thoracic Society. Guidelines for management of asthma in adults: I—chronic persistent asthma. *BMJ* 1990;**301**:651–3.

13 Chung KF. Role of inflammation in the hyperreactivity of the airways in asthma. *Thorax* 1986;**41**:657–62.

14 Barnes PJ. The changing face of asthma. *Q J Med* 1987;**63**:359–65.

15 Kerrebijn KF, von Essen-Zandvliet EEM, Neijens HJ. Effect of long-term treatment with inhaled corticosteroids and beta-agonists on bronchial responsiveness in asthmatic children. *J Allergy Clin Immunol* 1987;**76**:628–36.

16 Kraan J, Koeter GH, van der Mark TW, Sluiter HJ, de Vries K. Changes in bronchial hyperreactivity induced by four weeks of treatment with antiasthma drugs in patients with allergic asthma: a comparison between budesonide and terbutaline. *J Allergy Clin Immunol* 1985;**76**:628–36.

17 Barnes PJ, Greening AP, Neville L, Timmers J, Poole GW. Single dose slow-release aminophylline at night prevents nocturnal asthma. *Lancet* 1982;**i**:299–301.

18 Barnes PJ. Theophylline preparations. *Prescriber's Journal* 1986;**26**:26–31.

19 Scott PH, Tabachnik E, Macleod S, Correia J, Newth C, Levison H. Sustained-release theophylline for childhood asthma: evidence for circadian variation of theophylline pharmacokinetics. *J Pediatr* 1981;**99**:476–9.

20 Warren JB, Cuss F, Barnes PJ. Posture and theophylline kinetics. *Br J Clin Pharmacol* 1985;**19**:707–9.

21 Tabachnik E, Scott P, Correia J. Sustained-release theophylline: a significant advance in the treatment of childhood asthma. *J Pediatr* 1982;**100**:484–92.

22 Hendles L, Iafrate P, Weinberger M. A clinical and pharmacokinetic basis for the selection and use of slow release theophylline products. *Clin Pharmacokinet* 1984;**9**:95–135.

23 Neuenkirchen H, Wilkens JH, Oellerich M, Sybrecht GW. Nocturnal asthma and sustained release theophylline. *Eur J Respir Dis* 1985;**66**:196–204.

24 Arkinstall WW, Atkins ME, Harrison D, Stewart JH. Once-daily sustained-release theophylline reduces diurnal variation in spirometry and symptomatology in adult asthmatics. *Am Rev Respir Dis* 1987;**135**:316–21.

25 Rivington RN, Calcutt L, Child S, Macleod JP, Hodder RV, Stewart JH. Comparison of morning versus evening dosing with a new once-daily oral theophylline formulation. *Am J Med* 1985;**79**:(suppl 6A):67–72.

26 Johnston IDA, Ayesh R, Alton E, Essex EG, Cochrane GM, Hetzel MR. The pharmacokinetics of Uniphyllin in nocturnal asthma. *Br J Dis Chest* 1986;**80**:235–41.

27 Greening AP, Baillie E, Gribbin HR, Pride NB. Sustained release oral aminophylline in patients with airflow obstruction. *Thorax* 1981;**36**:303–7.

28 Weinberger M, Hendeles L. Slow-release theophylline. Rationale and basis for product selection. *N Engl J Med* 1983;**308**:760–4.

29 Zwillich CW, Sutton FD, Neff TA, Cohn WM, Matthay RA, Weinberger MM. Theophylline-induced seizures in adults. Correlation with serum concentration. *Ann Intern Med* 1975;**82**:784–7.

30 Rachelefsky GS, Wo J, Adelson J, *et al.* Behaviour abnormalities and poor school performance due to oral theophylline use. *Pediatrics* 1986;**78**:1133–8.

31 Koeter GH, Postma DS, Keyzer JJ, Meurs H. The effects of oral slow-release terbutaline on early morning dyspnoea. *Eur J Clin Pharmacol* 1985;**28**:159–64.

32 Ayres J, Fish DR, Wheeler DC, Wiggins J, Cochrane GM, Skinner C. Subcutaneous terbutaline and control of brittle asthma on appreciable morning dipping. *BMJ* 1984;**288**:1715–6.

33 Sykes AP, Higgins AJ, Ayres JG. Subcutaneous terbutaline is effective in the treatment of brittle asthma by achieving high serum terbutaline levels. *Thorax* 1987;**42**:231.

34 Pedersen VR, Laursen LG, Gnosspelius Y, *et al.* Bambuterol—effects of a new anti-asthmatic drug. *Eur J Clin Pharmacol* 1986;**31**:431–6.

35 Persson G, Wiren JE. The bronchodilator response from increasing doses of terbutaline inhaled from a multi-dose powder inhaler (Turbuhaler®). *Eur Respir J* 1990;**3**:24–6.

36 Cushley MJ, Lewis RA, Tattersfield AE. Comparison of three techniques of inhalation on the airway response to terbutaline. *Thorax* 1983;**38**:908–13.

37 Newman SP, Miller AB, Lennard-Jones TR, Moren F, Clarke SW. Improvement of pressurised aerosol deposition with Nebuhaler spacer device. *Thorax* 1984;**39**:935–41.

38 O'Reilly JF, Buchanan OR, Sudlow MF. Pressurised aerosol with conical spacer is an effective alternative to nebuliser in chronic stable asthma. *BMJ* 1983;**286**:1548.

39 Morgan MDL, Singh BV, Frame BH, Williams SJ. Terbutaline aerosol given through pear spacer in acute severe asthma. *BMJ* 1982;**285**:849–50.

40 Toogood JH, Baskerville J, Jennings B, Lefcoe NM, Johansson S-A. Use of spacers to facilitate inhaled corticosteroid treatment of asthma. *Am Rev Respir Dis* 1984;**129**:723–9.

41 Gunawardena KA, Smith AP, Shankleman J. A comparison of metered dose inhalers with nebulisers for the delivery of ipratropium bromide in domiciliary practice. *Br J Dis Chest* 1986;**80**:170–8.

42 Christensson P, Arborelius M, Lilja B. Salbutamol inhalation in chronic asthma bronchioles: dose aerosol vs jet nebuliser. *Chest* 1981;**79**:416–9.

43 Cayton RM, Webber B, Paterson JW, Clark TJH. Comparison of salbutamol given by pressure packed aerosol or nebulisation via IPPB in acute asthma. *BMJ* 1978;**72**:222–4.

44 Sears MR, Rea HH, Fenwick J, *et al.* Seventy five deaths in asthmatics prescribed home nebulisers. *BMJ* 1987;**294**:477–9.

45 Bradshaw J, Brittain RT, Coleman RA, *et al.* The design of salmeterol, a long acting selective beta$_2$-adrenocepter agonist. *Br J Pharmacol* 1987;**92**:590.

46 Ullman A, Svedmyr N. Salmeterol—a new long-acting inhaled beta$_2$-adrenoceptor agonist: comparison with salbutamol in adult asthmatic patients. *Thorax* 1988;**43**:674–8.

47 Lofdahl CG, Svedmyr N. Formoterol fumarate, a new beta$_2$-adrenoceptor agonist. Acute studies of selectivity and duration of effect after inhaled and oral administration. *Allergy* 1989;**44**:264–71.

48 Sykes AP, Ayres JG. A comparative study investigating the peak effect and duration of action of 12 mcg and 24 mcg of inhaled formoterol with that of 200 mcg of inhaled salbutamol. *Eur Respir J* 1988;**1**:195.

49 Becker AB, Simons FER, McMillan JL, Faridy T. Formoterol, a new long-acting beta$_2$-adrenergic receptor agonist. Double-blind comparison with salbutamol and placebo in selected children with asthma. *J Allergy Clin Immunol* 1989;**84**:891–4.

50 Cheung D, Timmers CM, Zwinderman AH, Bel EH, Dijkman JH, Sterk PJ. Long-term effects of a long-acting β$_2$-adrenoceptor agonist, salmeterol, on airway hyperresponsiveness in patients with mild asthma. *N Engl J Med* 1992;**327**:1198–1203.

51 Pearlman DS, Chervinsky P, Laforce C, *et al.* A comparison of salmeterol with albuterol in the treatment of mild-to-moderate asthma. *N Engl J Med* 1992;**327**:1420–5.

52 Riley PA, Mather ME, Keogh RW, Eady RP. Activity of nedocromil sodium in mast-cell-dependent reactions in the rat. *Int Arch Allergy Appl Immunol* 1987;**82**:108–10.

53 Wells E, Jackson CG, Harper ST, Mann J, Eady RP. Characterisation of primate bronchoalveolar mast cells. II. Inhibition of histamine, LTC4 and

PGD2 release from primate bronchoalveolar mast cells and a comparison with rat peritoneal mast cells. *J Immunol* 1986;**137**:3941–5.

54 Leung KBP, Flint KC, Brostoff J, Hudspith BN, Johnson NM, Pearce FL. A comparison of neodocromil sodium and sodium cromoglycate on human lung mast cells obtained by bronchoalveolar lavage and by dispersion of lung fragments. *Eur J Respir Dis* 1986;**96**:223–6.

55 Eady RP, Greenwood B, Jackson DM, Orr TSC, Wells E. The effect of nedocromil sodium and sodium cromoglycate on antigen-induced broncho-constriction in the ascaris-sensitive monkey. *Br J Pharmacol* 1985;**85**:323–5.

56 Youngchaiyud P, Lee TB. Effect of nedocromil sodium on the immediate response to antigen challenge in asthmatic patients. *Clin Allergy* 1986;**16**:129–34.

57 Moqbel R, Walsh GM, Kay AB. Inhibition of human granulocyte activation by nedocromil sodium. *Eur J Respir Dis* 1986;**69**(suppl 147):227–9.

58 Damon M, Chavis C, Crastes de Paulet A,, Michel FB, Godard P. Effect of nedocromil sodium on TxB2, LTB4 and LTD4 synthesis by alveolar macrophages from asthmatic subjects. *Eur J Respir Dis* 1986;**69**(suppl 147):206–9.

59 Joseph M, Capron A, Thorel T, Tonnel AB. Nedocromil sodium inhibits IgE dependent activation of rat macrophages and platelets as measured by schistosome killing, chemiluminescence and enzyme release. *Eur J Respir Dis* 1986;**69**(suppl 147):220–2.

60 Dahl R, Pedersen B. Influence of nedocromil solution on the dual asthmatic reaction after allergen challenge: a double-blind, placebo-controlled study. *Eur J Respir Dis* 1986;**69**(suppl 147):263–5.

61 Shaw RJ, Kay AB. Nedocromil, a mucosal and connective tissue mast cell stabiliser, inhibits exercise-induced asthma. *Br J Dis Chest* 1985;**79**:385–9.

62 Roberts JA, Thomson NC. Attenuation of exercise-induced asthma by pre-treatment with nedocromil sodium and minocromil. *Clin Allergy* 1986;**15**:377–81.

63 Del Bono L, Dente FL, Patalano F, Del Bono N. Protective effect of nedocromil sodium and sodium cromoglycate on bronchospasm induced by cold air. *Eur J Respir Dis* 1986;**69**(suppl 147):268–70.

64 Altounyan REC, Cole M, Lee TB. Inhibition of sulphur dioxide-induced bronchoconstriction by nedocromil sodium and sodium cromoglycate in non-asthmatic, atopic subjects. *Eur J Respir Dis* 1986;**69**(suppl 147):274–6.

65 Dixon CMS, Fuller RW, Barnes PJ. The action of nedocromil sodium on sulphur dioxide induced bronchoconstriction. *Thorax* 1986;**41**:246.

66 Robuschi M, Vaghi A, Simone A, Bianco S. Prevention of fog-induced bronchospasm by nedocromil sodium. *Clin Allergy* 1987;**17**:69–74.

67 Dorward AJ, Roberts JA, Thomson NC. Effect of nedocromil sodium on histamine airway responsiveness in patients allergic to grass pollen. *Clin Allergy* 1986;**16**:309–15.

68 Holgate ST. Clinical evaluation of nedocromil sodium in asthma. *Eur J Respir Dis* 1986;**69**(suppl 147):149–59.

69 Greif J, Fink G, Smorzik Y, *et al*. Nedocromil sodium and placebo in the management of bronchial asthma. A multicenter, double-blind, parallel group comparison. *Chest* 1989;**96**:583–8.

70 Goldin JG, Bateman ED. Does nedocromil sodium have a steroid sparing effect in adult asthmatic patients requiring maintenance oral corticosteroids? *Thorax* 1988;**43**:982–6.

71 Lal S, Malhotra S, Gribben D, Hodder D. An open assessment study of the acceptability, tolerance and safety of nedocromil sodium in long-term clinical

use in patients with perennial asthma. *Eur J Respir Dis* 1986;**69**(suppl 147):136–42.

72 Andersson K-E, Persson CGA. The clinical pharmacology of enprofylline and theophylline. In: Andersson K-E, Persson CGA, eds. *Anti-asthma xanthines and adenosine*. Amsterdam: Elsevier Science Publishers, 1985:41–55.

73 Persson CGA. Experimental lung actions of xanthines. In: Andersson K-E, Persson CGA, eds. *Anti-asthma xanthines and adenosine*. Amsterdam: Elsevier Science Publishers, 1985:61–82.

74 Maxwell DL, Fuller RW, Conradson TB, Dixon CMS, Hughes JMB, Barnes PJ. Opposing effects of theophylline and enprofylline on the cardiorespiratory effects of adenosine infusion in man. *Am Rev Respir Dis* 1987;**135**:A478.

75 Pauwels R, van Renterghem D, van der Straeten M, Johannesson N, Persson CGA. The effect of theophylline and enprofylline on allergen-induced bronchoconstriction. *J Allergy Clin Immunol* 1985;**76**:583–90.

76 Borga O, Andersson EK, Edholm LE, Fagerstrom PO, Lunell E, Persson CG. Enprofylline kinetics in healthy subjects after single doses. *Clin Pharmacol Ther* 1983;**34**:799–804.

77 Lunell E, Borga O, Larsson R. Pharmacokinetics of enprofylline in patients with impaired renal function after a single intravenous dose. *Eur J Clin Pharmacol* 1984;**26**:87–93.

78 Persson G, Andersson K-E, Persson CGA, Johannesson N, Nordlund P. Acute bronchodilator effects of single oral doses of an adenosine non-blocking xanthine and terbutaline. In: Andersson K-E, Persson CGA, eds. *Anti-asthma xanthines and adenosine*. Amsterdam: Elsevier Science Publishers, 1985:149–55.

79 Vilsvik JS, Persson CG, Amundsen T, *et al*. Comparison between theophylline and an adenosine non-blocking xanthine in acute asthma. *Eur Respir J* 1990;**3**:27–32.

80 Laursen LC, Eriksson G, Weeke B. Comparison of two weeks' treatment with enprofylline and theophylline in asthmatic patients. In: Andersson K-E, Persson CGA, eds. *Anti-asthma xanthines and adenosine*. Amsterdam: Elsevier Science Publishers, 1985:156–8.

81 Djukanovic R, Wilson JW, Britten KM, *et al*. The effect of an inhaled corticosteroid on airway inflammation and symptoms in asthma. *Am Rev Respir Dis* 1992;**145**:669–74.

82 Jeffery PK, Godfrey RW, Adelroth E, Nelson F, Rogers A, Johansson SA. Effects of treatment on airway inflammation and thickening of basement membrane reticular collagen in asthma: a quantitative light and electron microscopy study. *Am Rev Respir Dis* 1992;**145**:890–9.

83 Haahtela T, Jarvinen M, Kava T, *et al*. Comparison of a β$_2$-agonist, terbutaline, with an inhaled corticosteroid, budesonide, in newly detected asthma. *N Engl J Med* 1991;**325**:388–92.

84 Mullarkey MF, Blumenstein BA, Avidrade WP, *et al*. Methotrexate in the treatment of corticosteroid-dependent asthma. *N Engl J Med* 1988;**318**:603–7.

85 Shiner RJ, Nunn A, Chung KF, Geddes DM. Randomised double blind placebo-controlled trial of methotrexate in steroid dependent asthma. *Lancet* 1990;**336**:137–40.

86 Nierop G, Gijzel WP, Bel EH, Zwinderman AH, Dijkman JH. Auranofin in the treatment of steroid dependent asthma: a double blind study. *Thorax* 1992;**47**:349–54.

87 Alexander AG, Barnes NC, Kay AB. Cyclosporin A in corticosteroid-dependent chronic severe asthma. *Lancet* 1992;**339**:324–7.

88 Shapiro GG, Furukawa CT, Pierson WE, Gardiner R, Bierman CW. Double-blind evaluation of methylprednisolone versus placebo for acute asthma episodes. *Pediatrics* 1983;**71**:510–4.

89 Littenberg B, Gluck EH. A controlled trial of methylprednisolone in the emergency treatment of acute asthma. *N Engl J Med* 1986;**134**:150–2.

90 Deshpade A, McKenzie SA. Short course of steroids in home treatment of children with acute asthma. *BMJ* 1986;**293**:169–71.

91 Fanta CH, Rossino TH, McFadden ER. Glucocorticosteroids in acute asthma: a critical controlled trial. *Am J Med Sci* 1983;**74**:845–51.

92 Harrison BDW, Hart GJ, Ali NJ, Stokes TC, Vaughan DA, Robinson AA. Need for intravenous hydrocortisone in addition to oral prednisolone in patients admitted to hospital with severe asthma without ventilatory failure. *Lancet* 1986;**ii**:181–4.

93 Pierce RJ, Payne CR, Williams SJ, Denison D, Clark TJH. Comparison of intravenous and inhaled terbutaline in the treatment of asthma. *Chest* 1981;**79**:506–11.

94 Rossing TH, Fanta CH, Goldstein DH, Snapper JR, McFadden ER. Emergency therapy of asthma: comparison of the acute effects of parenteral and inhaled sympathomimetics and infused aminophylline. *Am Rev Respir Dis* 1980;**122**:365–71.

95 Siegel D, Sheppard D, Gelb A, Weinberg PF. Aminophylline increases the toxicity but not the efficacy of an inhaled beta-adrenergic agonist in the treatment of acute exacerbations of asthma. *Am Rev Respir Dis* 1985;**132**:283–6.

96 Coupe MO, Guly U, Barnes PJ. Comparison of nebulised adrenaline and salbutamol in acute severe asthma. *Clin Sci* 1986;**71**:80–1.

97 Spiteri MA, Millar AB, Pavia D, Clarke SW. Subcutaneous adrenaline versus terbutaline in the treatment of acute severe asthma. *Thorax* 1987;**42**:231.

98 Karpel JP, Appel D, Briedbart D, Fusco MJ. A comparison of atropine sulfate and metaproterenol sulfate in the emergency treatment of asthma. *Am Rev Respir Dis* 1986;**133**:727–9.

99 Ward MJ, MacFarlane JT, Davies D. A place for ipratropium bromide in the treatment of severe acute asthma. *Br J Dis Chest* 1985;**79**:374–9.

100 Flower RJ. Macrocortin and anti-phospholipase proteins. In: Weissman G, ed. *Advances in inflammation research*. Vol 8. New York: Raven Press, 1984.

101 Rafferty P, Holgate ST. Terfenadine (Seldane®) is a potent and selective histamine H1 receptor antagonist in asthmatic airways. *Am Rev Respir Dis* 1987;**135**:181–4.

102 Chan TB, Shelton DM, Eiser NM. Effect of an oral H1-receptor antagonist, terfenadine, on antigen-induced asthma. *Br J Dis Chest* 1986;**80**:375–84.

103 Barnes NC, Piper PJ, Costello JF. The effect of an oral leukotriene antagonist L-649,923 on histamine and leukotriene B4 induced bronchoconstriction in normal man. *Thorax* 1987;**42**:220.

104 Cloud ML, Enas GC, Kemp J, et al. A specific LTD4/LTE4-receptor antagonist improves pulmonary function in patients with mild, chronic asthma. *Am Rev Respir Dis* 1989;**140**:1336–9.

105 Cuss FM, Dixon CMS, Barnes PJ. Effects of inhaled platelet activating factor on pulmonary function and bronchial responsiveness in man. *Lancet* 1986;**ii**:189–92.

106 Chung KF, Dent G, McCusker M, Guinot PM, Page CP, Barnes PJ. Effect of a ginkgolide mixture (BN 52063) in antagonising skin and platelet responses to platelet activating factor in man. *Lancet* 1987;**i**:248–51.

107 Barnes PJ. Asthma therapy: basic mechanisms. *Eur J Respir Dis* 1986;**68**:217–65.

108 Lofdhal C-G, Barnes PJ. Calcium channel blockade and asthma—the current position. *Eur J Respir Dis* 1985;**67**:233–7.

109 Black JL, Barnes PJ. Potassium channel activators in asthma. *Thorax* 1990;**45**:213–8.

110 Williams AJ, Lee TH, Cochrane GM, *et al.* Attenuation of nocturnal asthma by cromakalin. *Lancet* 1990;**336**:334–6.

111 Richards DM, Brogden RN, Heel RC, Speight TM, Avery GS. Astemizole. A review of its pharmacodynamic properties and therapeutic efficacy. *Drugs* 1984;**28**:38–61.

112 Brandon ML, Weiner M. Clinical investigation of terfenadine, a non-sedating antihistamine. *Ann Allergy* 1980;**44**:71–5.

113 Laduron PM, Janssen PFM, Grommeren W, Legen JE. In vitro and in vivo binding characteristics of a new long-acting histamine H-1 antagonist, astemizole. *Mol Pharmacol* 1982;**21**:294–300.

114 Okerholm RA, Weiner DL, Hook RH. Bioavailability of terfenadine in man. *Biopharm Drug Dispos* 1981;**2**:185–90.

115 Howarth PH, Holgate ST. Comparative trial of two non-selective H1-antihistamines, terfenadine and astemizole, for hay fever. *Thorax* 1984;**39**:668–72.

116 Kemp JP, Buckley CE, Gershwin ME, *et al.* Multicenter, double-blind, placebo-controlled trial of terfenadine in seasonal allergic rhinitis and conjunctivitis. *Ann Allergy* 1985;**54**:502–9.

117 Girard JP, Sommacal-Schopf D, Bigliardi P, Henauer SA. Double-blind comparison of astemizole, terfenadine and placebo in hay fever with special regard to onset of action. *J Int Med Res* 1985;**13**:102–8.

118 Brostoff J, Lockhart JDF. Controlled trial of terfenadine and chlorpheniramine maleate in perennial rhinitis. *Postgrad Med J* 1982;**58**:422–3.

119 Mygind N. Topical steroid treatment for allergic rhinitis and allied conditions. *Clin Otolaryngol* 1982;**7**:343–52.

120 Varney VA, Gaga M, Frew AJ, Aber VR, Kay AB, Durham SR. Usefulness of immunotherapy in patients with severe summer hay fever uncontrolled by antiallergic drugs. *BMJ* 1991;**302**:265–9.

16 Chronic obstructive airways disease and respiratory infections

K FAN CHUNG, PETER J BARNES

Chronic obstructive airways disease

Chronic hypoxaemia in chronic bronchitis and emphysema may lead to the development of pulmonary hypertension, and the occurrence of cor pulmonale remains a bad prognostic sign. This stage of the disease may be associated with a reduced respiratory drive, leading to hypercapnia and hypoxaemia. Long term oxygen treatment improves tissue oxygenation, reduces pulmonary hypertension, and prolongs survival in hypoxic cor pulmonale. A controlled clinical trial by the Medical Research Council showed that 15 h of continuous oxygen treatment a day was necessary and that an improvement was observed only after 500 days of treatment.[1] The long term use of supplementary oxygen in this condition has been discussed previously.[2] The introduction of oxygen concentrators has made home treatment with oxygen cheaper and more convenient,[3] but it is essential that patients are adequately evaluated before this treatment is started and that they are supervised during treatment.[4]

Treatment of hypoxaemia solely with drugs, or in combination with oxygen treatment, remains a possibility. Interest has been shown in drugs that stimulate respiration and improve oxygenation in patients with hypoxaemia, one particular drug being the peripheral chemoreceptor stimulant almitrine. The use of pulmonary vasodilators to reduce the pulmonary hypertension of chronic obstructive airways disease is also being investigated.

ALMITRINE

Almitrine bismesylate (not marketed to date) is a triazine derivative that stimulates the carotid body[5] and therefore increases the ventilatory response of normal subjects to hypoxia, with little effect on the response to hypercapnia.[6 7] Almitrine also increases resting ventilation. Unlike stimulants such as doxapram, almitrine has little or no effect on the central nervous system. When given orally over weeks or months, it improves arterial oxygen pressure (Pao_2) and arterial carbon dioxide pressure ($Paco_2$) in patients who have chronic obstructive airways disease by increasing ventilation through an increase in hypoxic ventilatory stimulation.[8] An improvement in ventilation perfusion matching has also been reported,[9 10] the mechanism of which remains unclear. It may, however, be related to the observed increase in pulmonary vascular resistance and pulmonary artery pressure accompanied by a small decrease in cardiac output.[11] Potentiation of hypoxic pulmonary vasoconstriction by almitrine is short lived compared with its longer lasting effect on gas exchange.[11]

Almitrine may be administered orally or intravenously. Being highly soluble in lipids, it is absorbed from the gut within 2–3 h and is highly bound to albumin in the circulation.[12] It is extensively metabolised, and less than 20% is found unchanged. Because of a long plasma half life of about 2 days, steady state plasma concentrations occur after 2 weeks of oral treatment, reaching concentrations two to threefold higher than those on the first day. It has been recommended that treatment with almitrine should be stopped for 1 month after each 3 months of treatment with a daily dose of 100 mg/kg. Almitrine is not excreted in the urine because of high protein binding but is mostly lost through the bile. The physiological effect of a single dose of almitrine lasts for at least 6 h.

Almitrine has been recommended for use in both acute and chronic respiratory failure and for controlling hypoxaemia during sleep. The magnitude of the stimulatory effect of almitrine depends on the degree of hypoxaemia during resting, though worthwhile results have been observed in patients who were breathing 28% oxygen and had a mean Pao_2 of 9·2 kPa.[11] In a double blind study in France that lasted for 6 months, patients treated with almitrine (50 mg twice a day) compared with 200 stable hypoxic and hypercapnic patients treated with placebo showed a considerable increase in resting Pao_2 from 7·5 kPa to 8·5 kPa and a decrease in resting $Paco_2$ from 6·6 kPa to 6·0 kPa.[13] The patients felt less dyspnoeic, despite an increase in ventilation of 11%. There was a trend towards fewer admissions to hospital and improvement in pre-existing polycythaemia. A more recent study showed similar results after treatment with almitrine for 1 year.[14] Almitrine improves nocturnal oxygenation in patients with chronic bronchitis and emphysema in whom hypoxia is combined with hypercapnia. It also reduces the number of hypoxaemic episodes, presumably because of improved nocturnal oxygen saturation.[15]

A worrying feature of almitrine, however, is the occurrence of peripheral neuropathy with or without associated weight loss during prolonged treatment.[16 17] This sensory neuropathy usually occurs between the third and seventh month of treatment. One study of patients who had chronic obstructive airways disease reported that 7% spontaneously complained of paraesthesiae, 46% showed sensory disorders on clinical examination, and 74% showed electromyographic signs of peripheral neuropathy.[18] Treatment with almitrine may therefore merely unmask an underlying neuropathy. Nevertheless, the occurrence and persistence of paraesthesiae remain an indication for withdrawing the drug.

Whether almitrine will contribute appreciably to improving the prognosis of patients who have hypoxic cor pulmonale remains to be seen. It may reduce the early deterioration of hypoxaemia in chronic obstructive airways disease.[9] A potential synergistic effect of almitrine with oxygen treatment is also worth exploring, as this may mean that fewer hours of oxygen treatment are needed to achieve a beneficial effect. A recent study showed that the effects of almitrine and oxygen treatment were additive in increasing Pao_2 in patients with chronic obstructive lung disease.[20] Finally, the clinical importance of the pulmonary hypertension associated with almitrine in these patients at rest and during exercise[21] needs to be clarified.

PULMONARY VASODILATORS

The development of pulmonary hypertension in chronic obstructive airways disease is associated with a worse prognosis. Thus blue bloaters who have increased pulmonary artery pressure have a lower survival rate over 5 years than those whose pressure measurements are stable, despite similar degrees of hypoxaemia.[22] In an American study of long term oxygen treatment patients who had chronic obstructive airways disease and showed a greater decrease in pulmonary artery pressure in response to oxygen treatment had a considerably better survival rate.[23] The use of pulmonary vasodilators could therefore be important in treating patients with chronic obstructive airways disease and hypoxaemia.

Most studies of pulmonary vasodilators have been short term, and an examination of their long term use in chronic airways obstruction is needed, particularly to test the possibility of a synergistic effect on concomitant oxygen treatment. One possible problem with pulmonary vasodilatation is that arterial hypoxaemia may worsen as pulmonary vessels dilate to supply poorly ventilated units. In addition, most pulmonary vasodilators have a similar effect on the systemic vessels, so systemic hypotension may be a serious limiting problem.[24]

CALCIUM ANTAGONISTS

Reversal of the vasoconstriction induced by the entry of calcium can be achieved partly by blocking the voltage dependent calcium channels of vascular smooth muscle with calcium antagonists such as verapamil or nifedipine. Pulmonary vasoconstriction induced by hypoxia is inhibited in humans and animals by calcium antagonists.[25-27] Most studies of calcium antagonists in chronic obstructive airways disease have used nifedipine. In the short term nifedipine appreciably reduces pulmonary arterial pressure and increases cardiac output during rest and exercise in hypoxic patients who have chronic obstructive airways disease and who are breathing air or oxygen; there is, however, a small decrease in arterial PaO_2 in those breathing air.[28] When nifedipine was given for a longer term (6–9 weeks) to patients who had hypoxic cor pulmonale a sustained decrease in pulmonary haemodynamics was seen.[29] Headache, palpitations, ankle oedema, and systemic hypotension are the potential side effects of nifedipine.

Another calcium antagonist, felodipine, lowers pulmonary artery pressure in patients who have chronic bronchitis but has little effect in preventing the increase in pulmonary artery pressure during exercise when given for a longer period of 3–5 months.[30]

β_2 AGONISTS

Isoprenaline reduces the increased pulmonary vascular resistance in the pulmonary hypertension of hypoxic cor pulmonale.[31] In moderately hypoxic patients with chronic airways obstruction terbutaline, a β_2 adrenergic agonist, improves the right ventricular ejection fraction without reducing arterial oxygen tension.[32] More recently another β_2 adrenergic agonist, pirbuterol (15 mg orally), has been shown to reduce pulmonary artery pressure and pulmonary vascular resistance in similar groups of patients.[33][34] The decrease in pulmonary artery pressure and the increase in right ventricular ejection fraction after treatment with pirbuterol are also sustained with long term treatment for 6 weeks without a significant decrease in arterial Pao_2 or systemic blood pressure.[34] Thus, pirbuterol has appreciable inotropic action and vasodilatory effects on the pulmonary circulation, although there is no reason to believe that it is any different from other β_2 agonists such as salbutamol and terbutaline.

OTHER AGENTS

Hydralazine, theophylline, and ACE inhibitors such as captopril have also been shown to have a beneficial effect on pulmonary hypertension in chronic obstructive airways disease in short term studies.[35-37] Theophylline causes a sustained improvement in right ventricular function when given for 3 months.[38] Urapidil, a vasodilator that acts through the postsynaptic α_1 blockade while inhibiting the aortic pressure baroreceptor reflex and reducing central sympathetic tone, causes an appreciably greater decrease in pulmonary vascular resistance than in the systemic circulation in patients who have pulmonary hypertension of various aetiologies, including chronic obstructive airways disease.[39] By contrast, hydralazine has a much more appreciable effect on arterial blood pressure without affecting pulmonary artery pressures. Thus urapidil may be more selective in causing a greater reduction of resistance in the pulmonary vascular bed than in the systemic circulation.

Primary pulmonary hypertension

There is little effective treatment for most patients who have primary pulmonary hypertension, which usually runs a rapidly fatal course: there is, however, a substantial subgroup of these patients who may benefit from pulmonary vasodilators,[40][41] and it is important to identify these patients, whose deterioration may be slowed enough to make heart–lung transplantation possible.[42] In these patients considerable short term reductions in pulmonary vascular resistance can be shown at cardiac catheterisation, preferably using a short acting pulmonary vasodilator such as prostacyclin,[43] as its short half life avoids the dangers of prolonged systemic hypotension. Oral warfarin sufficient to maintain the prothrombin time at 2·0–2·5 times the normal range has been associated, in retrospective studies, with improved survival rates.

Secondary causes of pulmonary hypertension, such as thromboembolic disease, congenital heart disease, sleep apnoea syndromes, and fibrosing alveolitis, should be excluded as these conditions are not known to benefit from vasodilator treatment. It is unwise to use pulmonary vasodilator treatment in patients with primary pulmonary hypertension who do not respond in the short term, as complications of treatment are more likely to occur in this group, who have a fixed obstruction,[44] and may be deleterious.[24]

Calcium antagonists (nifedipine, verapamil, and diltiazem), hydralazine, diazoxide, captopril, and prostacyclin have all been used in primary pulmonary hypertension. In five patients in whom repeated haemodynamic assessment had been undertaken prostacyclin (by continuous intravenous infusion),[45] nifedipine,[46] diazoxide,[47 48] and isoprenaline[49] all induced a sustained reduction in pulmonary vascular resistance and improvement in clinical symptoms for 1–4 years. Which of these agents is the best vasodilator remains to be assessed.

Respiratory infections

Several new antibiotics that are useful for treating chest infections have been introduced. A more general discussion of these agents appears in chapter 30. Many different cephalosporins are currently available for prescription in the United Kingdom, including cefaclor, cefadroxil, cephamandole, cefotaxime, cefoxitin, cefsulodin, ceftazidime, and cefuroxime. These have been classified empirically as "first," "second," and "third generation" cephalosporins, based solely on the temporal sequence of their introduction on to the market. Thus the latest (third) generation drugs include ceftazidime, cefsulodin, and cefotaxime, which are mainly characterised by their increased resistance to β lactamases and by their broader range of activity against the Gram negative bacteria and limited activity against Gram positive bacteria. *Pseudomonas aeruginosa* is highly susceptible to ceftazidime and cefsulodin. Earlier cephalosporins (the second generation), such as cefoxitin, cefuroxime, and cephamandole, show a much broader range of antibacterial activity against Gram positive cocci and Gram negative bacilli such as *Escherichia coli*, *Klebsiella pneumoniae*, and *Proteus mirabilis*, with others being active also against pseudomonas, enterobacteria, and *Haemophilus influenzae*. Cefoxitin is active against *Bacteroides fragilis*.

Other antibiotics introduced recently that have chemical structures and antibacterial activities similar to third generation cephalosporins are latamoxef (moxalactam) and aztreonam. Latamoxef has a wider range of antibacterial activity, including *H influenzae*, all enterobacteria, and *B fragilis*.[50] Aztreonam, a monobactam (a single ringed β lactam), has a selective activity against enterobacteria and *P aeruginosa* but is inactive against Gram positive and anaerobic bacteria.[51] Imipenem, the first of a new β lactam class, the carbapenems, has been released recently and has a broader range of activity than the cephalosporins against anaerobic and Gram positive bacteria, including bacteroides. It is also stable to β lactamase.[52]

These cephalosporins (and latamoxef and aztreonam) are administered parenterally (intramuscular or intravenous routes). The most common adverse effects of these compounds are:

- local irritation at the site of injection;
- skin rashes;
- urticaria;
- diarrhoea occurs in only 3% of patients;
- infrequent bleeding due to hypoprothombinaemia may occur with cephamandole and latamoxef;
- at high doses latamoxef inhibits aggregation of platelets;
- eosinophilia, leucopenia, high plasma urea concentrations, and abnormal liver function test results may occur transiently after treatment with cephalosporins.

Newer macrolides have recently been introduced. Erythromcin has been widely used although nausea and vomiting are complications of therapy. Clarithromycin has greater activity against *H influenzae* and fewer gastric side effects. Clarithromycin and azithromycin have better pharmacokinetics than erythromycin, producing longer half lives and higher intracellular concentrations. Clarithromycin is approximately 100 times more acid stable and consequently has a higher bioavailability than erythromycin. The macrolides have a similar spectrum of activity to that of penicillin. They are useful as alternatives in penicillin allergic patients but are also active against *Mycoplasma pneumoniae, Legionella pneumophilia* and *Chlamydia pneumoniae*. The newer macrolides should be reserved for patients who can not tolerate erythromycin and for non-responders to erythromycin.

Ciprofloxacin is a 4-quinolone compound (an earlier derivative is nalidixic acid) that can be taken orally and is effective against staphylococci, streptococci, *H influenzae*, and, particularly, *P aeruginosa*.[53] It inhibits bacterial (but not human) DNA gyrase, which regulates the supercoiling of bacterial DNA and enables bacteria to accommodate their long chromosomes within the cell envelope. Because of this action ciprofloxacin does not seem to be susceptible to resistance mechanisms associated with the transfer of plasmids, and it has been suggested that the resistant strains are likely to develop only slowly, perhaps through chromosomal mutations.[54] When ciprofloxacin is administered to patients already taking theophylline, the doses of theophylline should be reduced and blood theophylline concentrations measured.

INFECTIONS OF THE LOWER RESPIRATORY TRACT

Cephalosporin concentrations achieved in bronchial secretions are only 2–20% of those in plasma. These are usually well above the minimum inhibitory concentrations for many bacterial species, as these antibiotics possess intrinsically high antibacterial activity and reach high serum concentrations. Similar penetration of aztreonam into sputum has been shown,[55] with increased penetration in patients who have respiratory failure.[56] Ciprofloxacin penetrates human lung tissue well, and tissue concentrations exceed serum concentrations.[57] Whether sputum concentrations of antibiotics are clinically relevant remains to be assessed, as concentrations in pulmonary tissue and airways are probably more essential in determining a favourable outcome of treatment than those in sputum.

The overall use and specific role of the newer cephalosporins and the other related antibiotics in treating infections of the respiratory tract remain to be established, as there have been no adequate comparisons with existing older antibiotics. Nevertheless, these antibiotics are extremely active and safe, possess a broad range of activity, and are of potential use in treating infections of the lower respiratory tract.

Infections with *Streptococcus pneumoniae* should still be treated with penicillin; the newer cephalosporins remain drugs of second choice. Strains of *H influenzae* that do not produce β lactamases should still be treated with ampicillin or co-trimoxazole; whether some of the third generation cephalosporins are as active remains to be seen. Strains of *H influenzae* resistant to ampicillin are sensitive to latamoxef and aztreonam, but whether these drugs will be therapeutically better than erythromycin or chloramphenicol also remains to be assessed. Bacteria producing β lactamase that are resistant to amoxycillin (such as *Staphylococcus aureus* and some strains of *H influenzae*) may be treated with a combination of amoxycillin and clavulanic acid. Clavulanic acid is an antibiotic with little useful activity, but it is a potent inhibitor of many β lactamases. It is also available in combination with ticarcillin. The newer cephalosporins are not the best drugs for treating the rare staphylococcal pneumonia, as they are inactive in vitro against *Staph aureus*. Infections with strains of staphylococcus that produce penicillinase should be treated with penicillins that are resistant to penicillinase, or with vancomycin. There has so far been little experience of treating staphylococcal infections with third generation cephalosporins.

PATIENTS WITH CYSTIC FIBROSIS

Respiratory infections in cystic fibrosis remain a great problem. *P aeruginosa* is now the most common organism colonising the respiratory tract of patients who have cystic fibrosis (70–90%) and is a great cause of acute exacerbations in this disease. Previously the main organism was *Staph aureus*; this change may have resulted from the use of effective antistaphylococcal drugs.

The most effective and established treatment for pulmonary infections in cystic fibrosis remains the combination of an antipseudomonal penicillin such as azlocillin or piperacillin with an aminoglycoside, as azlocillin or piperacillin given alone do not produce adequate results.[58] In patients who have been chronically infected with *P aeruginosa* carbenicillin and gentamicin administered by aerosol have produced subjective and objective improvement in lung function.[59] A reduced number of admissions to hospital has been shown in a similar group of patients treated with nebulised ticarcillin and tobramycin.[60]

The new antipseudomonal cephalosporins have been used to treat infective exacerbations of cystic fibrosis, and the most effective is probably ceftazidime followed by cefsulodin.[61 62] Clinical and bacteriological results obtained with these two cephalosporins

210

given alone do not seem to differ from those obtained when they are given in combination with an aminoglycoside.[62] Non-mucoid strains of *Pseudomonas* spp were eradicated in half or more of these patients, but much poorer results were obtained in those infected with the mucoid strain. With aztreonam fewer cases of eradication were seen, despite a favourable clinical outcome;[63] the addition of an aminoglycoside did not seem to improve the response to treatment.

In an open randomised study orally administered ciprofloxacin was as effective as intravenous azlocillin plus gentamicin against chest infections caused by *P aeruginosa* in adult patients with cystic fibrosis.[64] This may represent a useful advance in the treatment of cystic fibrosis, as ciprofloxacin is given orally and avoids the use of aminoglycosides, the dose of which can not be adjusted easily. The role of ciprofloxacin in long term chemotherapy of outpatients who have cystic fibrosis and who are infected with *P aeruginosa* remains, however, to be established: although no more resistance to ciprofloxacin than to conventional combination treatment was reported in that study,[64] there has been concern that pseudomonas may develop resistance to the antibiotic.[65] Similar fears have been raised about the use of ceftazidime.[66]

IMMUNOCOMPROMISED PATIENTS

One condition for which third generation cephalosporins may be extremely useful is pneumonia in immunocompromised patients, particularly that caused by Gram negative enterobacteriae or *P aeruginosa*. The most specific cephalosporin for treating *P aeruginosa* is cefsulodin; the most active is ceftazidime. Other potential drugs are aztreonam and latamoxef. It is probably wise to use these drugs in combination with an aminoglycoside to prevent the emergence of resistant strains and because of the synergistic effect of these two classes of antibotics.

In severe infections of unknown origin a broad spectrum cephalosporin may be used in combination with an aminoglycoside and an antianaerobic agent (for example, metronidazole). This cephalosporin or β lactam should preferably be resistant to β lactamase— for example, latamoxef, cefotaxime, or ceftazidime. The addition of the β lactamase inhibitor potassium clavulanate to ticarcillin (a broad spectrum penicillin effective against a wide range of Gram positive and Gram negative aerobic and anaerobic bacteria) may improve its effectiveness in treating suspected infection in immunosuppressed patients.[67]

As with all new antibiotics, care must be exercised in their selection for treating specific micro-organisms, as excessive indiscriminate use may lead to the emergence and spread of resistant bacteria. The third generation cephalosporins, β lactams, and 4-quinolones represent newer classes of antibiotics that are potentially useful to treat respiratory infections, particularly those caused by enterobacteriae, *P aeruginosa*, or strains of *H influenzae*, that produce β lactamase, especially in immunocompromised subjects. The indiscriminate prescription of these potent antimicrobials should be avoided.

AIDS pneumonia

Patients with AIDS often present with pulmonary complications. Up to 85% of these patients develop pneumonia due to *Pneumocystis carinii* at some stage of their illness, with a death rate ranging up to 35%.[68] The death rate during recurrent episodes is much higher. *P carinii* is most responsive to treatment with high dose co-trimoxazole (trimethoprim-sulphamethoxazole) and pentamidine isethionate. Neither drug is more effective or less toxic during the first episode of *P carinii* pneumonia,[69] but high dose co-trimoxazole is usually preferred as the initial drug. Inhaled pentamidine may be effective,[70] but the response is less rapid than with systemic pentamidine and carries a greater possibility of early relapse. Patients who do not respond to either co-trimoxazole or pentamidine may be treated with trimetrexate, methotrexate analogue eflornithine (an inhibitor of protozoal ornithine decarboxylase), or dapsone with trimethoprim.[71–73] The death rate in such patients is 90%. Aerosolised pentamidine is now being used as a prophylaxis against *P carinii* pneumonia, using nebulisers that can deliver particles 1–2 μm in diameter to maximise alveolar deposition.[74]

Although the pathological role of cytomegalovirus in the lungs of patients with *P carinii* pneumonia is not clear,[75] several antiviral agents, such as tribivarin, foscarnet (trisodium phosphonoformate), and ganciclovir (1,3 dihydroxy-2-propoxymethyl guanine, or DHPG) are being tried. Foscarnet, an inhibitor of DNA polymerase, may be useful in treating the early stages of cytomegalovirus pneumonia.[76 77]

The incidence of tuberculosis is on the increase in many countries, particularly in Africa, where the association of AIDS and tuberculosis is prevalent.

Despite the fact that no new antimycobacterial drugs have been introduced in the past 5 years, the chemotherapy of tuberculosis has been improved greatly. The combination of rifampicin and isoniazid initially allowed the total duration of treatment to be reduced from the usual 18 months to only 9 months, with the initial 2 months of treatment usually supplemented with ethambutol.[78] Several trials have shown that, by combining isoniazid and rifampicin with pyrazinamide and one other drug (usually streptomycin or ethambutol) during the first 2 months of treatment, the duration of treatment can be reduced further to only 6 months.[79–81] Thus, in the study by the British Thoracic Society both 6 month regimens supplemented for the first 2 months with streptomycin and pyrazinamide or with ethambutol and pyrazinamide were as effective as the traditionally recommended 9 month regimen, and relapse rates 3 years after stopping treatment were only 1·7% (streptomycin) and 3·2% (ethambutol) for the 6 month regimens. The British Thoracic Society has recommended both of these 6 month regimens as acceptable alternatives to the 9 month regimen, the completely oral ethambutol regimen being more convenient than the regimen requiring injections of streptomycin.

The 6 month regimen owes its success to the rediscovery of an old mycobacterial sterilising drug, pyrazinamide, and to the introduction of rifampicin in the 1970s. Pyrazinamide seems to be necessary in the first 2 months and rifampicin during the whole period of treatment for regimens using an initial phase of four drugs, though the continuous use of rifampicin seems to be more important.[82] The fears that the use of pyrazinamide would result in a large incidence of hepatotoxicity, as was shown when it was first used 50 years ago, were unfounded: used at the recommended dose of 35 mg/kg a day the addition of pyrazinamide for 2 months of the 6 month regimens of isoniazid and rifampicin did not increase the incidence of hepatitis (4%).[79] Arthralgia of the large and small joints was a minor problem that resulted from the increased serum concentration of uric acid (caused by the renal tubular secretion of uric acid being inhibited by pyrazinoic acid, the most important metabolite of pyrazinamide).

Despite these recent advances in short course chemotherapy for pulmonary tuberculosis, several problems still need to be tackled, particularly in poorer countries. The main problems, even with short course chemotherapy, are those of compliance, of inadequate chemotherapy resulting from ineffective drug regimens or from stopping treatment, and of the subsequent emergence of resistant strains. The use of supervised treatment two or three times a week for patients who cannot or will not administer drugs themselves may help to overcome some of these problems. A 6 monthly regimen containing isoniazid, rifampicin, pyrazinamide, and streptomycin or ethambutol given three times a week was effective against drug sensitive strains of tubercle bacilli and also in patients infected with bacilli that were resistant to isoniazid or streptomycin.[83] The supervision of treatment, however, is labour intensive and expensive.

The trials of short course chemotherapy have shown the effectiveness of several regimens, but it is important to realise that these were performed under strictly supervised study conditions. The realities of the problem are shown by a recent study in Peru, where up to one third of the patients abandoned a 12 month regimen and 14% an 8 month regimen.[84] In addition, a high rate of resistance of tubercle bacilli to the first line antituberculous drugs was observed, with only three quarters of previously untreated patients harbouring fully susceptible organisms.[85]

It seems that it is not possible to reduce the duration of effective antituberculous treatment to less than 6 months. In the studies undertaken in Singapore and east Africa daily regimens of streptomycin, isoniazid, rifampicin, and pyrazinamide for 2 months followed by isoniazid and rifampicin for 4 months, with or without pyrazinamide, resulted in an unacceptable level of relapse at 12%.[81 86] A further reduction in the duration of short course chemotherapy therefore seems to be limited.

There are several prospects for developing new antituberculous drugs. Ofloxacin, the new heterocyclic carbonic acid derivative similar to nalidixic acid is active *in vitro* against *Mycobacterium tuberculosis* as well as non-tuberculous mycobacteria such as *M kansasii*, *M xenopi*, *M fortuitum*, and *M mavinum*.[87] Ofloxacin may also be useful in treating resistant *M tuberculosis*.[88 89] In a preliminary study the drug was given for 6–8 months in combination with other antituberculous drugs to 19 patients who had chronic cavitating tuberculosis with bacilli resistant to isoniazid.[88]

Although the study showed that ofloxacin caused a decrease in the numbers of viable *M tuberculosis* bacilli and that five patients showed culture conversion, larger clinical trials are necessary.

The related compound, ciprofloxacin (discussed earlier), is also active against *M tuberculosis*.[90] Several derivatives of rifamycin also seem to be active against *M tuberculosis*, particularly strains that are resistant to rifampicin: ansamycin was active against *M tuberculosis* in animal models, achieving high tissue concentrations with a long half life;[91] cyclopentyl rifamycin has antimycobacterial properties similar to rifampicin in vitro,[92] but superior to rifampicin *in vivo* in mice.[93] These rifamycin compounds have a long half life and offer the possibility of intermittent treatment, particularly in non-compliant patients. The aminoglycoside antibiotic amikacin has *in vitro* activity against *M tuberculosis* and seems to be active against strains that are resistant to streptomycin. Cross resistance between amikacin, kanamycin, and capreomycin has been reported.[94]

1 Medical Research Council Working Party. Long-term domiciliary oxygen therapy in chronic hypoxic cor pulmonale complicating bronchitis and emphysema. *Lancet* 1981;**i**:681–6.

2 Flenley DC. New drugs in respiratory disease. *BMJ* 1983;**286**:871–5.

3 Howard P. Home oxygen. *Prescriber's Journal* 1986;**26**:115–22.

4 Evans TW, Waterhouse J, Howard P. Clinical experience with the oxygen concentrator. *BMJ* 1983;**287**:459–61.

5 Laubie M, Schmitt H. Long lasting hyperventilation induced by almitrine: evidence for a specific effect on carotid and thoracic chemoceptors. *Eur J Pharmacol* 1980;**61**:125–36.

6 Stradling JR, Barnes P, Pride NB. The effects of almitrine on the ventilatory response to hypoxia and hypercapnia in normal subjects. *Clin Sci* 1982;**63**:401–4.

7 Stanley NN, Galloway JM, Gordon B, Pauly N. Increased respiratory chemosensitivity induced by infusing almitrine intravenously in healthy man. *Thorax* 1983;**38**:200–4.

8 Maxwell D, Hughes JMB. Almitrine increases the steady-state hypotoxic ventilatory response in hypoxic chronic airflow obstruction. *Am Rev Respir Dis* 1985;**132**:1233–7.

9 Castaing Y, Manier G, Varene N, Guenard H. Effects of oral almitrine on the distribution of VA/Q ratios in chronic obstructive lung disease. *Bull Eur Physiopathol Respir* 1981;**17**:917–32.

10 Powles ACD, Tuxen DV, Mahood CB. The effect of intravenously administered almitrine, a peripheral chemoreceptor agonist, on patients with chronic airflow obstruction. *Am Rev Respir Dis* 1983;**127**:284–9.

11 Dull WL, Polu JM, Sadaul P. The pulmonary haemodynamic effects of almitrine infusion in men with chronic hypercapnia. *Clin Sci* 1983;**64**: 25–31.

12 Campbell DB, Gordon B, Taylor A, Taylor D, Williams J. The biodisposition of almitrine bismesylate in man: a review. *Eur J Respir Dis* 1983;**64**:337–48.

13 Arnaud F, Bertrand A, Charpin J, et al. Le bismesilate d'almitrine dans le traitement au long cours (6 mois) de l'insuffisance respiratoire chronique. Étude multicentrique à double insu. Bull Eur Physiopathol Respir 1982;18:373–82.

14 Howard P, Voisin C, Ansquer JC. Long term trial of almitrine bismesylate in chronic obstructive airways disease. Thorax 1987;42:222.

15 Connaughton JJ, Douglas NJ, Morgan AD, et al. Almitrine improves oxygenation when both awake and asleep in patients with hypoxia and carbon dioxide retention caused by chronic bronchitis and emphysema. Am Rev Respir Dis 1985;132:206–10.

16 Gherardi R, Benveniste C, Le Jonc JL, et al. Peripheral neuropathy in patients treated with almitrine bismesylate. Lancet 1985;i:1247–50.

17 Chedru F, Nodzenski R, Dunnard JF, et al. Peripheral neuropathy during treatment with almitrine. BMJ 1985;290:129–32.

18 Paramelle B, Vila A, Pollak P, et al. Frequence des polyneuropathies dans les bronchopneumopathies chroniques obstructives. Presse Med 1986;12:563–7.

19 Howard P. Almitrine bismesylate (Vectarion). Bull Eur Physiopathol Respir 1984;20:99–103.

20 Evans TW, Tweeney J, Waterhouse JC, Nichol J, Suggett AJ, Howard P. Almitrine bismesylate and oxygen therapy in hypnoxic cor pulmonale. Thorax 1990;45:16–21.

21 MacNee W, Connaughton JJ, Rhind GB, et al. A comparison of the effects of almitrine or oxygen breathing on pulmonary arterial pressure and right ventricular ejection fraction in hypoxic chronic bronchitis and emphysema. Am Rev Respir Dis 1986;134:559–65.

22 Weitzenblum E, Santegeau A, Ehrhart M, Mammoser M, Hirth C, Roegel E. Long-term course of pulmonary arterial pressure in chronic obstructive pulmonary disease. Am Rev Respir Dis 1984;130:993–8.

23 Timms RM, Khaja FV, Williams GW, Nocturnal Oxygen Therapy Trial Group. Hemodynamic response to oxygen therapy in chronic obstructive pulmonary disease. Ann Intern Med 1985;102:29–36.

24 Packer M, Greenberg B, Massie B, Cash H. Deleterious effects of hydralazine in patients with pulmonary hypertension. N Engl J Med 1982;306:1326–31.

25 Simonneau G, Escourrou P, Duroux P, Lockhart A. Inhibition of hypoxic pulmonary vasoconstriction by nifedipine. N Engl J Med 1981;304:1582–5.

26 Bishop MJ, Cheney FW. Comparison of the effects of minoxidil and nifedipine on hypoxic pulmonary vasoconstriction in dogs. J Cardiovasc Pharmacol 1983;5:184–9.

27 Young TE, Lundquist LJ, Chester E, Weir EK. Comparative effects of nifedipine, verapamil and diltiazem on experimental pulmonary hypertension. Am J Cardiol 1983;51:195–200.

28 Kennedy TP, Michael JR, Huang C-K, et al. Nifedipine inhibits hypoxic pulmonary vasoconstriction during rest and exercise in patients with chronic obstructive pulmonary disease. Am Rev Respir Dis 1983;129:544–51.

29 Sturani C, Bassein L, Schiavina M, Gunella G. Oral nifedipine in chronic cor pulmonale secondary to severe chronic obstructive pulmonary disease. Short and long-term effects. Chest 1983;84:135–42.

30 Bratel T, Hedeustierna G, Nyguist O, Ripe E. Long-term treatment with a new calcium antagonist, felodipine, in chronic obstructive lung disease. Eur J Respir Dis 1986;68:351–61.

31 Lockhart A, Lissar J, Salmon D. Effect of isoprotenerol on the pulmonary circulation in obstructive airways disease. Clin Sci 1967;32:177–87.

32 Stockley RA, Finnegan P, Bishop JM. Effect of intravenous terbutaline on arterial blood gas tensions, ventilation and pulmonary circulation in patients with chronic bronchitis and emphysema. *Thorax* 1977;**32**:601–5.

33 MacNee W, Wathen CG, Hannan WJ, Flenley DC, Muir AL. Effects of pirbuterol and sodium nitroprusside on pulmonary haemodynamics in hypoxic cor pulmonale. *BMJ* 1983;**287**:1169–72.

34 Peacock A, Busst C, Dawkins K, Denison DM. Response of pulmonary circulation to oral pirbuterol in chronic airflow obstruction. *BMJ* 1983;**287**:1180–3.

35 Rubin LJ, Peter RH. Hemodynamics at rest and during exercise after oral hydralazine in patients with cor pulmonale. *Am J Cardiol* 1981;**47**:116–22.

36 Jezek V, Ourednik A, Stephanek J, Boudik F. The effect of aminophylline on the respiration and pulmonary circulation. *Clin Sci* 1970;**38**:549–54.

37 Burke CM, Harte M, Duncan J, *et al.* Captopril and domiciliary oxygen in chronic airflow obstruction. *BMJ* 1985;**290**:1251.

38 Matthay RA, Berger HJ, Davies R, Loke J, Gottschalk A, Zaret BL. Improvement in cardiac performance by oral long-acting theophylline in chronic obstructive pulmonary disease. *Am Heart J* 1982;**104**:1022–6.

39 Adnot S, Defouilloy C, Brun-Buisson C, Abrouk F, Piquet J, Lemaire F. Hemodynamic effects of urapidil in patients with pulmonary hypertension: a comparative study with hydralazine. *Am Rev Respir Dis* 1987;**135**:288–93.

40 Reeves JT, Groves BM, Turkevich D. The case for treatment of selected patients with primary pulmonary hypertension. *Am Rev Respir Dis* 1986;**134**:342–6.

41 Packer M. Vasodilator therapy for primary pulmonary hypertension. *Ann Intern Med* 1985;**103**:258–70.

42 Higenbottom T. Primary pulmonary hypertension. *BMJ* 1986;**293**:1456–7.

43 Rubin LJ, Groves BM, Reeves JT, Frossolono M, Handel F, Cato A. Prostacyclin-induced acute pulmonary vasodilation in primary pulmonary hypertension. *Circulation* 1982;**68**:334–8.

44 Oakley CM. Management of primary pulmonary hypertension. *Br Heart J* 1985;**53**:1–4.

45 Higenbottom T, Wells F, Wheeldon D, Wallwork T. Long-term treatment of primary pulmonary hypertension with continuous epoprostenol (prostacyclin). *Lancet* 1984;**i**:1045–57.

46 Wise Jr JR. Nifedipine in the treatment of primary pulmonary hypertension. *Am Heart J* 1983;**105**:693–4.

47 Hall DR. Remission of primary pulmonary hypertension during treatment with diazoxide. *BMJ* 1981;**282**:1118.

48 Wang SWS, Pohl JEF, Rowlands DJ, Wade EG. Diazoxide in treatment of primary pulmonary hypertension. *Br Heart J* 1978;**40**:572–4.

49 Pietro DA, Labresh KA, Shulman RM, Folland ED, Parisi AF, Sasahara AA. Sustained improvement in primary pulmonary hypertension during six years of treatment with sublingual isoproterenol. *N Engl J Med* 1984;**310**:1032–4.

50 Moellering RC, Young LS. Moxalactam international symposium. *Rev Infect Dis* 1982;**1**(suppl 4).

51 Brogden RN, Heal RL. Aztreonam: a review of its antibacterial activity, pharmacokinetic properties and therapeutic use. *Drugs* 1986;**31**:96–130.

52 Kahan FM, Krapp H, Sundelof JG, Birnbaum J. Thiernamycin: development of imipenemcilastatin. *J Antimicrob Chemother* 1983;**12**:1–35.

53 King A, Phillips I. The comparative in-vitro activity of eight newer quinolones and nalidixic acid. *J Antimicrob Chemother* 1986;**18**:1–20.

54 Smith JT. The mode of action of 4-quinolones and possible mechanisms of resistance. *J Antimicrob Chemother* 1986;**18**:21–30.

217

55 Davies BI, Maesen FPV, Teengs JP. Aztreonam in patients with acute purulent exacerbations of chronic bronchitis: failure to prevent emergence of pneumococcal infections. *J Antimicrob Chemother* 1985;**15**:375–84.

56 Buchard DL, Hawkins SS, Dhruv R, Friedhoff LT. Penetration of aztreonam into human bronchial secretions. *Antimicrob Agents Chemother* 1985;**27**:263–5.

57 Schlenkhoff D, Knopf J, Dalhoff A. Penetration of ciprofloxacin into human lung tissue following a single intravenous administration. *Proc 14th Int Congr Chemother* 1985:1620–1.

58 Michaelsen H, Bergan T. Azlocillin with and without an aminoglycoside against respiratory tract infections in children with cystic fibrosis. *Scand J Infect Dis* 1981;**29**:88–97.

59 Hodson ME, Penketh ARL, Batten JC. Aerosol carbenicillin and gentamicin treatment of *Pseudomonas aeruginosa* infection in patients with cystic fibrosis. *Lancet* 1981;**ii**:1137–9.

60 Wall MA, Terry AB, Eisenberg J, McNamara M. Inhaled antibiotics in cystic fibrosis. *Lancet* 1983;**i**:1325.

61 Mastella G, Agostini M, Barcollo G, *et al.* Alternative antibiotics for the treatment of pseudomonas infections in cystic fibrosis. *J Antimicrob Chemother* 1983;**12**:297–311.

62 David TJ, Phillips BM, Conner PJ. Ceftazidime—a significant advance in the treatment of cystic fibrosis. *J Antimicrob Chemother* 1983;**12**:337–40.

63 Scully BE, Ores CN, Prince AS, Neu HC. Treatment of lower respiratory tract infections due to *Pseudomonas aeruginosa* in patients with cystic fibrosis. *Rev Infect Dis* 1985;**7**:709–14.

64 Hodson ME, Roberts CM, Butland RJA, Smith MJ, Batten JC. Oral ciprofloxacin compared with conventional intravenous treatment for *Pseudomonas aeruginosa* infection in adults with cystic fibrosis. *Lancet* 1987;**i**:235–7.

65 Roberts CM, Batten J, Hodson ME. Ciprofloxacin-resistant pseudomonas. *Lancet* 1985;**i**:1442.

66 Smith MJ, Fuller G, Hutchinson G, *et al.* Multiresistant *Pseudomonas aeruginosa* in cystic fibrosis patients treated with ceftazidime. *Thorax* 1987;**42**:235.

67 Bodey GP. Overview of the problem of infections in the immunocompromised host. *Am J Med* 1985;**79**:56–61.

68 Murray JF, Felton CP, Garay S, *et al.* Pulmonary complications of the acquired immunodeficiency syndrome: report of a National Heart, Lung and Blood Institute workshop. *N Engl J Med* 1984;**310**:1682–8.

69 Wharton JM, Coleman DL, Worsky CB, *et al.* Trimethoprim-sulfamethoxazole or pentamidine for *Pneumocystis carinii* pneumonia in the acquired immunodeficiency syndrome: a prospective randomized trial. *Ann Intern Med* 1986;**105**:37–44.

70 Golden JA, Hollander H, Conte JE. Inhaled pentamidine or low-dose intravenous pentamidine as novel therapy for *Pneumocystis carinii* pneumonia (PCP) in the acquired immunodeficiency syndrome (AIDS). *Am Rev Respir Dis* 1987;**135**:A168.

71 Leung GS, Mills J, Hopewell PC, Hughes W, Wofsy C. Dapsone-trimethoprim for *Pneumocystis carinii* pneumonia in the acquired immunodeficiency syndrome. *Ann Int Med* 1986;**105**:45–8.

72 Golden JA, Sjoerdsma A, Santi DV. *Pneumocystis carinii* treated with difluoromethylornithine. *West J Med* 1984;**141**:613–23.

73 McLees BD, Barlow JLR, Kuzma RJ, Baringtang DC, Schecter PJ, Sjoerdsma A. Successful eflornithine (DFMO) treatment of *Pneumocystis carinii* pneumonia (PCP) in AIDS patients failing conventional therapy. *Am Rev Respir Dis* 1987;**135**:A167.

74 Thomas J, O'Doherty M, Bateman N. *Pneumocystis carinii* pneumonia: aerosolised pentamidine gives effective prophylaxis. *BMJ* 1990;**300**:211–2.

75 Brodie HR, Broaddus C, Hopewell PC, Moss A, Mills J. Is cytomegalovirus a cause of lung disease in patients with AIDS? *Am Rev Respir Dis* 1985;**131**:227.

76 Apperley JF, Marcus RE, Goldman JM, Wardle DG, Gravett PJ, Chanas A. Foscarnet for cytomegalovirus pneumonitis. *Lancet* 1985;**i**:1151.

77 Farthing C, Dalgleish AG, Clarke A, McClure M, Chanas AC, Gazzard BG. Phosphonoformate (foscarnet): a pilot study in AIDS and AIDS related complex. *AIDS* 1987; **1**: 21–5.

78 British Thoracic Association. Short-course chemotherapy in pulmonary tuberculosis. *Lancet* 1980;**i**:1182–3.

79 British Thoracic Society. A controlled trial of 6 months' chemotherapy in pulmonary tuberculosis. Final report: results during the 36 months after the end of chemotherapy and beyond. *Br J Dis Chest* 1984;**78**:330–6.

80 Hong Kong Chest Service/British Medical Research Council. Controlled trial of four twice-weekly and a daily regimen all given for 6 months for pulmonary tuberculosis. *Lancet* 1981;**i**:171–4.

81 Singapore Tuberculosis Service/British Medical Research Council. Clinical trial of six-month and four-month regimens of chemotherapy in the treatment of pulmonary tuberculosis: the results up to 30 months. *Tubercle* 1981;**62**:95–102.

82 Coates ARM, Mitchison DA. The role of sensitivity tests in short course chemotherapy. *Bull Int Union Tuberc* 1983;**58**:110–4.

83 Hong Kong Chest Service/British Medical Research Council. Controlled trial of 4 three-times-weekly regimens and a daily regimen all given for 6 months for pulmonary tuberculosis. Second report: the results up to 24 months. *Tubercle* 1982;**63**:89–98.

84 Hopewell PC, Ganter B, Baron RB, Sanchez-Hernendez M. Operational evaluation of treatment for tuberculosis: results of 8- and 12-month regimens in Peru. *Am Rev Respir Dis* 1985;**132**:737–41.

85 Black W, Ganter B, Grzybowski S, Sanchez-Hernendez M, Hopewell P. Prevalence of initial bacillary resistance to antituberculous drugs in Peruvian patients with newly-discovered tuberculosis. *Am Rev Respir Dis* 1985;**131**:225.

86 East African/British Medical Research Council. Controlled clinical trial of five short-course (4-month) chemotherapy regimens in pulmonary tuberculosis: second report of the 4th study. *Am Rev Respir Dis* 1981;**123**:165–70.

87 Tsukamura M. In vitro antimycobacterial activity of a new antibacterial substance DL-8280—differentiation between some species of mycobacteria and related organisms by the DL-8280 susceptibility test. *Microbiol Immunol* 1983;**27**:1129–32.

88 Tsukamura M, Nakamura E, Yoshi S, Amano H. Therapeutic effect of a new antibacterial substance ofloxacin (DL 8280) on pulmonary tuberculosis. *Am Rev Respir Dis* 1985;**131**:352–6.

89 Stock JS, Wallace RJ. Preliminary data on the safety and efficacy of drug regimens containing ofloxacin in the therapy of multiple resistant mycobacterial infections. *Am Rev Respir Dis* 1987;**135**:A136.

90 Gay JD, DeYoung DR, Roberts GD. In vitro activities of ofloxacin and ciprofloxacin against mycobacterium tuberculosis, *M avium* complex, *M chelonei*, *M fortuitum*, and *M kansasii*. *Antimicrob Agents Chemother* 1984;**26**:94–6.

91 Della Bruna C, Schioppacassi G, Ungheri D, Jabes D, Marvillo E, Sanfilippo A. LM 427, a new spiropiperidyl rifamycin: in vitro and in vivo studies. *J Antibiot* 1983;**36**:1502–6.
92 Yates MD, Collins CH. Comparison of the sensitivity of mycobacteria to the cyclopentyl rifamycin DL 473 and rifampicin. *J Antimicrob Chemother* 1982;**10**:147–50.
93 Truffot-Pernot Ch, Grosset J, Bismuth B, Lecoeur H. Activite de la rifampicine administrée de maniere intermittente et de la cyclopentyl rifamycine (ou DL 473) sur la tuberculose experimentale de la souris. *Revue Française des Maladies Respiratoires* 1983;**11**:875–82.
94 Allen BW, Mitchison DA, Chan YC, Yew WW, Allan WGL. Amikacin in the treatment of pulmonary tuberculosis. *Tubercle* 1983;**64**:111–8.

17 Peptic ulceration

DONALD G WEIR

The pathogenesis of peptic ulcers is controversial. Nevertheless, our understanding and management of these disorders have been influenced by two aetiological factors: the organism *Helicobacter* (*Campylobacter*) *pylori*, which infects the antral and duodenal mucosa, and the use of non-steroidal anti-inflammatory drugs to relieve chronic musculoskeletal pain. Lesions caused by these drugs affect both the gastric and the intestinal mucosa and occur especially in elderly subjects and in patients with a history of peptic ulcer disease. In both instances acid secretion appears to play an important subsidiary role in causing and maintaining the ulcer. Accordingly, inhibiting acid secretion has always played an important part in our therapeutic endeavours.

Reducing acid secretion

Our understanding of the way in which gastric parietal cells function has increased in recent years.[1] The basolateral surfaces of the cells contain receptors for agents that stimulate them to produce acid, although a recent study has suggested that the receptors for these agents may in fact be on the submucosal macrophages.[2] Stimulating agents include histamine, muscarine, prostaglandins, and (possibly) gastrin. They are blocked respectively by the H_2 antagonists (cimetidine, ranitidine, famotidine, and nizatidine), antimuscarinic agents (atropine and pirenzepine), synthetic prostaglandins (misoprostol), and proglumide, a derivative of glutaramic acid that blocks gastrin production by canine parietal cells.

The apical mucosal surfaces of parietal cells contain the enzyme, hydrogen–potassium adenosine triphosphatase (H^+/K^+ ATPase), a proton pump which, with a carbonic anhydrase enzyme and a potassium chloride cotransporter, is responsible for the intravesicular secretion of hydrogen ions, which are then exported to the lumen of the stomach. By blocking the potassium chloride symport, using substituted benzimidazoles such as omeprazole, H^+/K^+ ATPase may be inhibited, and to a lesser extent by tricyclic antidepressant agents. The enzyme is stimulated by protein kinases, which are in turn activated by histamine through cyclic adenosine monophosphate, the stimulation of which is controlled by inhibitory processes derived from prostacyclin and prostaglandin E_2. By contrast, acetylcholine and gastrin may stimulate H^+/K^+ ATPase via calcium dependent mechanisms.

ANTACIDS

The oft repeated adage "no acid, no ulcer" accompanied the use of antacids to neutralise luminal gastric acid as the sole mechanism of symptomatic and therapeutic control of peptic ulcers until the development of the H_2 receptor antagonist cimetidine, in the mid 1970s. Nevertheless, antacids given in sufficient quantity heal duodenal ulcers at a rate comparable to that obtained using H_2 antagonist drugs. The frequency and dose of antacids consumed must be balanced to avoid the side effects (particularly diarrhoea) when using "non-absorbable" antacids, and to ensure adequate neutralisation of acidity so that the ulcer heals. Recent evidence suggests that a neutralising capacity of 200 mmol hydrochloric acid a day is effective in most patients.

The reason that low dose antacids are effective at healing duodenal ulcers, making the high doses previously recommended unnecessary, remains ill understood. The suggested modes of action include binding of bile acids, inactivation of pepsin, cytoprotection and binding epithelial growth factor.[3]

H_2 RECEPTOR ANTAGONISTS

The H_2 receptor antagonist drugs block the production of acid by parietal cells and, depending on the duration of action, produce gastric anacidity for varying periods up to 24 h. Multiple endoscopically controlled trials have shown that H_2 receptor antagonists heal 60–96% of duodenal ulcers in 4–8 weeks (compared with 35–45% with placebo plus antacids as required for the relief of pain).[4] Several studies have shown that single nocturnal doses of the H_2 antagonists cimetidine and ranitidine are as therapeutically effective as doses twice a day.

Since the introduction of cimetidine other more powerful H_2 antagonists with potentially fewer side effects have been introduced (table 17.1). The correct timing of the nocturnal dose is imperative if the maximum therapeutic effect is to be obtained: in general, the more powerful the agent the earlier in the day it should be taken. Also, the rate of healing of gastric and duodenal ulcers may be increased by more powerful H_2 antagonists. Treatment with cimetidine and other H_2 antagonists is associated with increased basal and postprandial gastrin concentrations, but the importance of this effect appears to be negligible.

Cimetidine has been prescribed to over 40 million patients and ranitidine to over 15 million, and the paucity of side effects is remarkable. The action of its non-parietal cell receptor blocking moiety also makes cimetidine compete for hepatic microsomal cytochrome P-450 and consequently delays the oxidative metabolism and excretion of toxins and alters the bioavailability of drugs such as warfarin, phenytoin, and theophylline that are cleared by this metabolic pathway. This effect occurs to a lesser extent with ranitidine when it is used at high doses to treat patients with Zollinger–Ellison syndrome, and not at all with famotidine or

TABLE 17.1—*Receptor and pump blockers*

	Healing doses (mg)	Maintenance dose (mg at night)	Strength compared with cimetidine
H_2 *Receptor antagonists*			
Cimetidine (Tagamet)	400 twice a day or 800 at night	400	× 1
Ranitidine (Zantac) Nizatidine (Axid) Roxatidine*	150 twice a day or 300 at night	150	× 4
Famotidine (Pepcid)	40 at night	20	× 20
Muscarinic receptor antagonist			
Pirenzepine (Gastrozepin)	50 twice a day or 25 twice a day and 50 at night	50	× 1
H^+/K^+ *ATPase inhibitor*			
Omeprazole (Lozec)	20–40 a day	20 or 20 on alternate nights	× 20
Lanzoprazole*	30 a day	?	× 20

* Not marketed to date.

nizatidine. Further interactions, including those with the tricyclic antidepressants desipramine, quinidine, fluorouracil, and procainamide have been recorded.

Cimetidine and ranitidine occasionally produce mental confusion, especially in the elderly and seriously ill patients; to date this has not been described with either famotidine or nizatidine. Hepatotoxicity, allergic reactions, bone marrow dyscrasias, rashes and gastrointestinal symptoms have been recorded sporadically without appreciable evidence of a causal relation. Impotence, gynaecomastia, and breast tenderness have been associated with cimetidine, and these effects have been supported by animal experiments. Such effects also occur to a mild degree with ranitidine at high doses, but do not seem to be a feature of the other H_2 antagonists.

Although bleeding gastric erosions associated with liver disease and stress in patients in intensive care have been prevented by treatment with cimetidine, multiple controlled studies of acutely bleeding peptic ulcers have shown treatment with cimetidine to have little beneficial therapeutic effect over placebo, though there was a favourable trend in cases of bleeding gastric ulcers.[5] This could relate to cimetidine's failure to produce adequate anacidity. However, recent research using the much more powerful drug omeprazole (an H^+/K^+ ATPase inhibitor) has shown no evidence that anacidity improves the mortality rate, incidence of bleeding or transfusion requirements of patients with acute upper gastrointestinal bleeding.[6]

Famotidine

Famotidine is an H_2 antagonist with a thiazole ring (rather than the furan ring of ranitidine or the imidazole ring of cimetidine).[7] On the basis of weight it is 20 times more potent than cimetidine and 7·5 times more powerful than ranitidine at inhibiting both basal and stimulated secretion of gastric acid in humans (table 17.1). The total output of pepsin, but not its concentration, is also reduced.

Peak plasma famotidine concentrations of 50–60 µg/l are attained 1–3·5 h after a 20 mg oral dose; a concentration of 13 µg/l is required for 50% inhibition of secretion of gastric acid. Famotidine is excreted in the urine (up to 30% being recovered unchanged) or metabolised to the sulphoxide derivative in the liver. The elimination half life is 2·5–4 h.

Clinical trials have shown that famotidine heals 71–92% of duodenal ulcers in 4–6 weeks. A dosage of 40 mg at night healed 91–97% of gastric ulcers after 8 weeks, and a nocturnal dose of 20 mg has been shown to reduce the rate of relapse of duodenal ulcers considerably and to control the manifestations of reflux oesophagitis. On a molar basis, famotidine is considerably more potent than either cimetidine or ranitidine at controlling the hypersecretion of gastric acid in the Zollinger–Ellison syndrome.

Famotidine seems to have no effect on the elimination of drugs metabolised by the liver. Animal studies have shown no evidence of teratogenic, mutagenic, or carcinogenic effects. Serum concentrations of gastrin increase only marginally, and the gastric mucosal changes described in experimental animals with other H_2 antagonists and omeprazole have not so far been seen. Toxic effects include altered bowel habits, dizziness, headaches, and (more importantly) occasional blood dyscrasia.

The potency, lack of toxic effects, and uniformity of uptake, bioavailability, and elimination make famotidine a potentially exciting new H_2 receptor antagonist.

Nizatidine

Like ranitidine, nizatidine contains a furan ring, and has a similar potency: it is four times as powerful as cimetidine by weight. Pharmacologically its actions are almost exclusively confined to the stomach, with little evidence of effects on the cardiovascular or central nervous systems. Absorption is only minimally affected by antacids; 90% is excreted in the urine, 65% unchanged. Accordingly, clearance is affected by renal, but not hepatic, failure. No evidence of hepatic or endocrine effects have been elicited by toxicology studies. No toxic effects were seen in 3500 patients who received nizatidine 300 mg a day for up to 8 weeks or 150 mg at night for a year. An evening dose of 300 mg suppressed nocturnal acid secretion without diurnal carry over, and there was no evidence of increased serum concentrations of gastrin.

Clinical studies have shown that nizatidine produces rates of healing of duodenal and gastric ulcers and a reduction in the rate of relapse comparable with those of ranitidine.

Ebrotidine

This is a new H_2 receptor antagonist that has been shown not only to effectively inhibit acid production, but also to have

225

remarkable gastroprotective effects. Whether this drug will find a significant place in clinical practice remains to be seen.[8]

H^+/K^+ ATPASE INHIBITORS

H^+/K^+ ATPase is found in the gastric fundal mucosa and possibly in the colon: only the stomach, however, generates a highly acid environment. As with sodium and calcium ATPase intestinal pump enzymes, H^+/K^+ ATPase relies on exchange of ions across the membrane and therefore depends on sufficient potassium ions being available in the gastric lumen.[1]

To inhibit this pump an antagonist is required that accumulates in an acid environment, is inactive at a neutral pH, and is activated by a pH lower than 3.

OMEPRAZOLE

Omeprazole, a substituted benzimidazole, meets these requirements, as it prevents the parietal cells from secreting acid even when stimulated by cyclic adenosine monophosphate and by the known gastric secretagogues. With a single daily dose of this drug it is possible to induce anacidity throughout the 24 h in most patients with duodenal ulceration. The drug is rapidly absorbed provided that enteric coating protects it from degradation by gastric acid: even then, its bioavailability varies, possibly because of its effect on the secretion of gastric acid, but even allowing for this, responses to a given dose still vary considerably among patients.

Omeprazole is eliminated as the sulphone and sulphide derivatives, and its half life is about 1 h. Omeprazole inhibits reactions mediated by cytochrome P-450 to the same extent as an equimolar dose of cimetidine: as the molar dose of omeprazole required for managing peptic ulceration successfully is 25 to 50 times lower than that of cimetidine, however, the effect is probably of little clinical importance, though delays in the elimination of aminopyrine and diazepam given intravenously have been reported.

A single dose of 20–40 mg omeprazole affects the secretion of gastric acid for 2–3 days and is independent of the plasma concentration of the drug. Dosage once a day results in increasing inhibition of gastric secretion for up to 5 days, after which it reaches a plateau.

Animal studies have shown a remarkable absence of toxic side effects. The main concern is that carcinoid lesions derived from

226

enterochromaffin like cells have been found in the gastric mucosa of rats. These lesions are thought to result from the hypergastrinaemia that results from the prolonged achlorhydria induced by the drug. Removal of the antral G cells by antrectomy prevents the lesions forming. Similar lesions have been recorded in other hypergastrinaemic states such as pernicious anaemia; the degree of hypergastrinaemia induced by omeprazole and the other H_2 antagonists, however, has never been shown to attain the levels found in pernicious anaemia. Another danger of prolonged achlorhydria is the development of increased counts of gastric bacteria, which in turn cause increased concentrations of nitrite and N-nitrosamines, which raises the theoretical spectre of gastric malignancy resulting from long term treatment with omeprazole.[9] These effects might be controlled by ensuring that gastric acid is secreted for short periods each week.

Controlled trials have shown unequivocally that omeprazole is superior to H_2 antagonists in its rate of healing and of relieving symptoms of duodenal, gastric, and oesophageal ulcers and is unquestionably the best drug for managing the Zollinger–Ellison syndrome, and in the long term management of elderly patients with resistant reflux oesophagitis. Toxicology studies have shown that it is safe for periods of up to 6 years. After treatment with omeprazole the serum gastrin concentration rises initially and then tends to fall with time. More importantly, there is no evidence of an increase in the number of argyrophilic cells in the oxyntic mucosa, which might be expected to occur if there was a predisposition to carcinoid tumour formation.

Lansoprazole

This is a new H^+/K^+ ATPase inhibitor, which has been demonstrated to be effective in the healing of peptic ulcers in 23 controlled trials. The doses used have varied from 7·5 to 60 mg per day, the usual dose being 30 mg. The results have demonstrated significantly better rate and completeness of peptic ulcer healing than that obtained using H_2 antagonist drugs, at least comparable to that of omeprazole. Ulcers that were resistant to H_2 antagonists were healed in 98% of patients within 4 weeks. The reported side effects included headache, diarrhoea and dizziness, but the incidence in all instances was less than 4%.

MUSCARINIC RECEPTOR ANTAGONISTS

The anticholinergic agent pirenzepine has a high affinity for the muscarinic receptors of parietal cells because of its ability to distinguish between the M_1 and M_2 muscarinic receptor sites. It specifically inhibits the M_1 site.[10] Pirenzepine reduces gastric basal and stimulated secretion of acid at doses that do not produce associated cholinergic effects in the central nervous system, heart, eye, bladder, colon or salivary system. This is due partly to its extremely limited penetration through the blood–brain barrier and partly to the specificity of muscarinic binding sites.

Pirenzepine 50 mg twice a day produces healing rates for duodenal ulcers similar to those achieved with cimetidine 400 mg twice a day. As a maintenance treatment in preventing the relapse of duodenal ulcer, pirenzepine 50 mg at night is nearly as effective as cimetidine 400 mg at night. Similar results have been obtained for gastric ulcers. Serious side effects such as urinary retention and glaucoma are rare, but one fifth of patients develop a dry mouth, blurring of vision, or both, at a dose of 50 mg twice a day.

This drug has a small therapeutic window between treatment and toxic side effects and is therefore not a front line agent for treating peptic ulceration. It may, however, be of value in managing the so called "flatulent dyspeptic syndromes", but this needs to be confirmed by controlled trials.

Mucosal protection

The pathogenesis of peptic ulceration is currently thought to be related to excessive secretion of acid and pepsin, or impaired mucosal defence mechanisms, or both. Anti-ulcer drugs may be categorised according to which of these processes they affect.

Drugs that enhance the mucosal protective mechanisms of gastroduodenal mucosa have been termed cytoprotective. This term embraces processes that:

● enhance mucosal thickness and secretion of mucus and bicarbonate;

● tighten the gastric intercellular mucosal barriers (thus inhibiting the back diffusion of hydrogen ions);

● promote the rate of regeneration of epithelial cells; and

● increase the flow of mucosal blood by a process that is independent of any effect on the secretion of gastric acid.

This concept has, however, been challenged, as H_2 antagonists have been shown to produce the same effects by inhibiting the secretion of acid. In addition, known gastric irritants can cause superficial mucosal damage even in the presence of excess prostaglandins, which are considered to be the ultimate cytoprotectors. Nevertheless, prostaglandins do seem to protect the deeper layers of the mucosa from damage and to enhance the rate at which superficial damage is healed. With these caveats in mind the term "cytoprotection" has been retained.

The process by which mild irritants may prepare the gastric mucosa to withstand the effects of more concentrated or powerful irritants is termed adaptive cytoprotection and is also thought to be related to the release of endogenous mucosal prostaglandins.

There is a considerable overlap in the activities of most of the effective anti-ulcer drugs: H_2 receptor antagonists produce appreciable cytoprotective effects, whereas colloidal bismuth (De-Nol), a known promoter of enhanced concentrations of mucosal prostaglandins, considerably depresses the concentration and output of pepsin,[11] in addition to its bactericidal effects on *H pylori*.

PROSTAGLANDINS

The gastric and intestinal mucosa both synthesise large amounts of prostaglandins, which have profound effects on intestinal function.[12] In particular, prostaglandins of the E and I series reduce the secretion of gastric acid and at lower concentrations promote cytoprotection rather than decreasing acid production.

Some studies suggest that the generation of prostaglandins by the cyclo-oxygenase pathway in the gastric (and possibly the duodenal) mucosa is defective in patients with duodenal ulcers. This in turn may reflect a shift to the products of the lipoxygenase pathway, such as leukotriene B_4, which is responsible for maintaining the inflammatory process. In particular, the secretion of bicarbonate by the duodenal mucosa has been shown to be defective in patients who have had ulcers that have healed.[13]

These reports led to the development of synthetic derivatives of prostaglandins E_1 and E_2 which, apart from their cytoprotective properties, also inhibit secretion from gastric parietal cells. Unlike their natural counterparts, which have a half life of only seconds, the synthetic derivatives are stable and thus can exert their effects on gastric secretion for hours rather than minutes. Table 17.2 lists the main varieties; to date only misoprostol has a product licence.

TABLE 17.2—*Prostaglandin analogues and surface agents*

	Usual healing doses (times/day)	Cyto-protec-tion	Inhibits gastric secretion	Inhibits gastrin
Prostaglandin analogues				
Misoprostil (PGE$_1$ derivative) (Cytotec)	200 µg × 4	+ +	Yes	No
Arbaprostil* (PGE$_2$ derivative)	100 µg × 4	+ +	Yes	Yes
Enprostil* (PGE$_2$ derivative)	50 µg × 4 or 70 µg × 2	+ +	Yes	Yes
Surface agents				
Sucralfate (Antipepsin)	1 g × 4	+	No	Not known
Tripotassium dicitrato-bismuthate (De-Nol)	120 mg × 4	+	Pepsin only	Not known

PGE = prostaglandin E.
* Not marketed to date.
+ = mildly, + + = strongly cytoprotective.

Trials suggest that synthetic prostaglandin E analogues are considerably more effective than placebo at healing both duodenal and gastric ulcers in 4–6 weeks and have effects similar to those of cimetidine in the same period. The potential of the prostaglandin analogues relates to their ability to inhibit gastric secretion and to enhance mucosal protection. It remains to be shown whether synthetic prostaglandins have any therapeutic advantage over the H$_2$ receptor antagonists (whose side effects are minimal) in managing peptic ulceration. Some evidence exists to suggest that they may be of value in managing gastrointestinal bleeding.

Experiments in animals and humans have shown that synthetic prostaglandin agents will protect against gastric mucosal lesions produced by alcohol, aspirin and other non-steroidal anti-inflammatory drugs, and lesions related to stress. The main clinical value of these agents is their ability to prevent ulceration and bleeding from the gastric mucosa in patients who take aspirin or non-steroidal anti-inflammatory drugs for chronic pain: ingestion of such drugs is one of the main causes of bleeding ulcers in elderly women in the United Kingdom today:[14] non-steroidal anti-inflammatory drugs are estimated to cause 30 000 acute gastrointestinal haemorrhages a year in the United Kingdom.[15] In the short term all ulcer healing drugs will reduce the mucosal damage induced by these agents. A series of controlled trials has shown that the synthetic prostaglandin analogue misoprostol (a prostaglandin E_1 derivative), is more effective than placebo, whereas similar trials with H_2 receptor antagonists have given conflicting results. One multicentre trial from the United States showed a dramatic reduction in the incidence of gastric ulcers when misoprostol was given in conjunction with non-steroidal anti-inflammatory drugs.[16] Two trials found that misoprostol was superior to sucralfate and one that it was better than cimetidine. In two small comparative trials with ranitidine one favoured ranitidine and one misoprostol. The cumulative effect of these results suggests that the protective effect of misoprostol is independent of its acid inhibitory properties and is probably more related to enhanced mucosal protection by its effects on mucus, bicarbonate secretion and increased mucosal blood flow.

Whether encouraging results will continue to be found after long term clinical use remains to be seen. It may well be that gastric mucosal protection is needed only for a relatively short initial period while adaptive cytoprotection mechanisms develop in the gastric mucosa. Evidence is accumulating that the major risk of non-steroidal anti-inflammatory drugs to the gastric mucosa occurs during the initial few months of exposure.[17] Misoprostol has been marketed for over 7 years and more than three million people have received it. The incidence of adverse drug reactions is 0·001%: dose related physiological side effects are the main therapeutic problems. Diarrhoea, usually temporary, occurs as a consequence of the effect of prostaglandins on the intestinal absorption of water and electrolytes. More seriously, prostaglandins are also uterotonic and therefore must not be prescribed to women who could become pregnant. The main remaining problem relates to the safety of long term use of misoprostol in conjunction with non-steroidal anti-inflammatory drugs.

Smoking has been shown to slow the rate of healing and to enhance the rate of recurrence of duodenal ulcers. Smoking inhibits tissue prostaglandins, thus inhibiting the healing process. Synthetic prostaglandin analogues reverse this imbalance and might have a place in treating the duodenal ulcers of smokers.

SURFACE AGENTS

Sucralfate

Sucralfate is the basic aluminium salt of sucrose, substituted with eight sulphate groups.[18] Its mode of action is not fully understood but seems to be related to enhanced production of endogenous prostaglandin and increased production of gastric mucus not induced by prostaglandin. When the drug reaches an acidic environment the molecule dissociates and becomes negatively charged and a viscous paste is formed from the polymerised product; this is the active form and selectively binds to the ulcer base. The barrier thus created protects the ulcer crater from autolysis induced by acid, pepsin and bile. The diffusion of hydrogen ions is inhibited and pepsin is adsorbed by the activated product. Acid and bile acid are both selectively bound by the compound. The activated product stimulates the secretion of bicarbonate and mucus and independently increases the production and release of prostaglandins by the gastric mucosa, thus enhancing cytoprotection.

Several controlled studies have shown that sucralfate 1 g four times a day is as effective as cimetidine 400 mg twice a day. The combination of cimetidine and sucralfate is synergistic and increases the rate of ulcer healing after 2 weeks, but not at 4 weeks. Theoretically, anacidity would interfere with the binding of sucralfate to the ulcer base and for that reason it is recommended that sucralfate is not taken with antacids. This may be a problem in patients who are accustomed to taking antacids for relief of pain, as pain relief is slower during healing with these agents.

Apart from causing constipation in a few patients, sucralfate has no toxic effects. Its main drawback is that doses are required every 6 h.

Bismuth compounds

Tripotassium dicitrato bismuthate (De-Nol) is the colloidal bismuth salt of citric acid. Like sucralfate, it forms an insoluble chelate with protein and mucoglycoproteins and results in a protective layer over the ulcer base in an acid milieu that acts as a barrier to the diffusion of acid. The precipitate has no effect on acid, but it absorbs and reduces the output of pepsin in the stomach for at least 24 h after the last oral dose.[10] The rate of healing of duodenal or gastric ulcers with this agent is reported to be comparable to that of cimetidine. In addition, colloidal bismuth is claimed to cure ulcers resistant to cimetidine.

The most important claim for tripotassium dicitrato bismuthate is that, like other bismuth compounds, it kills the organism H pylori.[19] This organism infects the antrum of the stomach, where it lives under the mucus layer close to the surface of the antral mucosal cells. The incidence of infection with *H pylori* in the overall population increases with age. Numerous studies have shown that infection with this organism is closely associated with non-autoimmune chronic gastritis, duodenitis and duodenal ulcers. A high incidence of gastric mucosal metaplasia in association with *H pylori* infection has been shown in the mucosa of the duodenal bulb of patients with duodenitis or duodenal ulcer. The hyperacidity associated with peptic ulceration may be caused by the *H pylori* urease enzyme, which splits gastric urea to produce ammonia. The ammonia alkalinises the environs of the antral G cells, with resulting enhanced gastrin and acid secretion. (This is a nice theory, but evidence of hypergastrinaemia associated with *H pylori* infection is lacking.) *H pylori* has been shown to produce antral gastritis, but not peptic ulceration, in normal volunteers.

Bismuth salts are bactericidal against *H pylori*, which is not true of H_2 receptor antagonists or sucralfate: clinical studies have shown, however, that the effect is often temporary and that the organism may persist, or recur, in up to half the patients infected, even after 6 weeks of treatment. Nevertheless, the patients who are treated successfully suffer relapse in the next year much less often (25%) than do those who remain infected after treatment (80%).[20] This has resulted in a search for an antibiotic that, either alone or in combination with a bismuth salt, will result in a greater degree of eradication of the *H pylori* organism. Ampicillin, tinidazole, metronidazole and others have been tried for varying time periods and in various combinations. To date no agent or combination of agents has been shown to consistently kill *H pylori* in all patients.[21]

The side effects of tripotassium dicitrato bismuthate include constipation and darkening of the faeces, tongue and teeth. Encephalopathy and neurotoxicity may occur in patients with renal failure. Accordingly, the drug should not be used for long term maintenance treatment.

Treatment options

Peptic ulcer healing rates with antacids, antimuscarinic agents, the available H_2 antagonists, synthetic prostaglandins, surface agents and H^+/K^+ ATPase inhibitors are greater than with placebo. The H^+/K^+ ATPase inhibitors are the most powerful and prolonged inhibitors of gastric acid secretion, and clinical trials have shown that their rates of healing and relief of symptoms are superior to those of conventional H_2 receptor antagonists. Furthermore, so called resistant duodenal ulcers, which cannot be healed by conventional H_2 receptor antagonists, are always amenable to treatment with H^+/K^+ ATPase inhibitors.[22] Accordingly the H^+/K^+ ATPase inhibitors are the best drugs for patients with peptic ulcers in whom a specific aetiological agent cannot be identified.

For patients with peptic duodenal ulcers associated with *H pylori* infection of the antral mucosa (and more particularly with metaplastic gastric mucosa in the duodenum), the preferred treatment is a bismuth salt with one or more of the antibiotics known to be active against the organism and, if necessary, an acid inhibitory drug for rapid ulcer healing and symptomatic relief. The ideal combination of drugs remains to be defined. However, it has been suggested that anacidity increases the effectiveness of some antibiotics against *H pylori*. Omeprazole, in association with amoxycillin, can eliminate *H pylori* in up to 82% of patients,[23] and the organism remains absent for up to a year.[21]

Whatever the relationship of *H pylori* to the initial production of peptic ulcer disease, there is now no doubt that if relapse is to be prevented, *H pylori* must be eradicated permanently.

For patients taking non-steroidal anti-inflammatory drugs for persistent skeletal pain, the synthetic prostaglandin agents seem currently to be most appropriate for prophylaxis and for managing erosions or ulcers induced by these drugs. The duration of treatment required, and their efficacy compared with the newer acid inhibitory drugs, remain to be assessed.

Whether any place remains for surgery in managing benign uncomplicated peptic ulcers is very doubtful.

Management of peptic related diseases

Chronic peptic ulceration should be considered not simply as the presence of an ulcer of prolonged duration but as a chronic remitting and relapsing disease that causes the intermittent appearance of an ulcer, with or without symptoms, for several years. The frequency of relapse and complications indicates the severity of the condition. The factors that favour aggressive, frequently relapsing duodenal ulcers rather than disease with a benign course, rare symptoms and no complications include:

- youth;
- male sex;
- a long history of ulcer symptoms;
- a strong family history of peptic ulcer disease;
- smoking;
- a low ratio of pepsinogen 1 to pepsinogen 2;
- initial resistance of the ulcer to healing; and
- the inability of nocturnal H_2 antagonist drugs to inhibit nocturnal gastric acidity to normal concentrations.

The role of smoking in the pathogenesis and healing of peptic ulceration is controversial. It has been suggested that smoking stimulates nocturnal secretion of acid, inhibits the rate of ulcer healing and enhances the rate of peptic ulcer recurrence, despite the treatment used to reduce the secretion of acid but a carefully controlled crossover trial failed to show that smoking had any appreciable effect on the inhibition of gastric secretion by H_2 antagonists,[24] suggesting that smoking affects primarily the mucosal defence mechanisms. Healing and recurrence of gastric ulcers relate to the size of the initial ulcer, the success or otherwise of initial treatment, smoking and the daily use of aspirin, indomethacin or other non-steroidal anti-inflammatory drugs. Up to four fifths of gastric ulcers have been attributed to smoking and the use of non-steroidal anti-inflammatory drugs.[25]

Reflux oesophagitis and oesophageal ulceration are caused by the mechanical effects of acid gaining access to the wrong place, and accordingly are more amenable to treatment that protects the lining of the oesophagus or inhibits gastric acid secretion. Long term treatment with H^+/K^+ ATPase inhibitors, especially in elderly patients, is probably the best single agent available today, although the cost of such treatment is considerable.

It is important to remember that not all peptic ulcers are associated with or caused by H $pylori$ infection: gastric ulcers associated with non-steroidal anti-inflammatory drugs are not related to H $pylori$ infection. A different strategy, using synthetic prostaglandin analogues with or without acid inhibitory drugs, is needed for patients who require intermittent or long term treatment with non-steroidal anti-inflammatory drugs.[26 27]

Management of persistent H $pylori$ positive disease

Because H $pylori$ cannot be eliminated from all patients, to maintain symptomatic remission either intermittent courses of treatment against *H pylori* or prolonged treatment with a low dose of an H_2 antagonist or an H^+/K^+ ATPase inhibitor will be required.

The dose of H_2 receptor antagonist drugs used for maintenance treatment and to prevent the relapse of duodenal ulcers is usually half the full therapeutic dose and is given as a single tablet at night. The cumulative rates of relapse are about 25% after 1 year's treatment and 50% after 2; this compares well with recurrence rates in excess of 80% in the first year after receiving placebo. The results of maintenance treatment for gastric ulcers are similar. A multicentre study from the Netherlands and Scotland suggests that omeprazole is capable of healing ulcers that resist treatment with conventional H_2 antagonist drugs and that maintenance with omeprazole (20–40 mg/day) keeps these patients in remission when they would have relapsed with high dose cimetidine or ranitidine maintenance treatment.[22]

The incidence, rather than the cumulative rate, of relapse is now seen to be a more appropriate criterion for assessing the progress of a chronic relapsing and remitting disease. Continuous maintenance treatment with cimetidine for 6 years reduced the incidence of symptomatic peptic ulcers to less than a quarter of that expected with placebo treatment and also reduced the incidence of complications of peptic ulcers (stenosis, haemorrhage, and perforation).[28]

The relapse of ulcers is often asymptomatic. The incidence of asymptomatic relapse varies from 21% to 30% a year in patients receiving placebo[29] and was 35% in patients receiving long term maintenance treatment with cimetidine for 6 years.[27] The relatively high incidence of asymptomatic ulcers seen in long term studies may explain the high incidence of peptic ulcer complications that occur, especially in patients taking non-steroidal anti-inflammatory drugs who have no history of ulcer symptoms. Asymptomatic ulcers in patients on long term maintenance with cimetidine are comparatively benign and are unlikely to produce complications.[30] Non-steroidal anti-inflammatory drugs are thought to mask the pain of mucosal damage while worsening the lesion, whereas H_2 receptor antagonists reduce the pain of ulcers while accelerating their healing.

1 Berglindh T, Sachs A. Emerging strategies in ulcer therapy: pumps and receptors. *Scand J Gastroenterol* 1985;20(suppl 108):7–14.

2 Mezey E, Palkovits M. Localisation of targets for anti ulcer drugs in cells of the immune system. *Science* 1992;**258**:1662–5.

3 Halter F. Review in depth: Antacids, an overview. *J Gastroenterol Hepatol* 1992;**4**:947–9.

4 Strum WB. Prevention of duodenal ulcer recurrence. *Ann Intern Med* 1985;**105**:757–61. (Review of preventing duodenal ulceration in America.)

5 Collins R, Langman M. Treatment with histamine H$_2$ antagonists in acute gastrointestinal hemorrhage: implications of randomized trials. *N Engl J Med* 1985;**313**:600–6.

6 Daneshmend TK, Hawkey CJ, Langman MJS, Logan RFA, Long RG, Walt RP. Omeprazole versus placebo for acute upper gastrointestinal bleeding randomised double blind controlled trial. *BMJ* 1992;**304**:143–7.

7 Campoli-Richards DM, Clissold SP. Famotidine: pharmacodynamic and pharmacokinetic properties and a preliminary review of its therapeutic use in peptic ulcer disease and Zollinger–Ellison syndrome. *Drugs* 1986;**32**:197–221.

8 Kowturcek SJ, Maczka J, Kaminski K, *et al.* Gastroprotective and antisecretory effects of Ebrotidine. *Scand J Gastroenterol* 1992;**27**:438–42. (Study demonstrating the effect of Ebrotidine in humans.)

9 Borg KO, Olbe L. Omeprazole: a survey of preclinical data. *Scand J Gastroenterol* 1985;**20**(suppl 108):5–120.

10 Carmine AA, Brogden RN. Pirenzepine: a review of its pharmacodynamic and pharmacokinetic properties and therapeutic efficacy in peptic ulcer disease and other allied diseases. *Drugs* 1985;**30**:83–126. (Full account of the pharmacological and clinical properties of pirenzepine reviewed by a group of international experts.)

11 Baron JH, Barr J, Batten J, Siderbotham R, Spencer J. Acid, pepsin and mucus secretion in patients with gastric and duodenal ulcer before and after colloidal bismuth subcitrate (De-Nol). *Gut* 1986;**27**:486–90.

12 Hawkey CJ, Rampton DS. Prostaglandins and the gastrointestinal mucosa: are they important in its function, disease or treatment? *Gastroenterology* 1985;**89**:1162–88.

13 Isenberg JI, Selling JA, Hogan DL, Koss MA. Impaired proximal duodenal mucosal bicarbonate secretion in patients with duodenal ulcer. *N Engl J Med* 1987;**316**:374–9.

14 Somerville K, Faulkner G, Langman M. Non-steroidal anti-inflammatory drugs and bleeding peptic ulcer. *Lancet* 1986;**i**:462–4. (Evidence that non-aspirin, non-steroidal, anti-inflammatory drugs were taken over twice as often by patients with bleeding ulcers than by matched community controls. Elderly women seem to be especially at risk.)

15 Blower AL. NSAID gastropathy—a growing problem. *Gastroint Futures Clin Pract* 1989;**4**:4–7.

16 Graham DY, Agrawal NM, Roth SH. Prevention of NSAID-induced gastric ulcer with misoprostol: multicentre, double-blind placebo-controlled trial. *Lancet* 1988;**ii**:1277–80.

17 Hawkey CJ. Non-steroidal anti-inflammatory drugs and peptic ulcers. *BMJ* 1990;**300**:278–84.

18 Brogden RN, Heel RC, Speight TM, Avery GS. Sucralfate: a review of its pharmacodynamic properties and therapeutic use in peptic ulcer disease. *Drugs* 1984;**27**:194–209.

19 Misiewicz JJ, Lacey L. *Campylobacter pylori*: clinical aspects. *Gastroenterol Int* 1989;**2**:160–71.

20 Coghlan JG, Humphries H, Dooley C, *et al. Campylobacter pylori* and recurrence of duodenal ulcers—a 12 month follow-up study. *Lancet* 1987;**ii**:1109–11.

21 Labenz J, Gyenes E, Ruhl GH, Borsch G. *Helicobacter pylori* re-infection and clinical course of peptic ulcer disease in the first year post-amoxicillin/omeprazole treatment. *Eur J Gastroenterol Hepatol* 1992;**4**:893–7.

22 Tytgat GN, Lamers CBHW, Hameetman W, Jansen JMBJ, Wilson JA. Omeprazole in peptic ulcers resistant to histamine H_2-receptor antagonists. *Aliment Pharmacol Ther* 1987;**1**:31–8.

23 Bayerdorffer E, Mannes GA, Sommer A, *et al.* High dose omeprazole treatment combined with amoxicillin eradicates *Helicobacter pylori*. *Eur J Gastroenterol Hepatol* 1992;**4**:697–702.

24 Baurfeind P, Cilluffo T, Fimmel CJ, *et al.* Does smoking interfere with the effect of histamine on intragastric acidity in man? *Gut* 1987;**28**:549–56.

25 McIntosh JH, Byth K, Piper DW. Environmental factors in aetiology of chronic gastric ulcer: a case control study of exposure variables before the first symptoms. *Gut* 1985;**26**:789–98.

26 Nunes D, Kennedy NP, Weir DG. Treatment of peptic ulcer disease in the arthritic patient. *Drugs* 1989;**3**:451–61.

27 Watkinson G, Hopkins A, Akbar FA. The therapeutic efficacy of misoprostol in peptic ulcer disease. *Postgrad Med J* 1988;**64**(suppl):60–73.

28 Bardhan KD, Anglo–Irish Cimetidine Long Term Study Group. Six years of continuous cimetidine treatment in peptic ulcer disease: efficacy and safety. *Aliment Pharmacol Ther* 1988;**2**:395–407.

29 Boyd EJ, Wilson JA, Wormsley KG. The fate of asymptomatic recurrences of duodenal ulcer. *Scand J Gastroenterol* 1984;**19**:808–12.

30 Underwood DD, Amos JC, Venables CW, *et al.* Three computer models for the calculation of prevalence of peptic ulcer disease during long-term treatment. *Aliment Pharmacol Ther* 1988;**2**:407–19.

18 Gall stones

IAN A D BOUCHIER

The first operation on the gall bladder was performed in 1867 by John Stough Bobbs, since when cholecystectomy has become the accepted method of treating patients with cholelithiasis. The recent introduction of agents that can safely dissolve gall stones and the advent of lithotripsy have added new dimensions to managing this common and economically important disorder. The development of laparoscopic cholecystectomy has been an important advance in therapy. Gall bladder stones may be removed by surgery, systemically dissolved with bile acids, crushed by extracorporeal shock waves, or locally dissolved with methyl *tert*-butyl ether; endoscopic sphincterotomy has been successful in managing common bile duct stones. Doctors can now offer several treatment options to patients with gall stones; and though this has enhanced the scope for manoeuvre it has created new difficulties in making decisions.

Diagnosis

Gall stones may present in various ways. The most common and characteristic is either acute cholecystitis or obstruction of the common bile duct. Only 5% of patients with acute cholecystitis do not have coexistent gall stones. Gall stones may rupture into the bowel, obstruct the terminal ileum, or cause pancreatitis. Gall stones and cancer of the bladder may coexist. A few patients with cholecystitis may have jaundice but not choledocholithiasis, but most patients with gall stones who are jaundiced have stones obstructing the common bile duct. Cholangitis is diagnosed when, in addition to cholestasis, there are chills, fever and pain and tenderness in the right upper quadrant. Flatulence, intolerance of fatty food, and vague right upper quadrant and epigastric pains are often ascribed to gall stones and chronic cholecystitis: however, such complaints are equally often related to other common gastrointestinal disorders, and one of the main difficulties for the clinician is to decide what treatment to offer a patient with gall stones who presents with these symptoms alone. Because only 15% of gall stones are radio-opaque plain abdominal radiography is often unhelpful: ultrasonography or oral cholecystography (or both) are the basic diagnostic tools. When choledocholithiasis is suspected endoscopic retrograde cholangiopancreatography or percutaneous transhepatic cholangiography may be performed in addition to ultrasonography and computed tomography.

Stones in the gall bladder

Gall stones and acute cholecystitis are an indication for cholecystectomy, which is the major abdominal operation most often performed in the United Kingdom. Because choledocholithiasis occurs in 10–15% of patients, often with no overt symptoms, the common bile duct should be investigated for gall stones. Operative cholangiography is no longer considered to be essential in a patient undergoing cholecystectomy: other techniques exist for evaluating the bile ducts, such as preoperative ultrasonography and peroperative choledocoscopy, which have the advantage of avoiding an operative cholangiogram. The routine examination of the bile ducts has the advantage of reducing unnecessary bile duct exploration; of diagnosing gall stones that would otherwise have been overlooked by palpation, thereby reducing the number of residual gall stones in the common bile duct; and of demonstrating unsuspected disease.

The consensus has moved towards early operation for patients with acute cholecystitis. On admission to hospital they receive appropriate medical support. Intravenous fluids are given if the patient is vomiting and an adequate urinary flow is maintained; it is seldom necessary to use a nasogastric tube. Analgesics recommended include morphine, pethidine and pentazocine, although the last may cause hallucinations in the elderly. Non-steroidal anti-inflammatory agents are used in some centres to control pain. Appropriate treatment is provided for associated cardiac or pulmonary disease. There is no evidence that anticholinergic agents are of value.

Only half of the patients coming to operation will have infected bile, from which various aerobic and anaerobic organisms may be cultured. The yield of bacteria increases if there is obstruction of the cystic duct or cholangitis. A correlation exists between the incidence of positive bile cultures and the development of wound infection, intra-abdominal sepsis, and death. The choice of antibiotic may be governed by the degree to which it is concentrated in the bile or the probable bacterial sensitivity: liver dysfunction or obstruction of the cystic or common bile duct, however, make therapeutic concentrations of antibiotics in the bile unlikely. Recommended antibiotics include a cephalosporin given intravenously or orally—for example, parenteral cefuroxime (750 mg–1·5 g intravenously every 8 h, or 500 mg orally twice a day), gentamicin (2–4 mg/kg/day), ampicillin (4 g/day), or tetracycline (2–4 g/day). Some authorities recommend Gram staining uncentrifuged bile obtained at cholecystectomy to help make the choice of antibiotic, thereby avoiding unnecessary treatment. Metronidazole (800 mg initially then 400 mg every 8 h for 7 days by mouth; 500 mg every 8 h by intravenous infusion) is used in severe infections, in elderly patients, and when an empyema is present.

It is general surgical practice to perform a cholecystectomy as soon as the patient is fit enough, usually within 12–72 h of admission. Thus, although emergency operations are occasionally indicated, urgent cholecystectomy is the procedure performed most often. After 14 days, organisation and fibrosis become more prominent, making a cholecystectomy much more difficult and necessitating a wait of 2–3 months before an elective operation is possible.

Emergency surgery of the biliary tract is seldom needed because the average patient is not critically ill. For patients with toxaemia, a perforation, spreading infection, or severe cholangitis immediate intervention is necessary. In such circumstances a cholecystectomy may not be possible, and the wiser decision is to undertake a cholecystostomy. Gall bladder stones may be removed in this way, but they will recur unless the gall bladder is excised later. The management of choledocholithiasis and ascending cholangitis has been revolutionised by the widespread use of oral endoscopic sphincterotomy. This may be performed before an abdominal operation to remove the gall stones and drain an infected biliary system, thereby reducing the degree of toxaemia and infection and making the subsequent cholecystectomy much safer.

At present conventional cholecystectomy is being replaced by a mini-incision cholecystectomy or laparoscopic cholecystectomy.

241

The precise place that these undoubtedly valuable procedures will have in gall bladder surgery remains to be established.

GALL BLADDER DISEASE IN THE ELDERLY

Acute cholecystitis in patients over 65 years old can be a serious disease; clinical signs are not always typical and there is a high complication rate. The patient frequently has intercurrent illnesses such as heart or lung disease or diabetes mellitus, which increase the postoperative morbidity and mortality. The risk of operation, however, is not greatly increased in elderly patients who are otherwise medically fit. The death rate in patients under 50 years of age undergoing cholecystectomy is about 0·1%, but it rises to nearly 3% in patients who are elderly and may approach 8% if such patients are operated on for complications associated with gall stones. Most perforated or gangrenous gall bladders are found in this age group. Elderly patients tolerate emergency operations on the biliary tract poorly. A cholecystostomy may often be the most advantageous operation for an elderly patient because it can be performed rapidly through a small incision under local anaesthesia if necessary. Once the patient has recovered, the biliary tree is evaluated by ultrasonography, and if normal no further operation is necessary; the wisest course may be not to undertake any additional operation. If stones are shown in the gall bladder or in the bile duct system, cholecystectomy may be warranted or endoscopic sphincterotomy and removal of bile duct stones may be necessary. The decision will depend largely upon the patient's age and state of health.

Cholelitholytic drugs

Oral drugs may be used to dissolve cholesterol rich gall stones as an alternative to elective cholecystectomy. In western communities about 75–80% of all gall stones are composed mainly of cholesterol and are theoretically amenable to dissolution using drugs that increase cholesterol solubility in bile. The outstanding biochemical abnormality in patients forming cholesterol gallstones is the secretion of hepatic bile that is saturated or supersaturated with cholesterol. The main factor is the increased secretion of biliary cholesterol which occurs in obesity, aging and females.

The two main drugs used are chenodeoxycholic acid and

ursodeoxycholic acid. Both are naturally occurring bile acids. Ursodeoxycholic acid is the 7-β-hydroxy epimer of chenodeoxycholic acid. They are absorbed to some extent by passive non-ionic diffusion in the jejunum, but most absorption occurs in the distal ileum where an active transport system ensures the conservation of free and conjugated bile acids. After returning to the liver via the portal system the bile acids are conjugated as glycine and taurine derivatives and are excreted in bile.

DOSE OF DRUGS AND SELECTION OF PATIENTS

Chenodeoxycholic acid is effective at doses of 10–15 mg/kg/day; the dose of ursodeoxycholic acid is 8–10 mg/kg/day. Ursodeoxycholic acid is more expensive than chenodeoxycholic acid and to provide more cost effective treatment the two should be combined in doses of 6 mg/kg/day of each drug,[1] given at bedtime in a single dose for best effect.

Patients suitable for cholelitholytic treatment should have a functioning gall bladder as shown by oral cholecystography; if stones are radiolucent they are probably formed mainly of cholesterol. The stones should be less than 15 mm in diameter and the patient should not be suffering from acute symptoms. Women who are fertile should be using adequate contraceptive precautions. The likelihood of success in compliant patients is about 60%. "Floating stones" seen on oral cholecystograms have a high cholesterol content and are successfully dissolved in 80–90% of patients. Large stones that occupy much of the volume of the gall bladder are less likely to respond to bile acid therapy. Contraindications to bile acid treatment include a non-functioning gall bladder and gall stones that are calcified.

About one third of the stones that appear to be radiolucent on conventional radiography contain appreciable mixtures of calcium salts and pigment. Calcium and pigment gall stones do not generally respond to dissolution with bile acid, which is probably why response rates are so slow in some patients with apparently radiolucent stones. Computed tomography is more effective than oral cholecystography in determining the presence of calcium salts. It is cost effective to submit patients to computed tomography before embarking on a course of oral bile acid therapy.[2]

MODE OF ACTION

Although chenodeoxycholic acid and ursodeoxycholic acid are both effective in dissolving gall stones that contain cholesterol, their effects on cholesterol and bile acid metabolism and their mechanisms for dissolving cholesterol in bile differ. Both reduce cholesterol saturation in bile, both reduce the proportion of biliary cholesterol in the vesicular phase, both prolong the time required for precipitation of cholesterol crystals (nucleation time).[3] Chenodeoxycholic acid reduces the secretion and synthesis of cholesterol but has no effect on its absorption; ursodeoxycholic acid reduces cholesterol secretion, has little effect on cholesterol synthesis and reduces its absorption. Hepatic synthesis of bile acids from cholesterol is moderately increased or unchanged by therapeutic doses of ursodeoxycholic acid, whereas chenodeoxycholic acid reduces it.

Chenodeoxycholic acid and ursodeoxycholic acid differ greatly in their mode of cholesterol solubilisation: chenodeoxycholic acid solubilises cholesterol in micelles whereas ursodeoxycholic acid enhances the transport of cholesterol in liquid crystalline form, which is why the bile acids have been combined to treat cholesterol gall stones.

ADVERSE EFFECTS

Both drugs have proved to be safe in clinical practice. Chenodeoxycholic acid causes moderate changes in liver biochemistry, minor increases in serum low density lipoprotein cholesterol concentration, and diarrhoea. In contrast, ursodeoxycholic acid has been shown to be very safe and causes no adverse effects or signs of toxicity. For this reason, ursodeoxycholic acid has tended to replace chenodeoxycholic acid as a single agent when treating gall stones.

RESPONSE TO TREATMENT

Stones of 5–10 mm in diameter usually dissolve within 1–2 years, and smaller stones within 6–12 months. A low cholesterol diet may enhance complete dissolution. Obese patients are more resistant to treatment and may require larger doses of the bile acid for a longer period. Regular 6 monthly follow up with ultrasonography or cholecystography is required. It takes at least 6 months' treatment before there is any change in the size of gall stones, but treatment is unlikely to be effective if no reduction in size is observed after 1 year of consistent therapy. The risk of complications is not increased during stone dissolution.

Cholelitholytic drugs have not proved popular in clinical use for several reasons. Firstly, fewer than 30% of all patients with gall stones fulfil the criteria for oral dissolution treatment, and when such factors as obesity and compliance are considered the figure may be as low as 10%. Secondly, the duration of treatment is a problem because stones in most patients take 18–24 months to dissolve. Furthermore, radiolucent stones sometimes calcify during bile acid therapy, more commonly with ursodeoxycholic acid than with chenodeoxycholic acid.

Recurrence is a problem, because the abnormality of cholesterol metabolism returns once drug treatment is discontinued and within 4–6 weeks the patient secretes bile that is once again supersaturated with cholesterol; thus gall stones tend to recur when treatment stops. The recurrence rate is 10% a year for the first 5 years, after which stones do not recur. There is therefore an overall recurrence rate of 50% or, put another way, treatment is effective in half of all patients treated. Unfortunately there is no way of predicting or preventing recurrence. Initial suggestions that non-steroidal anti-inflammatory drugs might be of value have yet to be confirmed and they are not recommended at present. Low dose bile acid treatment or a low cholesterol diet, or high fibre diets are not effective. Newly formed stones are identified more readily by ultrasonography than cholecystography. Single stones tend to recur as single stones, and multiple stones as multiple. Recurrent stones are no more likely to cause symptoms than the original stones.

The management of patients once stones have been completely dissolved has yet to be established, but patients should probably be followed up every 6 months with ultrasonography so that small stones can be identified; a further course of ursodeoxycholic acid treatment will usually dissolve any newly formed stones very rapidly. The alternative is to wait until symptoms develop and then offer a course of bile acid treatment to dissolve the stones. Patients receiving bile acid therapy therefore require long term surveillance even after their stones have dissolved. This is one of the major drawbacks of this form of treatment compared with cholecystectomy.

Cholelitholysis has not found favour although it is safe, convenient, and is not associated with death or disease. It is useful in patients with chronic respiratory or cardiac disease for whom other treatments are unsuitable. It can also be offered as an alternative to patients who wish to avoid surgery, such as those who do not want to take time off work and those awaiting an operation for another reason. All patients with radiolucent gall stones should be offered at least the opportunity of considering cholelithiasis as an alternative to cholecystectomy when being counselled about treatment for their gall stones. At present the main use of cholelitholytic drugs is as adjuvant therapy to extracorporeal shock wave lithotripsy.

Contact dissolutions: methyl *tert*-butyl ether

Methyl *tert*-butyl ether is an ether with a boiling point of 52·2°C and is liquid at body temperature. It is highly effective at dissolving cholesterol gall stones when infused into the gall bladder via a percutaneous transhepatic 5 Fr pigtail catheter inserted under ultrasonic control. Treatment should start with 2 ml of the agent. Gall stones can be dissolved within hours after repeated cycles of hand infusion of methyl *tert*-butyl ether followed by complete aspiration. A microprocessor assisted solvent transfer system has been developed that can simultaneously infuse solvent into and aspirate solvent from the gall bladder at high flow rates through a multilumen catheter, thereby enhancing the efficacy and safety of contact dissolution therapy. The procedure is performed without anaesthesia. Nausea, vomiting, duodenal erosion, pain, haemolysis, and inadvertent anaesthesia may be encountered. The symptoms of nausea and vomiting can be reduced if the treatment time is kept short and the profusion volume as low as possible. Dissolution is often incomplete and small residual stones may remain to form a nidus for new stone formation. Only patients with cholesterol gall stones can be treated this way; calcium or pigment stones are not dissolved.

Treatment with methyl *tert*-butyl ether is likely to remain confined to specialist centres and be offered to patients who are unsuitable for open cholecystectomy. It is an invasive procedure that can be performed safely by skilled radiologists accustomed to percutaneous transhepatic cannulation of the gall bladder, but it is unlikely to find a wide role in clinical practice. Contact dissolution therapy has the advantage that neither stone load nor a non-functioning gall bladder influence the outcome of dissolution.

Other methods of dissolving gall stones

ROWACHOL

Rowachol is an inexpensive preparation of six cyclic monoter-pines (menthol, menthone, pinene, borneol, camphene, and cineol) in olive oil, which has chlororetic and spasmolytic properties. It may be used to treat cholesterol stones in the gall bladder and the bile ducts at a dose of one capsule/10 kg/day. The duration of treatment is similar to that for bile acids. Rowachol has not found general acceptance in the management of gall stones.

HMG COA REDUCTASE INHIBITORS

The rate limiting enzyme in cholesterol biosynthesis is microso-mal 3-hydroxy-3-methylglutaryl-coenzyme A (HMG CoA) reduc-tase. Two competitive inhibitors of this enzyme, pravastatin and simvastatin, which have been introduced to lower serum choles-terol levels, also reduce the cholesterol content of bile. There are reports that cholesterol gall stones have been dissolved in patients who were receiving these agents for their lipid lowering effects, but no formal evaluation of the role of HMG CoA reductase inhibitors for gall stone dissolution are available at present.

EXTRACORPOREAL SHOCK WAVE LITHOTRIPSY

Since their introduction in 1986, the lithotripsy machines have undergone considerable development and refinement. The first generation machines generated shock waves by discharging a spark underwater, which was painful and the patient required general or spinal anaesthesia, or at least parenteral opiate analgesia. Second and third generation systems have been developed with varying combinations of approaches for shock wave generation and target imaging apparatus. The techniques include electrostatic spark discharge, electromagnetic shocks, and pulse piezoelectric shock generation.

The criteria for selecting patients suitable for extracorporeal shock wave lithotripsy include

- a history of biliary colic;
- a solitary radiolucent gall bladder stone with a diameter of no greater than 30 mm or up to three radiolucent stones with a similar total stone mass;
- gall bladder visualisation on oral cholecystography;

- identification of the stones and the gall bladder by ultrasonography;
- a shock wave path that avoids lungs and bones, and no complications from the gall stones;
- patients who are pregnant or receiving any treatment that may result in a coagulopathy are unsuitable for lithotripsy.

As with bile acid therapy, only 30% of all patients with gall bladder stones are suitable for lithotripsy. Stones may be fragmented at one procedure but patients may require a second or many procedures in order to fragment the stones. Ultrasonographic examination of the gall bladder is performed immediately before, and again on the day after, the lithotripsy procedure. All subjects require sedation with intravenous diazepam and pethidine.

The successful treatment of patients with gall stones requires a combination of mechanical fragmentation plus chemical solvent dissolution. This is because the spiral valves of Heister represent a barrier to the expulsion of fragments from the gall bladder lumen, gall bladder contractility is probably impaired during the formation of stones and certainly remains so after the stones have been fragmented, and the choledochoduodenal sphincter presents a second potential barrier to the passage of small fragments. Patients should receive either oral ursodeoxycholic acid or a combination of ursodeoxycholic acid and chenodeoxycholic acids in doses indicated above, administered as a single dose at bedtime. This treatment is started on the day before lithotripsy and should continue for at least 3 months after the stones are no longer demonstrable on ultrasonography. Extracorporeal shock wave lithotripsy shatters large stones into smaller fragments which are easier to pass or dissolve. Recent data suggest that most stones disappear by dissolution and not expulsion; hence the importance of adjuvant dissolution therapy.[4] Thus, lithotripsy and bile acid treatment are more effective than bile acid therapy alone.[5]

Although the rate of adverse effects is claimed to be low, minor side effects are common and are not without their problems. These include cutaneous petechiae, transient haematuria, mild leucocytosis, hypertransaminasaemia, and 35% of patients will have some degree of biliary colic; occasional symptomatic pancreatitis may occur after stone fragmentation. The post-dissolution management of patients treated with lithotripsy will probably be similar to that of patients treated with cholelitholytic agents. Furthermore, stones also recur in patients treated by lithotripsy. Thus, the issues of recurrent medical surveillance and further courses of treatment will need to be faced.

Lithotripsy is as cost effective as conventional cholecystectomy in patients with a small load of stones, but less cost effective if the bulk of stones (size and number) is large. It is important to consider the need for bile acid therapy and the nature of the post dissolution surveillance programme when attempting to compare the cost of surgery against lithotripsy.[6]

DIET

No evidence exists that any particular diet influences gall bladder or gall stone disease. A low fat diet is frequently prescribed but has not been evaluated satisfactorily: how much such a diet benefits the symptoms or the underlying disorder of hepatic metabolism or gall bladder function remains to be assessed. Similarly, the results of treatment with a high fibre diet have been disappointing and the careful observation of patients who have undergone gall stone dissolution during bile acid therapy suggests that a high fibre diet does not prevent the recurrence of gall stones. Epidemiological evidence indicates that patients ingesting two units of alcohol daily are less likely to develop gall stones, but alcohol has no therapeutic role in their treatment.

Asymptomatic gall stones

The management of patients with asymptomatic gall stones is controversial: debate exists over whether the stones should be left alone or whether they should be treated by cholecystectomy or the newer forms of non-operative treatment. The issues have been clarified with the publication of several studies of patients with asymptomatic gall stones who have been followed up for long periods. Stones that have been present for a long time do not give rise to symptoms or complications as often as had previously been believed: in one study the cumulative probability of developing biliary pain was only 18% after 20 years. The risk of developing pain seems to diminish with increasing duration of follow up.

Furthermore, biliary complications are always preceded by episodes of biliary pain, and the initial development of a symptomatic illness is not as severe as had been feared. Many authorities therefore believe that asymptomatic stones should not be treated. Another approach is to offer the patient bile acid or some other form of non-operative therapy for the gall stones, although this may lead to more cholecystectomies because patients in whom litholysis is unsuccessful or whose stones recur may eventually press for an operation. For these reasons I do not treat stones that are truly asymptomatic. However, this advice cannot be extrapolated to stones in all parts of the world: in Chile, for example, where gall bladder cancer complicates gall stones, it is advisable that all gall bladders containing asymptomatic stones are removed.

Stones in the common bile duct

The introduction of endoscopic sphincterotomy has revolutionised the treatment of stones in the common bile duct. Before endoscopy was used to remove such stones their presence was generally accepted as an indication for laparotomy, cholecystectomy, and the exploration of the common bile duct. Pre-operative preparation included the administration of parenteral vitamin K if jaundice was present (5–10 mg daily for 3 days) and antibiotics. An operative cholangiogram is always recommended. The usual procedure is a supraduodenal choledochotomy drained with a T tube that is left for 7–10 days; and a cholangiogram is usually obtained before its removal. Transduodenal sphincterotomy may be attempted if the stones are impacted at the lower end of the common bile duct, in which case T tube drainage may be unnecessary.

Endoscopic sphincterotomy has replaced operations on the common bile duct in most centres. It is simpler and cheaper than an abdominal operation and is preferred by patients; it is of particular value in frail and elderly patients with stones remaining after a cholecystectomy. In experienced hands, success rates of over 95% are regularly reported. Sphincterotomy may be difficult to achieve when the papilla is within a large diverticulum or if a Billroth II partial gastrectomy has been performed. Stones may not be extracted when sphincterotomy is followed by an immediate complication such as bleeding or perforation or, most frequently, if the stones are too large. Stones smaller than 10 mm in diameter are usually easily removed but difficulty increases with stones larger than 15–20 mm in diameter. Smaller stones may pass spontaneously once a sphincterotomy has been performed or may be extracted using a balloon catheter or metal basket.

Complications of endoscopic sphincterotomy are rare; they include bleeding, pancreatitis, cholangitis and retroperitoneal perforation. Open abdominal surgery is required in under 2% of patients with complications and the overall mortality rate is around 1%. This compares favourably with the outcome of operations on the common bile duct, which may carry a death rate of 5–12%. Long term complications include stenosis and, occasionally, cholangitis. About two thirds of patients have air in the biliary tree and free reflux of barium into the bile duct, but this does not cause difficulty. Debate continues as to whether the technique should be restricted to elderly and frail patients. The outcome for young and fit patients remains uncertain and many authorities prefer to remove stones by an abdominal operation in young patients rather than by endoscopic sphincterotomy.

Endoscopic sphincterotomy is being used with increasing frequency in patients who have a gall bladder. In particular, those with acute biliary disorders such as cholangitis or gall stone pancreatitis may be treated initially with an endoscopic duct decompression followed by an elective cholecystectomy when their general medical condition has become satisfactory. A second group of suitable patients are elderly and frail individuals with stones in the common bile duct as well as the gall bladder whose bile duct stones have been cleared by sphincterotomy. A decision can then be made whether the stones in the gall bladder warrant treatment or can be left alone. In one study only 10% of such patients required cholecystectomy for biliary pain or cholecystitis during a follow up period of up to 6 years.

Endoscopic treatment of gall stones is cheaper than abdominal surgery, the procedure can be completed in 30 min, and the patient is usually discharged from hospital in 2–6 days. Most patients prefer this form of treatment to surgery. In the future, bile duct stones will probably be managed increasingly by endoscopic sphincterotomy, and abdominal surgery will be used only in selected circumstances or if endoscopic sphincterotomy is not available.

OTHER ENDOSCOPIC TECHNIQUES

About 90% of all bile duct stones can be removed using an endoscopic sphincterotomy, but very hard stones or those that are impacted at the terminal bile duct may not be amenable to this treatment. Alternative developments include electrohydraulic, ultrasonographic, or mechanical lithotripsy. Even laser technology has been applied to fragmenting common bile duct stones, but this is available in very few centres. The development of laser systems is improving, however, and with modifications of endoscopic equipment laser technology may well become more economical, efficient and safe.

LITHOTRIPSY

Stones in the common bile duct are amenable to fragmentation by extracorporeal shock wave lithotripsy. At present this form of therapy is unlikely to be used in preference to endoscopic sphincterotomy. Care must be exercised in locating the stone and avoiding shock trauma to the head of the pancreas. Lithotripsy is unlikely to be of value in patients who require urgent treatment such as those with cholangitis, pancreatitis or jaundice. In any event, endoscopic sphincterotomy will be required from time to time to facilitate the passage of stone fragments in those patients who have undergone lithotripsy, and it seems reasonable to offer lithotripsy only to patients who have been treated unsuccessfully by endoscopic sphincterotomy or who require shock wave fragmentation of a large stone.

DISSOLUTION OF COMMON BILE DUCT STONES

Bile acids may be used to dissolve stones in the common bile duct but are not recommended because the course of treatment is prolonged and the outcome uncertain. Any form of dissolution is undertaken on the basis of direct infusion of a cholelitholytic agent into the common bile duct via a T tube or a catheter positioned by endoscopic sphincterotomy or transhepatic placement. The earlier agents used were heparin and sodium cholate, the success of which almost certainly depended simply on a mechanical flushing effect. Direct infusion of ursodeoxycholic acid or chenodeoxycholic acid is not therapeutically effective.

At present only the semisynthetic vegetable oil mono-octanoin has found favour as a potential solvent for dissolving cholesterol stones in the biliary tract. Mono-octanoin (Capmul, Moctanin) consists of about 70% glyceryl mono-octanoate and 30% glyceryl dioctanoate with traces of glyceryl trioctanoate and caprylic acid. Before use mono-octanoin is diluted with water in a ratio of 10 parts water to 90 parts oil. The solution is infused at a rate of 3–5 ml/h using a drip or infusion pump, and an overflow manometer is placed in the tubing between the pump and the patient to ensure that the pressure in the system does not exceed 12 cm of mono-octanoin. The drug is not toxic to the liver. Treatment is usually given for 7 days, but some clinicians have continued the infusion for up to 2 weeks.

Despite initial enthusiasm for intraductal infusion of mono-octanoin, recent reports suggest that it is not particularly effective. A large study demonstrated unequivocal success in only 26% of patients; in a further 20% the calculi became smaller but remained in the biliary tree. Overall, mono-octanoin was useful in only 54% of patients. The drug is safe but side effects encountered include abdominal pain, nausea, vomiting and diarrhoea. These are related to the dose and can be reduced or abolished by diminishing the rate of infusion or amount of mono-octanoin.

Mono-octanoin is unlikely to become widely established in clinical practice. The increased use of endoscopic sphincterotomy will almost certainly replace this agent, which will be reserved mainly for dissolving residual fragments of stones.

The emulsifiability of mono-octanoate is limited and can be improved by using glycerol mono-octanoate modified by adding N-(2-hydroxyethyl)-palmitamide (Palmidrol) and the poloxamer Pluronic F-68. Some reports suggest that this modified solution is clinically more effective than mono-octanoin alone.

Treatment of calcium and pigment stones

No effective method exists for dissolving calcium gall stones or those composed primarily of brown or black bile pigment. Glyceryl mono-octanoate, Palmidrol, Pluronic F-68, and bile salts may all contribute to the disruption of the organic matrix and may be infused via a catheter placed in the biliary tree, but clinical successes are few and side effects such as nausea and diarrhoea occur in up to 40% of patients, comparable with the incidence of side effects to mono-octanoin. Other agents that have been used include methylhexyl ether and urea-EDTA (ethylenediamine-tetra-acetic acid) solutions, but the problems with these treatments are that the solutions are not readily available, the regimens are complicated, and experience has thus far been limited only to one or two centres. It is therefore too early to say whether such forms of treatment will replace conventional endoscopic sphincterotomy or surgery of the common bile duct. Although data presented from time to time suggest that extracorporeal shock wave lithotripsy may be used successfully for calcium or pigment stones, the bulk of evidence is that lithotripsy is ineffective against such stones, whether in the gall bladder or the bile duct.

Conclusion

Cholecystectomy presently remains the best treatment for stones in the gall bladder. In good hands the operation is safe, effective and, if properly indicated, is associated with very few postoperative problems. At present the role of laparoscopic cholecystectomy is being vigorously debated. Under certain circumstances litholysis with bile acids may be offered as an alternative to cholecystectomy. Extracorporeal shock wave lithotripsy, although attractive, remains an expensive option. Non-operative management of stones in the gall bladder requires surveillance after dissolution and further treatment may be necessary if stones recur. Many patients will therefore feel that the best option is cholecystectomy unless an operation is contraindicated for medical reasons.

Choledocholithiasis is managed best in the first instance by endoscopic sphincterotomy, at least in older patients or those in whom abdominal surgery is contraindicated. Sphincterotomy alone may be sufficient, but mechanical extraction of the stones may be necessary. In certain circumstances infusion of a litholytic agent may be required to dissolve a stone or a fragment of a stone; extracorporeal shock wave lithotripsy may also be used. No effective drug treatment is available for stones composed primarily of calcium or bile pigment: these are removed either by an operative procedure or, when present in the common bile duct, by endoscopic sphincterotomy. Mechanical procedures may facilitate the removal of a stone that does not pass spontaneously.

The variety of procedures available has greatly increased the range of options when deciding which treatment to offer patients.

Treatment must be tailored to each individual and will depend on the site and nature of the stones, the age of the patient, and the presence of any associated diseases that might increase the risks of anaesthesia and operation. Clinicians are encouraged to discuss all the therapeutic options with their patients before selecting a particular form of therapy.

1 Jazrawi RP, Pigozzi MG, Galatola G, et al. Optimum bile acid treatment for rapid gall stone dissolution. Gut 1992;33:381–6.
2 Walters JRF, Hood KA, Gleeson D, et al. Combination therapy with oral ursodeoxycholic and chenodeoxycholic acids: pretreatment computed tomography of the gall bladder improves gall stone dissolution efficacy. Gut 1992;33:375–80.
3 Sahlin S, Ahlberg J, Angelin B, et al. Nucleation time of gall bladder bile in gall stone patients: influence of bile acid treatment. Gut 1992;32:1554–7.
4 Tint GS, Dyrszka H, Sanghavi B, et al. Lithotripsy plus ursodiol is superior to ursodiol alone for cholesterol gall stones. Gastroenterology 1992;102:2042–9.
5 Erton A, Hernandez RE, Campeau RJ, et al. Extracorporeal shock-wave lithotripsy and ursodiol versus ursodiol alone in the treatment of gall stones. Gastroenterology 1992;103:311–16.
6 Nicholl JP, Brazier JE, Milner PC, et al. Randomised control trial of cost-effectiveness of lithotripsy and open cholecystectomy as treatments for gallbladder stones. Lancet 1992;340:800–7.

19 Insulin

J NIALL MacPHERSON, JOHN FEELY

Since insulins were reviewed in *New Drugs* in 1983, human insulins have become the most commonly prescribed preparations. Their advent has stimulated further assessment of insulin pharmacokinetics and of insulin regimens for achieving good control of diabetes. Intense controversy has been occasioned recently by the suggestion that the counterregulatory hormone response to hypoglycaemia may be less in patients taking human insulin.

Research is being directed to the feasibility of using alterations in the structure of the insulin molecule to produce preparations with therapeutic advantages over existing insulins. Disposable plastic syringes and needles and blood glucose concentration testing strips have become prescribable by general practitioners in the United Kingdom, and pen devices are being used more for subcutaneous insulin administration. The remaining uncertainties about whether near normoglycaemia can prevent complications in type I diabetes have stimulated the long term study phase of the diabetes control and complications trial. The use of insulin for non-insulin dependent diabetes has attracted interest, and the United Kingdom prospective diabetes study will include an assessment of the effect of this treatment on outcome. The importance of educating diabetic patients about their self care and the complexities of this education process have also been increasingly recognised.

Insulin preparations

FORMULATIONS

Table 19.1 summarises insulin preparations currently available. Soluble insulins consist of insulin in simple solution and are absorbed rapidly when injected subcutaneously. These are the only insulins available for intravenous administration. The insulin zinc suspensions use the relative insolubility of insulin combined with zinc in acetate buffer to retard absorption from the injection

TABLE 19.1—*Currently available insulins*

Types and species	Proprietary name	Peak activity (h)	Duration (h)
	Short acting neutral soluble insulins		
Human	Actrapid (pyr)		
	Human Velosulin (emp)		
	Pur-In Neural (emp)		
	Humulin S (prb)	2–5	5–8
Porcine	Velosulin		
Bovine	Hypurin Neutral		
	Intermediate acting		
Isophane (NPH) insulins			
Human	Human Insulatard (emp)		
	Pur-In Isophane (emp)		
	Protaphane (pyr)		
	Humulin I (prb)	4–12	12–24
Porcine	Insulatard		
Bovine	Hypurin Isophane		
Biphasic insulins			
Human	Humulins M1, M2, M3, and M4 (10% soluble 90% NPH to 40% soluble 60% NPH) (prb)		
	Penmix 30/70 (pyr)		
	Pur-In Mix 25/75 (emp) — (30% soluble 70% NPH)		
	Actraphane (pyr)	3–8	12–24
	Human Mixtard (emp)		
	Human Initard (emp) (50% soluble 50% NPH)		
Porcine	Mixtard		
	Initard		
Mixed species	Rapitard MC (25% porcine soluble 75% bovine IZS)		
Insulin zinc suspensions (IZS)			
Porcine amorphous	Semitard MC	5–10	12–16
Human lente	Monotard (pyr)	6–14	16–22
(30% amorphous 70% crystalline)	Humulin Lente (prb)		
	Long acting		
Insulin zinc suspensions (IZS)			
Mixed species lente	Lentard MC (porcine amorphous, bovine crystalline)	6–14	18–30
Bovine lente	Hypurin Lente		
Human ultralente	Human Ultratard (pyr)	8–24	24–28
(IZS crystalline)	Humulin ZN (prb)		
Protamine zinc insulin (PZI)			
Bovine	Hypurin Protamine Zinc	10–20	20–36

emp = enzymatic modification of porcine insulin; prb = proinsulin recombinant bacterial; pyr = precursor yeast recombinant.
The range of Penmix and Pur-In and hypodermic equipment is continuously expanding.

257

site. As amorphous suspensions (semilente insulins) have small particles they are absorbed rapidly and have a duration of action somewhat longer than that of soluble insulin, whereas crystalline suspensions (ultralente insulins) have larger particles, are more slowly absorbed, and have a duration of action of more than 24h. Lente insulins comprise a 30% amorphous 70% crystalline mixture. Isophane (NPH) and protamine zinc (PZI) insulins use the relative insolubility of a combination of protamine zinc and insulin to retard absorption.

Soluble and isophane insulins may be mixed in the syringe without the quick action being lost, whereas mixing soluble insulin with zinc suspensions leads to some loss of quick action, probably by soluble insulin interacting with excess zinc. Mixing soluble with protamine zinc insulin also gives rise to loss of some quick action. Biphasic insulins are marketed as mixtures of soluble and isophane (Mixtard, Actraphane Initard, Penmix 30/70, and Humulins M1-M4) or a mixture of 25% porcine soluble with 75% bovine ultralente (Rapitard MC). All insulins are marketed in U100 strength (100 units/ml). Bovine insulins remain available as the Hypurin series of neutral, soluble, isophane, lente, and protamine zinc insulins.

DURATION OF ACTION

For clinical use insulins have been classified traditionally into short, intermediate, and long acting. The rate of absorption of the same insulin, however, shows considerable variation and decreases with the size of the dose. Thus, large doses of "intermediate" acting insulins can have a long duration of action. Insulin absorption tends to be fastest from the abdomen and slowest from the resting thigh. Antibodies to insulin can also affect absorption. The classification in the table should therefore be interpreted in this light.

Administration of insulin

INSULIN SYRINGES

Most diabetic patients use disposable plastic insulin syringes available in 0·5 ml (up to 50 units) and 1 ml (up to 100 units) sizes for subcutaneous injection. Since September 1987 combinations of syringes and needles for this purpose have been prescribable.

Instructions from the DSS and National Pharmaceutical Association have been that needle and syringe should be used once only: extensive studies have shown, however, that the reuse of disposable insulin syringes and needles by the same person is safe. The British Diabetic Association has advised that plastic syringes may be used up to six times in total, although if patients wish to use their syringes only once they are free to do so.[1] A needle clipping device to remove needles from their hubs is prescribable, which ensures their safe disposal.

PEN DEVICES

Increasing numbers of patients are using pen devices in place of insulin syringes for injection. The NovoPen I is a robust device like a fountain pen and uses cartridges of insulin, Human Actrapid Penfills, that can deliver measured doses of insulin in 2 unit increments. Studies have shown a high level of acceptance of the device, which is particularly suitable for facilitating regimens incorporating Actrapid injections before each of the three main meals. The cartridge insulin, but not the pen or its special needles, is available on prescription. Other currently available pen devices are Penject, which incorporates a disposable insulin syringe, Autopen, and Accupen. Further pen devices have become available. NovoPen II now provides a device for injecting Protaphane and Penmix 30/70 formulations.

JET INJECTION

Jet injectors are high pressure devices that eject insulin through a fine nozzle.[2] The high velocity generated permits insulin to penetrate the skin without a needle being used. Jet injectors appear to be able to deliver accurate and reliable amounts of insulin to subcutaneous tissue. The greater dispersion obtained gives more rapid absorption of short and intermediate acting insulins and consequently reduces the total duration of action. Although the initial pain of injection may be reduced, delayed pain and bleeding may be greater. Denaturation of some insulin by the jet, and consequently increased immunogenicity, is a theoretical possibility. Despite having been available for some years jet injectors have not yet achieved wide usage.

Insulin species

As recombinant DNA technology has become the usual mode of

insulin manufacture, most diabetics in the United Kingdom are now treated with human insulins.[34] Human insulin differs from bovine in that the alanine of A8 and valine of A10 of the bovine A chain are threonine and isoleucine respectively in the human A chain, and the C terminal (B30) amino acid of the B chain (which is alanine in the cow) is threonine in the human molecule. Human and porcine insulins differ only in that the B30 amino acid is alanine in the pig.

To date, human insulin has been produced on an industrial scale by four different processes. The Novo/Nordisk company has previously produced human insulin by enzymic modification of porcine insulin (emp) but the Novo division now uses recombinant DNA technology in yeasts to produce human insulin (pyr) derived from proinsulin. Lilly originally made insulin from the combination of separate A and B chains produced by recombinant DNA technology using fermentation in *Escherichia coli* with subsequent chemical combination of the chains (crb). This process has been superseded by production from proinsulin in *E coli* (prb).

Human insulin is slightly more soluble than porcine and bovine insulins, and a more rapid subcutaneous absorption, particularly of long acting formulations, might therefore be predicted. Pharmacokinetic studies of human ultralente insulin confirm that it is more rapidly absorbed than the bovine formulation, has earlier and more definite peak insulin concentrations, but has a sufficiently long duration of action to make human ultralente a suitable preparation to provide basal insulin requirements by injection once a day.[5] Most studies of intermediate acting isophane and lente human insulin formulations and of human soluble insulins show that they have a slightly shorter action than porcine preparations when subcutaneously injected.

THE CONTROVERSY ABOUT HUMAN INSULIN AND HYPOGLYCAEMIA

From 1985 to 1989 the proportion of British diabetic patients treated with human insulin increased from around 6% to more than 75%.[4] As with changes in the 1970s to highly purified (monocomponent) insulins and in the early 1980s to U100 insulin, some patients reported changes in their warning symptoms of hypoglycaemia on transfer to human insulin.[6] The possibility that human and animal insulins might cause different counterregulatory hormone responses to hypoglycaemia, however, and media coverage of the further suggestion that change to human insulin had been associated with an increase in sudden unexplained deaths, led to the current intense interest in possible relations between human insulin and hypoglycaemic unawareness.[4 7]

Several cases of altered experience of hypoglycaemia after transfer to human insulin can be explained fairly readily. Bovine insulin is more immunogenic than human or porcine insulin, and a lower antibody titre on transfer to human insulin may alter dose requirements and duration of action. The change to human insulin may be made when the regimen is altered to improve control. Such improvement in glycaemic control has been associated with a lowered glucose threshold for the release of counterregulatory hormones,[8] with a consequent delay in experiencing adrenergic symptoms. The more rapid absorption of human insulin may also on occasion give rise to quicker changes in blood glucose concentrations, thus altering symptoms of hypoglycaemia.

These factors operating when there has been change from bovine insulin or an alteration in insulin regimen may account for much of the altered symptoms of hypoglycaemia on transfer to human insulin. More difficult to explain are suggestions of altered hypoglycaemic awareness after transfer from highly purified porcine insulins to the same regimens of human insulin, when the altered pharmacokinetics might be expected to cause only minor differences. Several crossover trials have shown no difference in hypoglycaemic experiences between human and porcine insulin,[9] but other studies suggest a high incidence of hypoglycaemic unawareness on transfer to human insulin:[10 11] these, however, have been criticised for inappropriate questionnaire design and implausibly high rates of severe hypoglycaemia.[7] Surveys of experience of hypoglycaemia after change to human insulin are similarly conflicting: a British Diabetic Association questionnaire showed that 24 of 158 patients changing to human insulin experienced less hypoglycaemic warning,[12] whereas in the Netherlands Heine and van de Veen recorded a steady reduction in the number of patients with severe hypoglycaemia admitted to hospitals during 1983–8, when the use of human insulin was increasing.[13] About a third of diabetic patients usually lose adrenergic symptoms of hypoglycaemia during the first 20 years. Gale has pointed out how this could lead to attribution bias,[7] so 1500 of 100 000 patients a year can be expected to report altered symptoms even if their treatment is not changed.

Studies of the counterregulatory hormone response to experimental hypoglycaemia in normal subjects are similarly conflicting: some show no difference between insulins[9] and others show reduced responses of noradrenaline or altered symptoms when human insulin is taken.[14] Although the trigger to counterregulatory hormone response is hypoglycaemia, insulin affects the release of noradrenaline independently of its effects on blood glucose concentrations. This leads to suggestions that porcine insulin (which is slightly more lipophilic than human insulin) could have a quicker action because it penetrates the blood–brain barrier more quickly. The relevance of those mechanisms to the hypoglycaemia experienced by diabetic patients is not known.

While controversy over human insulin and hypoglycaemia continues certain policies seem to be appropriate. Newly diagnosed patients should be given human insulin, and those who have been taking human insulin since their diagnosis are very unlikely to gain benefit from a transfer to animal insulin. Tight control of diabetes is associated with increased hypoglycaemia and reduction in warning symptoms whatever insulin is used, so treatment objectives should not be unrealistically high. During the past six years many patients have been successfully transferred from bovine to human insulins, so those in the United Kingdom still taking bovine insulins are increasingly likely to be a small group of patients with long standing diabetes, the course of which has been particularly favourable. The only indications for transfer from bovine insulins—lipoatrophy or allergy to insulin—are unlikely to apply to these patients, and as long as suitable bovine preparations remain available doctors may deem it wise to avoid unnecessary change. When change is required an initial dose reduction of 10% has been suggested for patients taking less than 0·9 units/kg and a 25% reduction for those taking higher doses. Return to original animal insulins should be considered for patients who have experienced problems on transfer from animal to human insulin that cannot be explained by changes in regimen or control and for patients who have lost confidence in human insulin.

Indications for and objectives of treatment with insulin

By definition, insulin is indicated for type I (insulin dependent)

diabetes. Regimens sufficient to avoid primary diabetic manifestations of thirst, polyuria, weight loss, and ketosis are easily
achieved. The aim for most patients, however, is to normalise their
metabolism sufficiently to prevent the long term complications of
diabetes developing. A wealth of data and results of recent trials to
maintain near normoglycaemia for relatively short periods provide
encouragement that this may prove possible. Current evidence is
not conclusive, however, which justifies the investment in the
currently running diabetes control and complications trial of
intensified versus conventional glycaemic control.[15][16] This follows
up a primary prevention group as well as patients with early
retinopathy and assigns adolescents as well as adults for randomisation. The numbers enrolled give hope for clear conclusions.
Meanwhile, for young type I patients it is reasonable to aim for the
best glycaemic control possible within the following constraints.
Sudden near normoglycaemia after mediocre control of diabetes
can cause acute deterioration in retinopathy, so monitoring optic
fundi is particularly important during acute improvement in
control. Near normoglycaemia is associated with a significant
incidence of hypoglycaemic episodes,[16] and for most patients can
only be achieved at the expense of considerable time and effort.
Near normal glycated haemoglobin concentrations achieved in
clinical trials are not representative of the general diabetic population, in whom concentrations several standard deviations above
normal are the norm. For many patients, achievements in diabetic
control are perhaps most realistically measured against improvement over this norm rather than an unrealistic goal of normality.

Insulin has a place in the management of some type II (non-
insulin dependent) diabetic patients. The dominance of hyperglycaemia as the major risk factor determining outcome is perhaps
more controversial for type II than type I diabetes. In populations
with early onset of type II diabetes (such as Pima Indians and
Asians in Britain) the clinical course and the role of hyperglycaemia in determining outcome may be similar to that in type I
patients. In European populations presenting with type II diabetes
in middle or later life, however, the outcome is heavily influenced
by an excess of cardiovascular disease, which may as plausibly be
related to the interaction of hyperglycaemia with hypertension,
hyperlipidaemia, hyperinsulinaemia, and a postulated genetic association between type II diabetes and cardiovascular disease as to
hyperglycaemia alone. The only major prospective trial of insulin

treatment in type II diabetes, the university group diabetes programme, showed no better outcome with insulin than with diet
alone, despite better glycaemic control with insulin.[17] The United
Kingdom prospective diabetes study has enrolled a substantial
cohort of type II patients treated with insulin[18] but has not as yet
produced any reports on outcome. Pending these results it is
reasonable to aim for as good glycaemic control as possible in type
II diabetic patients who are not old and whose life expectancy is
not limited by other medical conditions. Most type II patients are
overweight, and strenuous efforts should be made to achieve good
control through dietary measures before considering the use of
insulin. Underweight or normal weight patients receiving maximum oral treatment but who have poor glycaemic control are
severely insulin deficient and should be treated with insulin.

For insulin dependent and non-insulin dependent diabetic
patients the control of hypertension, smoking, and hyperlipidaemia are increasingly recognised as being important to prevent
macrovascular disease. Control of hypertension also substantially
slows the rate of progression of diabetic nephropathy.

Insulin regimens

In normal subjects insulin is secreted at two rates: a basal rate
during fasting to exert an inhibitory control on the catabolic
processes of glycogenolysis, gluconeogenesis, lipolysis, and the
breakdown of proteins; and a rapid rate in response to meals to
promote the storage of absorbed fuels. Insulin regimens should
mimic this pattern to achieve good control.

INTENSIFIED CONTROL REGIMENS

In continuous subcutaneous insulin infusion a battery powered
pump infuses soluble insulin through a subcutaneous cannula to
provide the basal rate and boluses are given before meals through
the pump. In one form of intensified conventional treatment
soluble insulin is given three times a day before meals, often using
a pen device for convenience of injection; the basal insulin concentration is provided by an injection of ultralente insulin, usually
given at night before bed, as this preparation's prolonged absorption time provides fairly consistent background insulin concentrations once a steady state has been reached. Alternatively, an
intermediate acting insulin given at bedtime can be used to provide

overnight basal insulin concentrations. If patients are carefully selected, motivation is maintained, and intense supervision is applied then both these techniques can produce near normal glucose and glycated haemoglobin concentrations, though continuous subcutaneous insulin infusion tends to give slightly better results.[19 20] It is equally clear, however, that if these conditions do not apply continuous subcutaneous insulin infusion or frequent injections give results no better than less intense regimens. Patients most suitable for these approaches to self management are likely to be those who have already shown high motivation and the ability to obtain good glycaemic control with conventional regimens. Patients with brittle diabetes or who on psychological testing perceive the pump or pen technology as externalising the responsibility for their diabetes are unlikely to do well. Continuous subcutaneous insulin infusion carries the possible disadvantage that if the pump fails the onset of ketoacidosis may be more rapid and more likely to be associated with dangerous hyperkalaemia because there is no continuing depot of subcutaneous insulin. For these reasons continuous subcutaneous insulin infusion has not achieved widespread use in the United Kingdom. By contrast, the use of frequent injection regimens using pen devices is increasing because even when good diabetic control is not achieved, they may help patients achieve flexibility of mealtimes and activities and the psychological benefit of the feeling that they have more control over their diabetes.

The recent Diabetes Control and Complications Trial Research Group[21] clearly demonstrated that intensive treatment (external insulin pump or three or more insulin injections and four home blood glucose assessments a day) over 6·5 years markedly delays the onset and slows the progression of retinopathy, neuropathy, and nephropathy compared with conventional insulin treatment. While there was a two- to threefold increase in severe hypoglycaemia such intensive regimens are likely to be offered to more patients in the future.

TWICE DAILY INSULIN REGIMENS

The insulin regimen used by most type I diabetic patients remains the combination of short and intermediate acting insulin injected twice a day, before breakfast and before the evening meal. The morning short acting insulin is intended to produce a rise in insulin concentration after breakfast, and the intermediate acting insulin injected in the morning reaches its peak action in the afternoon. Insulin action after the evening meal and during the night is similarly provided by the evening injection of short and intermediate acting insulins. Soluble and isophane or lente formulations are used. A common difficulty with these regimens is morning fasting hyperglycaemia because the duration of action of the evening intermediate acting insulin is insufficient.[22] Increasing the dose of evening intermediate acting insulin tends to produce hypoglycaemia (often asymptomatic) around 0300. Delaying the intermediate insulin injection to before bedtime may help. Substituting ultralente formulations for the intermediate acting insulin can also be tried, but may produce more hypoglycaemia in the hours before waking.

In the adjustment of twice daily regimens patients have been asked traditionally to adjust the dose of medium acting insulin given before breakfast according to the blood glucose concentration before the evening meal and the evening dose according to the blood glucose concentration before breakfast. The variability of absorption of medium acting insulins is such, however, that these adjustments can only logically be made on the basis of a trend in blood glucose concentrations for several days. The lack of need for fine adjustment of dose in these regimens justifies the use of premixed biphasic soluble isophane combinations and adjusting the mix and dose to long term trends in blood glucose concentrations. The pharmacokinetics of subcutaneous soluble insulin injections are more favourable for rapid adjustments in dose and provide further justification for the use of soluble insulin three times a day and intermediate acting insulin at bedtime by patients seeking flexibility and good glycaemic control.

INSULIN REGIMENS FOR NON-INSULIN DEPENDENT DIABETES

When insulin is used to treat non-insulin dependent diabetic patients[23] regimens for patients with dominant insulin deficiency need not differ from those used for type I subjects, and twice daily biphasic insulins are a reasonable choice. Insulin requirements will be increased, often substantially, in obese patients. In subjects with less pronounced insulin deficiency the relief of fasting hyperglycaemia caused by overnight insulin deficiency will probably improve endogenous insulin response to meals, thereby also reducing postprandial glycaemic excursions. Regimens using a single daily injection of bedtime ultralente or isophane insulins at a dose adjusted to the fasting morning blood glucose concentration have therefore been proposed for those with moderate insulin deficiency.

Using the insulins

Unlike most other drug treatments, achieving good metabolic control of diabetes is not simply a matter of adjusting insulin dose to response. This is because of the very imprecise relation between effect and the dose of subcutaneous insulin and because many variables other than insulin affect the control of diabetes. In normal physiology insulin is secreted in a pulsatile manner into the portal circulation, and its secretion is finely regulated from minute to minute through stimulation by gut derived factors and the prevailing blood glucose concentration, which is in turn influenced by the processes of feeding, fasting, exercise, prevailing level of insulin sensitivity, and counterregulatory hormone levels.

Current replacement treatment is an attempt to imitate this physiological activity with subcutaneous injections of insulin that have coefficients of variation for half time of absorption of about 25% in individual patients. Insulin is then absorbed into the systemic, as opposed to portal, circulation to act on tissues with a sensitivity to insulin that varies considerably from day to day. The whole system is administered by the patient, for whom treating and monitoring diabetes is only one of life's many daily tasks. This dominance of variability in determining the effect of subcutaneous insulin injections implies that insulins cannot be used as "precision tools," that attention to factors other than insulin is important in determining diabetic control, and that any regimen producing near normoglycaemia must carry a certain incidence of hypoglycaemia.

Newly diagnosed insulin dependent diabetic patients presenting with hyperglycaemia but not ketosis may be introduced to insulin treatment as outpatients provided that regular adequate contact with a diabetic specialist nurse is available. Restoration of normoglycaemia is not required urgently for such patients, and the initial insulin requirement may be found empirically in a period of days. Those seeking a guide to determining initial insulin requirements may find the tables published by Holman and Turner helpful.[24] All patients who are capable of benefiting should be instructed in monitoring blood sugar concentrations at home.

For patients already taking insulin who encounter problems with poor or unstable diabetic control, the basic practicalities of diabetic self care should be assessed before considering complexities in the insulin regimen. Some recently diagnosed patients may intermittently stop taking insulin because in their remission phase they believe they no longer have diabetes, or as a form of denial of the condition, or simply because they forget an injection, particularly those using multiple injection regimens. Problems of this type will be detected only if a suitably relaxed listening environment, in which the patient's views and feelings may be expressed, is provided. Lipohypertrophy caused by repeated injection into the same site may cause pronounced variability in insulin absorption and must be looked for. Chaotic life styles of teenagers, particularly regarding the times of sleeping, waking, and eating, may severely disrupt control. Conversely, obsessional patients may generate diabetic instability by overfrequent and excessive adjustment of insulin dose in response to home monitoring of blood sugar concentrations.

Even when adherence to treatment is good, fasting hyperglycaemia is a common problem.[21] Three conceptually separate but interacting phenomena probably contribute to this.[25] The waning of free insulin concentrations in the early hours of the morning after taking intermediate acting insulins in the evening has already been referred to. The dawn phenomenon is an increase in insulin requirement in the few hours before wakening, which may be caused by a rise in growth hormone concentration among other factors. In theory continuous subcutaneous insulin infusion regimens that increase the basal rate at about 0400 to 0800 might overcome this problem. When a decrease in sensitivity to insulin is caused by the counterregulatory hormone response to preceding hypoglycaemia the resultant hyperglycaemia is commonly referred to as the Somogyi phenomenon. Hypoglycaemia at about 0300 is common with twice daily insulin regimens and can give rise to fasting hyperglycaemia through the Somogyi effect. This phenomenon and other effects of excess insulin may possibly operate at other times of the day. When insulin requirements exceed 1 unit/kg/day the possibility that the insulin dose is too high should be considered if recognised causes of high insulin requirement (such as adolescence, obesity, or pregnancy) are absent. An increase in the insulin requirement of a previously well controlled patient may be caused by the onset of hyperthyroidism, which is more prevalent in type I diabetes. Decreased requirements may also be caused by hypothyroidism, Addison's disease, or advancing diabetic nephropathy. Concurrent illness of any type may increase the insulin requirement.

The need to educate insulin dependent patients about their self care has long been recognised. The limitations of simply imparting information, however, have increasingly been apparent,[26] and attention is being directed to ways of changing the attitudes to diabetes that impede self care. Such techniques start with patients' concepts of their diabetes and encourage their exploration of these concepts. Although opinions about educational methods may vary, patients should reasonably expect to attend a centre where an active interest in education is maintained.

Future developments

The advent of recombinant DNA technology in the manufacture of human insulin has resulted in the availability of effective insulins of lower immunogenicity but with relatively few obvious therapeutic advantages over the highly purified porcine insulins that they replace. The technology has, however, permitted the creation of new amino acid substitutions that favourably alter the pharmacokinetics or pharmacodynamics of the molecules of what have been called "designer insulins."

Commercially available soluble insulin preparations exist in the form of hexamers, and the delay in absorption from subcutaneous tissue is contributed to by the time required for dissociation into dimeric or monomeric forms. Substituting aspartate for the B9 serine and glutamate for the B27 threonine residues of human insulin alters the interaction between insulin monomers and results in monomeric insulins with normal receptor binding. Recent studies show quicker subcutaneous absorption of this insulin analogue and more rapid hypoglycaemic effect, which promises better matching between rises in glycaemia after meals and insulin concentrations.[28]

The insulin molecule has also been modified to change the isoelectric point towards neutral values while preserving stability, thus producing insulin that, when injected as a slightly acid solution, crystallises at neutral pH in the tissues and delays absorption. Such insulins may be able to combine less variable absorption than current suspensions with long absorption times.[29] The possibility of insulins with greater activity on hepatic glucose output than on peripheral glucose disposal has also been raised. Proinsulin was at one time thought to be such a substance but has now been withdrawn from clinical trials.

1 Alexander WD, Tattersall R. Plastic insulin syringes: reuse or waste £8m a year. *BMJ* 1988;**296**:877–8. (Summarises evidence for the safe reuse of syringes, current regulations, and British Diabetic Assocation advice.)
2 American Diabetic Association task force on jet injectors. Position statement on jet injectors. *Diabetes Care* 1988;**11**:600–1.
3 Pickup J. Human insulin. *BMJ* 1986;**292**:155–7.
4 Pickup J. Human insulin—problems with hypoglycaemia in a few patients. *BMJ* 1989;**299**:991–3.
5 Hildebrandt P, Berger A, Vøland Aa, Kuhl C. The subcutaneous absorption of human and bovine ultralente formulations. *Diabetic Med* 1985;**2**:355–9. (Absorption rate of human ultralente, though faster than that of bovine ultralente, makes it suitable as the basal insulin preparation for multiple injection regimens.)
6 Anonymous. Transferring diabetic patients to human insulin. *Lancet* 1989;**i**:762–3.
7 Gale EAM. Hypoglycaemia and human insulin. *Lancet* 1989;**ii**:1264–6.
8 Amiel S, Sherwin RS, Simonson DC, Tamborlane WV. Effect of intensive insulin therapy on glycaemic thresholds for counter-regulatory hormone release. *Diabetes* 1988;**37**:901–7.
9 Berger M. Human insulin, much ado about hypoglycaemic (un)awareness. *Diabetologia* 1987;**30**:829–33.
10 Teuscher A, Berger WG. Hypoglycaemia unawareness in diabetics transferred from beef/porcine insulin to human insulin. *Lancet* 1989;**ii**:382–5.
11 Berger W, Keller U, Honegger B, Jaeggi E. Warning symptoms of hypoglycaemia during treatment with human and porcine insulin in diabetes mellitus. *Lancet* 1989;**i**:1041–4.
12 Redmond S. Changing to human insulin. *Balance* 1988;**Aug/Sept**:66–7.
13 Heine RJ, van de Veen FA. Human insulin and hypoglycaemia. *Lancet* 1990;**335**:62.
14 Heine RJ, van der Heyden EAP, van de Veen FA. Responses to human and porcine insulin in healthy subjects. *Lancet* 1989;**ii**:946–8.
15 Diabetes Control and Complications Trial (DCCT) Research Group. Are continuing studies of metabolic control and microvascular complications in insulin dependent diabetes mellitus justified? *N Engl J Med* 1988;**218**:246–50. (Review of evidence that good glycaemic control may prevent diabetic complications, with conclusion that case is not yet proved. References for contrary view cited.)
16 DCCT Research Group. Diabetes control and complications trial (DCCT). Results of feasibility study. *Diabetes Care* 1987;**10**:1–19. (Structure of the important DCCT trial. Evidence of increased hypoglycaemia with intensified control.)
17 University Group Diabetes Programme. Effects of hypoglycaemic agents on vascular complications in patients with adult onset diabetes. VIII. Evaluation

of insulin therapy: final report. *Diabetes* 1982;**31**(suppl 5): 1–81. (Insulin treatment did not reduce death rate or improve outcome of microvascular disease in type II diabetic patients.)

18 Multicentre study. UK prospective study of therapies of maturity onset diabetes. I. Effects of diet, sulphonylurea, insulin or biguanide therapy or fasting plasma glucose and body weight over one year. *Diabetologia* 1983;**24**:404–11. (Structure of UK prospective trial that will include assessment of role of insulin treatment on outcome of type II diabetes.)

19 Marshall SM, Home PD, Taylor R, Alberti KGMM. Continuous subcutaneous insulin versus injection therapy: a randomized cross-over trial under usual diabetic conditions. *Diabetic Med* 1987;**4**:521–5. (One comparison of continuous subcutaneous insulin infusion and optimised injection treatment showing comparable control. References to other continuous subcutaneous insulin infusion trials cited.)

20 Saurbrey N, Arnold Larsen S, Møller Jensen B, Kuhl C. Comparison of continuous subcutaneous insulin infusion with multiple insulin injections using the NovoPen. *Diabetic Med* 1988;**5**:150–3. (Trial showing slightly better control with continuous subcutaneous insulin infusion but patient preference for multiple injections with NovoPen. Other studies cited.)

21 Diabetes Control and Complications Research Group. The effect of intensive treatment of diabetes on the development and progression of long-term complications in insulin-dependent diabetes mellitus. *N Engl J Med* 1993; **329:** 977–86.

22 Francis AJ, Home PD, Watford S, Alberti KGMM, Mann N, Reeves WG. Prevalence of morning hyperglycaemia, determinants of fasting blood glucose concentrations in insulin treated diabetics. *Diabetic Med* 1985;**2**:89–94.

23 Tattersall B, Scott AR. When to use insulin in the maturity onset diabetic. *Postgrad Med J* 1987;**63**:859–64.

24 Holman RR, Turner RC. A practical guide to basal and prandial insulin therapy. *Diabetic Med* 1985;**2**:45–53. (Guidelines for insulin doses in patients starting insulin treatment.)

25 Gerich JE. Glucose counter-regulation and its impact on diabetes mellitus. *Diabetes* 1988;**37**:1608–17.

26 Anderson RM. The personal meaning of having diabetes. Implications for patient behaviour and education or kicking the bucket theory. *Diabetic Med* 1986;**3**:85–9.

27 Pickup J. The pursuit of perfect control in diabetes. Better insulin better delivered. *BMJ* 1988;**297**:929–31. (Description of possibilities in modifying insulin molecules as well as new ways of delivering insulin.)

28 Vora JP, Owens DR, Dolben J, *et al.* Recombinant DNA derived monomeric insulin analogue: comparison with soluble human insulin in normal subjects. *BMJ* 1988;**297**:1236–9. (Shows more rapid subcutaneous absorption of monomeric insulin analogue.)

29 Jørgensen S, Vaag A, Langkjaer L, Hougaard P, Markussen J. NovoSol Basal: pharmacokinetics of a novel soluble long acting insulin analogue. *BMJ* 1989;**299**:415–9. (Long acting soluble insulin analogue shows less variability in absorption than Ultratard.)

20 Oral antidiabetic agents

NORMAN R PEDEN

Non-insulin dependent diabetes is a heterogeneous disorder characterised by fasting hyperglycaemia (which results from increased hepatic glucose output), reduced sensitivity of peripheral tissues to the effects of insulin, and varying degrees of insulin deficiency that affects particularly the first phase of insulin secretion. It is commonly associated with obesity (particularly of upper body distribution), hypertension, and hyperlipidaemia. Thus patients with non-insulin dependent diabetes have a high incidence of disability and death from cardiovascular disorders.

As most patients are overweight, the main thrust of management should be aimed at weight reduction, which reduces the metabolic disorder by increasing the patient's sensitivity to insulin; it also has beneficial effects on the associated hypertension and hyperlipidaemia.[1] Unfortunately, many patients fail to implement or persist with the changes of lifestyle necessary to reduce weight adequately and oral antidiabetic agents and insulin should be considered for such patients. Oral antidiabetic agents and insulin will usually lower blood glucose concentrations, but there is a lack of satisfactory evidence that such treatment improves the long term outlook for patients with non-insulin dependent diabetes. Neither do we know which is the most appropriate treatment for such patients in reducing long term morbidity and mortality. The ongoing United Kingdom Prospective Diabetes Study is expected to clarify some of these issues.

As hyperglycaemia is only one of several major cardiovascular risk factors in these patients, the importance of detecting and treating hypertension and hyperlipidaemia has received recent emphasis, and cigarette smoking should be actively discouraged.

Dietary management

Current British,[2] European and north American dietary recommendations for patients with non-insulin dependent diabetes

272

generally agree and aim to reduce weight in overweight patients, maintain body weight in normal weight patients, and reduce hyperglycaemia. Diets should be relatively high in carbohydrates (providing 50–55% of total energy), the carbohydrate being complex, unrefined, and high in dietary fibre (of low glycaemic index). Fat content should be restricted to 30–35% of total energy intake with saturated fats in particular being restricted to 10% or less of total calorie intake, while monounsaturated fats should comprise 10–15% and polyunsaturated fats 10% of total calorie intake. Alcohol intake should be restricted because of its energy content and hypertensive effects, and if sweeteners are necessary then "non-calorific" agents such as saccharin and aspartame should be used.

It is important that diets prescribed conform to the patient's cultural, ethnic, and economic expectations, and the acceptability in the United Kingdom of diets containing up to 50% of energy as complex carbohydrate has been questioned. Indeed, one of the more successful long term dietary strategies in managing patients with non-insulin dependent diabetes in Britain was based on a more traditional diet containing 38% fat and 42% carbohydrate, averaging 6·27 MJ a day.[3]

The various aspects of these general recommendations have been reviewed in detail,[2 4] but several contentious issues remain. Not all studies agree that high carbohydrate diets improve glycaemic control in patients with non-insulin dependent diabetes (this particularly applies to patients whose diabetes is poorly controled).[5] Some evidence also exists that high carbohydrate diets may exacerbate the hypertriglyceridaemia characteristic of non-insulin dependent diabetes, which may be undesirable as hypertriglyceridaemia seems to be an important risk factor for coronary heart disease in these patients. The applicability of the glycaemic index of individual foods when consumed as part of a mixed meal has also been questioned.

In short term metabolic ward studies, very low energy liquid formula diets are effective in achieving weight loss and correcting the metabolic abnormalities of patients with non-insulin dependent diabetes, but the place, if any, of such diets in managing obese outpatients with diabetes has yet to be assessed, particularly given the propensity to silent ischaemic heart disease in these patients.

Diets remain easy to prescribe and dietary advice easy to impart (at least superficially), but the problem of ensuring compliance,

273

particularly in the long term, remains. A study of patients followed up for 6 years showed that 60% were considered to comply well with dietary advice in the long term:[3] a 3 year follow up study, however, showed that normal weight patients tend to keep to the prescribed energy intake more conscientiously than do overweight patients, though most patients did increase their intake of dietary fibre and unrefined carbohydrate. In a general diabetic clinic population only three of 92 patients achieved a greater than 50% of daily energy intake as carbohydrate, and only four achieved less than 30% of daily energy intake as fat.[6]

Agents modifying nutrient digestion and absorption

FIBRE

Water insoluble fibres such as the hemicelluloses seem to reduce gastrointestinal transit times and increase faecal bulk. Water soluble viscous fibres such as pectins and guar gum seem to slow gastric emptying, intestinal transit, and carbohydrate absorption by many complex and ill understood mechanisms. Diets that are high in fibre and complex carbohydrates seem to improve glycaemic control better than do diets supplemented with fibre such as guar gum and bran.

Nevertheless there has been considerable interest in the potential use of guar gum in patients with non-insulin dependent diabetes. Several studies have been reported, which give conflicting results. It seems, however, that a useful reduction in postprandial glycaemia occurs if guar is intimately mixed with food—for example, by sprinkling granules on the food[7] or incorporating them into food during its preparation. To overcome the unpleasant intestinal effects that may occur, it has been recommended that guar should be started at a low dose and gradually increased—for example, a half sachet (2·5 g) guar granules a day building up to 15 g a day. In contrast with the conflicting evidence for a hypoglycaemia effect of guar, evidence exists that guar supplementation lowers serum cholesterol by about 10% in patients with diabetes.

GLYCOSIDE HYDROLASE INHIBITORS[8]

These compounds diminish carbohydrate absorption by inhibiting glycoside hydrolases, including sucrase, maltase and γ amylase, in the upper small intestine and thus slowing hydrolysis and absorption of disaccharides and more complex carbohydrates. These compounds reduce postprandial glycaemia in short term studies and when used continuously for up to 1 year. Acarbose in smaller doses (50 mg) decreases the glycaemic response to food without causing malabsorption, while larger doses cause varying degrees of malabsorption in patients with both non-insulin dependent and insulin dependent diabetes. The resulting malabsorption delivers increased amounts of carbohydrates to the colon where it undergoes bacterial breakdown that can result in unpleasant flatulence and bloating. The best investigated of these compounds is acarbose, which is now marketed in the United Kingdom, and newer compounds are now being assessed. This form of treatment will find a place in managing patients with non-insulin dependent diabetes in association with diet and other oral antidiabetic agents.

Sulphonylureas

Sulphonylureas are indicated for patients who fail to achieve an adequate reduction in hyperglycaemia after trying dietary treatment, typically for 3 months. What proportion of patients are given these drugs will depend on the aims of treatment. The aim of the United Kingdom Prospective Diabetes Study is normoglycaemia (fasting plasma glucose concentration below 6·0 mmol/l) but only 30% of patients achieved that target by dietary treatment alone and the rest required oral hypoglycaemic agents or insulin.[9] By contrast, in a 6 year follow up study of a large group of patients with non-insulin dependent diabetes, 71% were receiving dietary treatment alone after 6 years and only 12% needed oral hypoglycaemic agents. The mean fasting plasma glucose concentration in these patients was 9–10 mmol/l, but this was not associated with a higher death rate than expected.[3] In patients who had only partially responded to 3–4 months of dietary management, treatment with sulphonylurea (chlorpropamide or glibenclamide) reduced the mean (s.d.) concentration of fasting plasma glucose from 8·3(1·9) to 6·7(1·3) mmol/l and of glycosylated haemoglobin from 9·1(2·1)% to 7·8(1·2)%. The effect occurred irrespective of whether patients were obese.[9] Patients with higher fasting plasma glucose concentrations (more than 10 mmol/l) have been shown to

275

require larger doses of sulphonylurea and to be less likely to achieve normal fasting plasma glucose concentrations. The use of sulphonylurea drugs is associated with weight gain (4% in 1 year), which is unfortunate in patients who are mostly above ideal body weight at diagnosis.

A proportion of patients will fail to have an adequate initial response to sulphonylurea treatment (primary failure) and a further group, perhaps 5% of patients a year, will cease to respond to these drugs in the longer term (secondary failure). Some evidence exists that such patients have lower insulin secretory capacity than do good responders, and have more severe hepatic and peripheral resistance to insulin.[10] Evidence also exists that an appreciable proportion of patients with secondary failure probably comply poorly with diet or medication, or both. Patients failing to respond to a first generation sulphonylurea may occasionally improve when given a second generation agent.[11]

For many years considerable controversy has existed about the mode of action of sulphonylureas. Short term studies show that they undoubtedly sensitise the β cells to glucose and stimulate first and second phase insulin secretion. Longer term studies, however, often show a reduction in hyperglycaemia with no increase in plasma insulin concentrations, and the hypoglycaemic action has therefore been ascribed to "extrapancreatic" effects.[12] Improved β cell function may generate the extrapancreatic effects that maintain normoglycaemia, and hence lessen the need for an increase in insulin secretion. Hyperglycaemia itself, however, is known to reduce insulin secretion; comparisons of insulin secretion before and after treatment are therefore not straightforward. Glucose clamp studies have clarified this issue by demonstrating that at a given glucose level sulphonylurea therapy stimulates insulin secretion.[13]

Several studies in vitro have clarified the mechanism of the stimulatory effects of sulphonylurea on insulin secretion. Sulphonylurea drugs seem to bind to high affinity receptors on the plasma membranes of β cells, thus decreasing potassium permeability and causing membrane depolarisation. Calcium ion influx then occurs through voltage dependent channels, and the increase in cytosolic calcium triggers insulin secretion.[11] There is also evidence to suggest that, in some second generation sulphonylurea drugs, two distinct binding sites for hypoglycaemic activity may reside in the sulphonylurea and non-sulphonylurea portions of the molecule.

PHARMACOKINETICS

The absorption of some sulphonylureas is affected by food and it appears that tolbutamide, glipizide and glibenclamide are more effective when taken 30 min before food. Likewise hyperglycaemia itself can affect the absorption of sulphonylurea drugs, probably by causing a glucose concentration dependent slowing of gastric emptying. Sulphonylureas are in general well absorbed from the intestine and are highly bound to protein in the blood, which makes them subject to drug binding interactions. The binding sites on albumin for glibenclamide and glipizide are different from those for first generation agents, and displacement interactions with drugs such as phenylbutazone, salicylates and warfarin—which increase the hypoglycaemic response to tolbutamide and chlorpropamide—may therefore perhaps be less likely with these newer agents. Oral hypoglycaemics that are extensively metabolised are susceptible to hepatic enzyme induction (phenytoin and rifampicin) or inhibition (cimetidine). The second generation drugs are generally metabolised extensively in the liver, and some of the older drugs—acetohexamide (Dimelor) in particular—have active metabolites that are excreted unchanged in the urine and may be responsible for much of the hypoglycaemic activity of the parent compound. The differing pharmacokinetic properties of these drugs give doctors a group of agents with a wide range of elimination half lives and durations of hypoglycaemic effect from which to choose (table 20.1). Elimination half-lives do not correlate well with duration of hypoglycaemic effect, which is often longer than expected and may reflect the binding of drug to B cell receptors.

Considerable (up to 20-fold) variation exists in the steady state concentrations of sulphonylurea between patients during long-term treatment. Some variation is undoubtedly caused by poor drug compliance, although for tolbutamide genetic factors may control the rate of drug metabolism. In general there is no simple relation between drug and blood glucose concentrations. Care must be exercised in giving these drugs to patients with chronic liver disease: not only may drug metabolism be affected and the amount of carrier protein reduced, but such patients are also particularly likely to develop hypoglycaemia. Renal insufficiency may also have profound effects on the excretion of acetohexamide and of unchanged chlorpropamide

TABLE 20.1—*Comparison of established and newer sulphonylurea hypoglycaemic agents*

Drug	Elimination and approximate half life (h)	Duration of action (h)	Daily dose range (mg/day)
First generation			
Tolbutamide (Pramidex, Rastinon)	Hepatic (4–8)	6–12	500/2000 (divided doses)
Chlorpropamide (Diabinese, Glymese Melitase)	Hepatic/Renal (36)	24–72	100/500 (once a day)
Second generation			
Glibenclamide (Daonil, Euglucon)	Hepatic (6–12)	12–16	2·5–15 (once or twice daily)
Glibornuride (Glutril)	Hepatic (6–10)	8–16	12·5–75 (once or twice daily)
Gliclazide (Diamicron)	Hepatic (12)	12–18	40–320 (once daily)
Glipizide (Glibenese, Monodiab)	Hepatic (3–5)	6–10	2·5–30 (above 10 mg twice daily)
Gliquidone (Glurenorm)	Hepatic (1–2)	2–4	45–180 (divided doses)

INDIVIDUAL SULPHONYLUREA AGENTS

Tolbutamide

This is absorbed fairly rapidly (glucose concentration dependent), is extensively metabolised and has a relatively short elimination half-life, generally 4–8 h, so that it is administered twice or three times daily. It remains a useful, relatively safe drug for elderly patients.

Chlorpropamide

As well as being excreted unchanged from the kidneys chlorpropamide is extensively metabolised in the liver. Because of its very long elimination half life it accumulates in 7–10 days, so the dosage should not be adjusted more often than every fortnight and the drug should not be given more than once a day. Its use should be avoided in elderly patients. Chlorpropamide alcohol flushing, which may be a dominantly inherited condition, is not a problem with the second generation sulphonylureas. Acute ingestion of alcohol may, however, potentiate the action of sulphonylureas.

Glibenclamide

Glibenclamide was the first of the second generation high potency drugs to become available. Some accumulation of glibenclamide occurs during long term treatment, and the duration of action extends for more than 12 h. If blood sugar concentrations are not controlled the drug should be given twice a day in larger doses. Hypoglycaemia may be a problem, particularly after meals, as glibenclamide prolongs insulin release that is stimulated by glucose. The bioavailability of different glibenclamide formulations may vary considerably. The reported elimination half life varies between studies, perhaps because of methodological problems with certain assays.

Glipizide

This drug is totally absorbed and peak serum concentrations occur 2 h after a dose. Although absorption may slow if a dose is taken with food—because of delayed gastric emptying—the hypoglycaemic effect is enhanced by administering the drug before meals. Glipizide has a shorter duration of hypoglycaemic effect than glibenclamide. When the daily dosage exceeds 10 mg it is best given in two doses about 30 min before the morning and evening meals: this also provides better glycaemic control in the evening than does one dose a day.

Gliquidone

This is the most extensively metabolised of the sulphonylureas, and the metabolites are inactive. It has a short duration of hypoglycaemic action, and should therefore be given twice or three times a day before meals. No evidence exists of gliquidone accumulating in patients with renal failure but severe hypoglycaemia has been well documented in this condition. Gliquidone may be useful in patients with impaired renal function and may be an alternative to tolbutamide in managing elderly patients.

Gliclazide

Gliclazide may have beneficial effects on platelet aggregation and haemostasis. Unlike other sulphonylureas, and for reasons that are not clear, gliclazide does not seem to cause weight gain. It has a long duration of hypoglycaemic effect, however, and is therefore usually given once a day. Renal mechanisms seem to be unimportant in the elimination of gliclazide, which seems to be relatively safe when used for elderly patients and those with renal impairment.

Glibornuride

This is a drug of moderate potency; the duration of its effect (in terms of insulin release and reduction in blood sugar concentration) is similar to that of tolbutamide and much shorter than that of glibenclamide. Larger doses of glibornuride should be divided and given twice daily.

Although all the second generation drugs are eliminated primarily by hepatic metabolism, some evidence suggests that all, with the possible exception of gliclazide, may have their hypoglycaemic effect potentiated in patients in renal failure.

UNWANTED EFFECTS

The principal unwanted effect of sulphonylurea drugs is hypoglycaemia. Mild hypoglycaemia seems to be relatively common: it may be slightly more common with glibenclamide than chlorpropamide, and appreciably less so with glipizide and particularly tolbutamide. Factors predisposing to severe sulphonylurea induced hypoglycaemia include advanced age (in one study 77% of episodes were in patients aged 70 years or more), impaired renal function, drug interactions, reduced food intake, and intercurrent illness.[14] Glibenclamide and chlorpropamide may cause severe protracted hypoglycaemia that carries a death rate of up to 10%, and an additional 3% of patients have serious neurological sequelae.

The conclusions of the University Group Diabetes Program in the United States, which recorded high cardiac death rates in patients being treated with tolbutamide, have been widely criticised. They have, nevertheless, been responsible for a reappraisal of the place of drugs and diet in non-insulin dependent diabetes. There has also been a trend to discontinue sulphonylurea drugs in patients with non-insulin dependent diabetes who experience acute myocardial infarction and to control with insulin the blood glucose during the peri-infarct period, which has improved outcome in uncontrolled studies. In vitro evidence suggests different effects of tolbutamide and glibenclamide on myocardial metabolism: tolbutamide has inotropic effects, increases oxygen consumption, stimulates glycogenolysis, and inhibits calmodulin binding to rabbit heart membranes. These effects are shared by tolazamide, another first generation sulphonylurea, but not by glibenclamide.

COMBINED SULPHONYLUREA/INSULIN THERAPY

Because of the apparent importance of extrapancreatic effects in the long term control of hyperglycaemia in patients with non-insulin dependent diabetes, the combined use of sulphonylureas and insulin has been investigated again in patients with non-insulin dependent diabetes and those with insulin dependent diabetes. The use of combination therapy in non-insulin dependent diabetes has recently been the subject of a meta-analysis of 17 published, randomised controlled clinical trials:[15] compared with insulin therapy alone, combined sulphonylurea/insulin therapy produced a modest improvement of glycaemic control with lower insulin doses, and it appears that more obese patients with higher residual C-peptide secretion are more likely to benefit.

CHOICE OF A SULPHONYLUREA DRUG

A longer acting drug such as glibenclamide, glipizide, gliclazide, or chlorpropamide is usually chosen for younger patients. For elderly patients or those with renal impairment a shorter acting drug is generally preferable; tolbutamide is the best tested and cheapest, and gliquidone, glipizide, or gliclazide are alternatives. In view of the risk of hypoglycaemia, which may occur with any sulphonylurea drug, the need for continued use of the drug should always be considered when reviewing patients with near normoglycaemia.

Metformin[16]

Metformin is an effective drug which requires the presence of insulin for its effect and does not stimulate insulin secretion. Metformin is indicated as an adjunct to dietary treatment for patients who are overweight, but it may also be used to supplement sulphonylurea treatment of patients failing to achieve adequate control of hyperglycaemia.

Metformin reduces basal hepatic output by reducing hepatic gluconeogenesis, and enhances insulin stimulated peripheral glucose disposal including glucose metabolism by muscle. High concentrations of metformin accumulate in the intestinal mucosa and are associated with a reduced rate of glucose absorption and an increase in intestinal glucose utilisation. Increased glucose utilisation in the intestinal wall probably increases lactate production and hence the supply of this gluconeogenic precursor to the liver; this may, in turn, partially reduce the antigluconeogenic effect of metformin on the liver. Metformin probably has some anorectic properties. The use of metformin therefore tends to lead to weight reduction, albeit modest, which is likely to be beneficial in patients who are primarily overweight. Nevertheless, the important effects of metformin probably relate to a reduction in hepatic glucose output and increased peripheral glucose utilisation, as an appreciable reduction in fasting plasma glucose concentrations has been reported in patients with no significant weight reduction. Although metformin has been reported to increase insulin binding to low affinity receptors, its effects are probably mediated at postreceptor level.

Clinical studies have shown that, when used as an adjunct to dietary treatment in patients with non-insulin dependent diabetes, metformin produces useful reductions (about 20%) in concentrations of fasting plasma glucose and glycosylated haemoglobin, perhaps a little less than sulphonylureas. When given to patients whose hyperglycaemia is inadequately controlled with sulphonylurea treatment metformin will produce a modest further reduction in fasting plasma glucose concentration—for example, from 8·9 to 7·3 mmol/l—although such combined treatment does not usually produce normoglycaemia. Postprandial hyperglycaemia, particularly after midday and evening meals, is often reduced by a greater degree than the fasting glucose.

Metformin often causes gastrointestinal upset, particularly nausea and diarrhoea. This can be avoided by starting treatment at a low dose, 500 mg once or twice a day taken after breakfast and the evening meal, and then increasing the dose by 500 mg at weekly intervals. Although the recommended maximum dose is 1500–2000 mg a day, several workers have usefully and gradually increased the dose up to 2500–3000 mg a day. Metformin is not appreciably metabolised in humans, is rapidly eliminated via the kidneys by glomerular filtration and active tubular secretion, and has a plasma half life of 2–4 h. Absorption, however, is slow and variable. Excretion is thus less rapid in patients with impaired renal function, which results in accumulation.

The main concern about the use of biguanide drugs has been the development of lactic acidosis, which resulted in the withdrawal of phenformin some years ago. Metformin is structurally different from phenformin, it does not bind to plasma proteins, and has a much shorter plasma half life. It also binds much less readily to biological membranes, particularly mitochondrial membranes, than does phenformin, so does not show the same strong inhibitory effect on oxidative phosphorylation. Accordingly, the use of metformin is not usually associated with fasting hyperlactataemia, although mild postprandial hyperlactataemia may occur. There seems to be no appreciable risk of lactic acidosis developing in patients treated with metformin provided that they do not have impaired renal function, liver disease, severe cardiorespiratory disease, severe peripheral vascular disease, do not abuse alcohol, and are not old.

When used as the only adjunct to dietary treatment, metformin does not stimulate insulin secretion and hence does not cause hypoglycaemia. Metformin does appear to be concentrated in the intestinal mucosa, and this may be related to another observed adverse effect, the malabsorption of vitamin B12. Metformin appears to have beneficial effects of lowering triglycerides, and to a lesser extent cholesterol, particularly in hypertriglyceridaemic patients.

Other approaches and future developments

The antiobesity agent fenfluramine and its active D isomer dexfenfluramine have been studied in obese diabetic patients. By their effect on stimulating serotonin receptors they appear to have useful appetite suppressing effects (particularly on carbohydrate craving), promote weight loss and improve glucose tolerance. There has also been interest in the use of serotonin reuptake inhibitor antidepressants such as fluoxetine and sartraline for their appetite suppressant and probable glucose lowering effects in obese diabetics. Atypical β adrenoceptor agonist drugs showing a high degree of selectivity for stimulating thermogenesis (compared with β_1 cardiac and β_2 bronchial smooth muscle effects) appear to be potent antiobesity agents, and improve insulin sensitivity in non-insulin dependent diabetic rodents and insulin sensitivity and plasma glucose concentration in obese humans.

There is evidence that elevated free fatty acid concentrations contribute to the hyperglycaemia of non-insulin dependent diabetes.[17] The lipid lowering agent acipimox (an antilipolytic drug) and bezafibrate in some studies lower blood glucose levels in patients with this disease.[18] The area of inhibition of fatty acid oxidation is being investigated with a range of novel compounds. Etomoxir, an inhibitor of long chain fatty acid oxidation, is one such drug which is demonstrated to have glucose lowering, triglyceride lowering, and antiketonaemic effects in patients with non-insulin dependent diabetes and is under investigation.

Because insulin resistance plays a significant part in the pathophysiology of non-insulin dependent diabetes, therapeutic agents that would sensitise the tissues to the effects of insulin by novel mechanisms, overcoming insulin resistance, could be of therapeutic value. One such group of agents, the oral thiazolidinediones, are now under intensive investigation. Drugs in this class include ciglitazone (the best studied), proglitazone and englitazone. These drugs lower plasma glucose, insulin and triglycerides in animal models of non-insulin dependent diabetes and are now being evaluated in patients.[19]

1 Alberti KGMM, Gries FA. Management of non-insulin dependent diabetes mellitus in Europe: a consensus view. *Diabetic Med* 1988;5:75–81.
2 Nutrition Sub-Committee of the British Diabetic Association's Professional Advisory Committee. Dietary recommendations for people with diabetes: an update for the 1990s. *Diabetic Med* 1992;9:189–202.
3 Hadden DR, Blair AT, Wilson EA, *et al*. Natural history of diabetes presenting age 40–69 years: a prospective study of the influence of intensive diet therapy. *Q J Med* 1986;59:579–98.
4 Anonymous. Report of the American Diabetes Association's Task Force on Nutrition. *Diabetes Care* 1988;11:127–211. (Nine review articles covering in detail the debate of the task force about various important aspects of nutrition and exercise in diabetes mellitus. Subjects of particular relevance to this review include fat, glycaemic index of strachy foods, dietary fibre, alternative sweeteners, and diet in obesity.)
5 Scott AR, Attenborough Y, Peacock I, Fletcher E, Jeffcoate WJ, Tattersall RB. Comparison of high fibre diets, basal insulin supplements, and flexible insulin treatment for non-insulin dependent (Type II) diabetics poorly controlled with sulphonylureas. *BMJ* 1988;297:707–10. (Provocative paper that questions the efficacy and practicability of high fibre diets in typical English patients.)
6 Close EJ, Wiles PG, Lockton JA, Walmsley D, Oldham J, Wales JK. Diabetic diets and nutritional recommendations. What happens in real life? *Diabetic Med* 1992;9:181–8. (An interesting read in relation to reference 2.)
7 Fuessl HS, Williams G, Adrian TE, Bloom SR. Guar sprinkled on food: effect on glycaemic control, plasma lipids, and gut hormones in non-insulin

dependent diabetic patients. *Diabetic Med* 1987;**44**:63–8. (Study of 18 patients with non-insulin dependent diabetes; showed that guar granules sprinkled on food had useful effect on postprandial glycaemia and other variables.)

8 Hillebrand I. Pharmacological modification of digestion and absorption. *Diabetic Med* 1987;**4**:147–50. (Review of the pharmacology of α glucosidase inhibitors and their clinical use.)

9 Multicentre study. UK prospective diabetes study. II. Reduction in HbA_{1c} with basal insulin supplement, sulphonylurea, or biguanide therapy in maturity-onset diabetes. *Diabetes* 1985;**34**:793–8. (Very useful interim analysis of the UK Prospective Diabetes Study containing data about the different effects of diet, sulphonylureas, metformin, and insulin in non-insulin dependent diabetes.)

10 Groop L, Schalin C, Franssila-Kallunki A, Widen E, Ekstrand A, Eriksson J. Characteristics of non-insulin dependent diabetic patients with secondary failure to oral antidiabetic therapy. *Am J Med* 1989;**87**:183–90. (Detailed analysis of metabolic aspects of secondary sulphonylurea failure.)

11 Gerich JE. Oral hypoglycaemic agents. *N Engl J Med* 1989;**321**:1231–45. (Comprehensive review of sulphonylureas and metformin.)

12 Beck-Nielson H, Hother-Nielson O, Pedersen O. Mechanism of action of sulphonylureas with special reference to the extrapancreatic effects: an overview. *Diabetic Med* 1988;**5**:613–20. (Useful review article concentrating on the various potential extrapancreatic sites of action of sulphonylureas and clinical implications.)

13 Hosker JP, Burnett MA, Davies EG, Turner RC. Sulphonylurea therapy doubles β cell response to glucose in Type II diabetic patients. *Diabetologia* 1985;**28**:809–14.

14 Ferner RE, Neil HAW. Sulphonylureas and hypoglycaemia (Editorial). *BMJ* 1988;**296**:949–50. (Summarises current information on incidence, severity, causes, and management of hypoglycaemia due to sulphonylureas.)

15 Pugh JA, Wagner ML, Sawyer J, Rameris G, Tuley M, Friedberg SJ. Is combination sulphonylurea and insulin therapy useful in NIDDM patients? A meta-analysis. *Diabetes Care* 1992;**15**:953–9.

16 Bailey CJ. Biguanides in NIDDM. *Diabetes Care* 1992;**15**:775–82. (A detailed and current review of biguanides and their use in non-insulin dependent diabetes.)

17 Foley JE. Rationale and application of fatty acid oxidation inhibitor treatment of diabetes mellitus. *Diabetes Care* 1992;**15**:773–84.

18 Jones IR, Swai A, Taylor R, Miller M, Laker MF, Alberti KGMM. Lowering of plasma glucose concentrations with bezafibrate in patients with moderately controlled NIDDM. *Diabetes Care* 1990;**13**:855–63.

19 Hoffman CA, Colca JR. New oral thiazolidinedione antidiabetic agents as insulin sensitisers. *Diabetes Care* 1992;**15**:1075–8. (Brief review of this new class of antidiabetic drug.)

21 Vitamin D metabolites and analogues, bisphosphonates, and other endocrine drugs

COLIN R PATERSON, JOHN FEELY

One consequence of our increased understanding of the physiology of vitamin D has been the development of considerably more potent analogues for the treatment of hypoparathyroidism and the bone disease of renal failure. The treatment of symptomatic patients with Paget's disease of bone with calcitonin and etidronate has been augmented with the availability of the new bisphosphonates. These newer drugs have also proved valuable in the management of the hypercalcaemia of malignant disease. One bisphosphonate, etidronate, has become available for use in a cyclical régime in certain patients with osteoporotic fractures of vertebrae.

Vitamin D analogues and metabolites

Vitamin D (calciferol) is the precursor for the production by the kidney of a hormone, calcitriol (1,25-dihydroxycholecalciferol), which is responsible for active calcium absorption in the gut. Calcitriol (Rocaltrol) is effective in promoting calcium absorption and raising the plasma calcium concentrations in patients whose endogenous calcitriol production is impaired. This is the case in renal failure, in hypoparathyroidism (parathyroid hormone is required for the 1-hydroxylation step in vitamin D metabolism), and in one form of a rare inherited disorder, vitamin D dependent rickets. In these disorders calcitriol is effective in microgram doses compared with the milligram doses needed with native vitamin D.

A useful analogue of calcitriol is alfacalcidol, 1α-hydroxycholecalciferol (One-alpha). This is hydroxylated at the 25 position in the liver to give calcitriol; as with calcitriol, microgram doses are effective in patients with hypoparathyroidism or with renal failure. Both drugs increase the plasma calcium concentration in a few days in patients newly diagnosed as having hypoparathyroidism.

The speed of action of calcitriol and alfacalcidol is an advantage compared with that of calciferol itself, but this very speed may contribute to the ease with which patients can be poisoned by unwary doctors. As with poisoning with vitamin D, hypercalcaemia may cause permanent renal damage and soft tissue calcification. All patients taking these preparations must have regular checks of their serum calcium concentrations. As the half life of calcitriol in the plasma is about 3 h, appreciable fluctuations in plasma calcium concentrations are likely to occur; for most patients alfacalcidol is the preparation of choice.

CHRONIC RENAL FAILURE

Some patients with chronic renal failure have bone pain, muscle weakness, increased plasma alkaline phosphatase activity, and histological evidence of osteomalacia, all of which are due largely to a failure to produce calcitriol from calciferol. Symptomatic relief in such cases can be obtained with microgram doses of calcitriol or alfacalcidol. In childhood growth may improve. Calciferol itself is no longer used in renal failure because of its long half life and the fact that, if toxicity occurs, hypercalcaemia may persist for weeks. Calcitriol and alfacalcidol, however, may also readily cause hypercalcaemia and several reports have indicated that, even without hypercalcaemia, these drugs may be associated with increased loss of renal function. For these reasons caution is needed in managing patients with skeletal symptoms.

The place of any of these drugs in managing symptomless patients not undergoing dialysis is uncertain. Symptomless patients already undergoing haemodialysis, and who have radiological and biochemical evidence of osteodystrophy (subperiosteal erosions and increased plasma alkaline phosphatase activity), respond to treatment with alfacalcidol within a year, but hypercalcaemia is common and difficult to prevent. Long term treatment is less effective; the bone disease in some patients worsens despite continuing treatment. Secondary hyperparathyroidism may be prevented in patients with normal hand radiographs who are undergoing regular haemodialysis by giving small doses (0·25–0·5 µg a day) of calcitriol.

HYPOPARATHYROIDISM

The newer preparations, particularly alfacalcidol, are indicated for the initial treatment of symptomatic patients in whom speed in correcting the hypocalcaemia is needed. For patients already well controlled with calciferol no change should be made; the long half life of calciferol in the tissues means that, if a patient has to be transferred from calciferol to alfacalcidol, there should be a gap of perhaps 1 month without treatment followed by cautious and carefully monitored introduction of alfacalcidol in an initial dose of 0·5 µg daily.

Satisfactory results in long term management are obtained with calciferol, dihydrotachysterol, or alfacalcidol. With all three drugs constant vigilance—including estimating serum calcium concentrations at least every 4 months—is essential. More frequent checks are needed during, and just after, pregnancy and it is particularly important that serum albumin is taken into account when serum calcium concentrations are measured. Calciferol and its metabolites are passed into breast milk and breast feeding is generally not advisable. Glucocorticoid treatment may alter greatly the therapeutic dose of calciferol or alfacalcidol.

OSTEOMALACIA AND RICKETS

Calcitriol and alfacalcidol are not indicated for treating nutritional osteomalacia or rickets. Vitamin D, either by mouth or by a single depot injection of 7·5 or 15 mg, remains the best drug; this dose should not be repeated more often than once every 6 months. In patients with osteomalacia caused by malabsorption (including patients with long standing obstructive jaundice) parenteral vitamin D, with a single depot injection every 6–12 months, is indicated if the malabsorption cannot be relieved.

In patients with X linked hypophosphataemic rickets the most common form of rickets resistant to vitamin D, the best treatment is currently phosphate supplements together with either calcitriol at a dose of 0·25–1·0 µg a day or alfacalcidol at a similar range of doses. One form of vitamin D dependent rickets is caused by deficiency of 1α-hydroxylase, and the disorder is fully corrected by administering calcitriol 1–2 µg a day.

Bisphosphonates

The bisphosphonates (formerly diphosphonates) are a group of analogues of pyrophosphate that are adsorbed on to hydroxyapatite crystals and inhibit bone resorption and formation. The only bisphosphonates currently marketed are etidronate disodium (Didronel, formerly EHDP), pamidronate disodium (Aredia, formerly APD) and sodium clodronate (Bonefos, Loron). These drugs have a definite role in the management of symptomatic Paget's disease of bone and in the control of hypercalcaemia of malignancy. They may have a place in the treatment of some patients with osteoporosis.

PAGET'S DISEASE OF BONE

No case exists for giving bisphosphonates (or calcitonin) to symptomless patients with Paget's disease. The patients for whom medical treatment is most clearly indicated are those with bone pain (particularly if the serum alkaline phosphatase activity is appreciably increased) and those with progressive neurological impairment. In some cases bone pain due to Paget's disease may be indistinguishable from that due to osteoarthropathy. In such cases a trial of treatment is appropriate. Treatment with etidronate should be stopped if the symptoms have not started to resolve within 2 months.

The usual dose of etidronate is 5–10 mg/kg/day continuing, if a symptomatic or biochemical response is seen, for about 6 months. Higher doses of about 20 mg/kg/day are also effective if given for 1 month only; more prolonged treatment with such doses may be associated with troublesome side effects such as bone pain and spontaneous fractures. With either regimen prolonged remissions may follow a single course.

Only 5% of etidronate is absorbed from the intestine, the remainder being excreted in the faeces. Absorption is impaired by food, particularly foodstuffs containing calcium and antacids, so the drug is best given once a day while fasting (such as at bedtime). The drug is rapidly removed from the blood by renal excretion and adsorption on to bone surfaces. Etidronate should not be given to patients with renal failure or enterocolitis. In some patients nausea or diarrhoea can occur as side effects. Bisphosphonates other than etidronate are not yet licensed in the United Kingdom for treating Paget's disease, but intravenous pamidronate and oral clodronate appear to be effective.

Most patients with symptomatic Paget's disease of bone should be treated in the first instance with oral etidronate. Patients with predominantly lytic Paget's disease, however, and those with fractures and infractions, are probably best treated with salmon calcitonin (salcatonin, Calsynar, Miacalcic) at an initial dose of 100 units a day. With calcitonin most patients have a symptomatic response, but some suffer relapse even while treatment continues. Remissions after a course of calcitonin may be short, and maintenance treatment (often 100 units a week) may be helpful. Calcitonin is more expensive than etidronate and must be given by injection. Flushing occurs after injections in about a quarter of the patients.

HYPERCALCAEMIA OF MALIGNANT DISEASE

As many patients with severe hypercalcaemia are depleted of sodium and water, the first line of management in such cases consists of rehydration, generally with saline. Various drugs of limited value, including calcitonin, glucocorticoids, mithramycin and phosphate, have been used in the past. In recent years the management of these patients has been transformed by the availability of the newer bisphosphonates (notably pamidronate and clodronate). These drugs are given, initially at least, by infusion but clodronate is also available in an oral preparation for maintenance therapy.

Pamidronate can be given as a single infusion of 30 mg in not less than 250 ml saline over 4 h. Larger doses or repeated infusions may be needed for severe or persistent hypercalcaemia. Serum calcium concentrations fall after about 24 h and may remain low for many days after a single infusion.

Clodronate is administered as daily intravenous infusions of 300 mg in at least 500 ml saline over at least 2 h. These are continued until the serum calcium is normal, usually between 3 and 5 days. The oral maintenance therapy is generally with 800 mg twice daily; as with etidronate it is important that this is taken at least 2 h before and 2 h after meals.

OSTEOPOROSIS

Etidronate has recently become available in a cyclical regimen also including calcium supplements (Didronel PMO) for the management of patients with established vertebral fractures. This leads to a small decrease in vertebral fracture rate and a modest increase in bone density. The overall value of this treatment remains controversial and there is no evidence to support its continuation for more than 3 years. The treatment has not been shown to prevent fractures of the peripheral skeleton. Its main indication is thought to be the management of patients with one or two symptomatic vertebral crush fractures to diminish the chance of further fractures. The long term effects of this regimen are not known, and for patients in whom hormone replacement therapy is appropriate this is to be preferred.

Other endocrine drugs

Experience with bromocriptine confirms its place in the treatment of the prolactinomas, and its list of indications includes parkinsonism and the suppression of lactation. The medical treatment of endometriosis has advanced recently with the use of danazol, gestrinone and gonadorelin analogues, which may be given to suppress gonadal function.

Danazol

Danazol (Danol) is a synthetic steroid, a derivative of ethisterone, which suppresses the hypothalamic–pituitary–ovarian axis by inhibiting the output of gonadotrophins from the pituitary. It may also act by inhibiting the binding of sex steroids to cellular receptors and has therefore been used to reduce hormonal stimulation of the endometrium and breasts in endometriosis and cystic disease respectively. Although expensive, it is an effective form of medical treatment for endometriosis as it acts partly by temporarily suppressing gonadal function. Side effects are common and predictable in view of its androgenic and anabolic activity.

Danazol is well absorbed and peak concentrations occur after 2 hours. It is metabolised in the liver and excreted in bile and urine. As with many hormones, the half life of its biological activity does not correlate with the plasma half life, and it should be given two to four times a day.

ENDOMETRIOSIS

When endometriosis is treated with danazol dysmenorrhoea is usually the first symptom to be relieved as menstruation is suppressed: relief of pain and dyspareunia occurs in over 75% of patients within 3 months. Increased conception rates may possibly follow treatment with danazol in infertile women with endometriosis. Those with severe or ovarian endometriosis do not have a complete response, but danazol is still valuable if given before and after operation to promote healing of some lesions and to limit the extent of the operation. After treatment the average annual recurrence rate is about 15%. Most patients with mild to moderate disease have a prolonged remission, and second courses of treatment may be given if necessary. Dosage (200–800 mg a day) depends on the severity of the condition. Treatment should be started on the first day of a menstrual cycle to reduce the risk of irregular bleeding and unrecognised pregnancy. The initial daily dose is 400–600 mg; this is reduced monthly to 200 mg (or to a higher figure if amenorrhoea is not maintained). Treatment is continued for 6 months in patients with mild disease and up to a year in those with severe disease.

MENORRHAGIA

Danazol appreciably reduces blood loss in the first month, producing amenorrhoea usually by the third month of treatment. Long term treatment with 200 mg a day commonly reduces menstrual loss to acceptable amounts with continuing menstruation in most patients. In most patients an effect continues for some months after treatment has been stopped.

FIBROADENOSIS OF THE BREAST

More than 75% of patients with cyclical symptoms in fibroadenosis (or mammary dysplasia—painful nodular benign breast disease) respond to treatment with danazol. Pain, tenderness, and premenstrual engorgement are relieved or abolished within 3 months of starting treatment (usually 400 mg a day reducing to 200 mg a day after 1 or 2 months). Nodularity usually reduces within 6 months. Some patients have a prolonged remission after the end of treatment. The possibility of coexisting malignant disease of the breast should be borne in mind. At present treatment is usually given only to patients with severe symptoms.

OTHER USES

Danazol has proved valuable in managing gynaecomastia in men for whom underlying causes have been excluded. In about two thirds of such patients a dose of 200–600 mg a day relieves the severe and painful symptoms. Danazol has also been used in precocious puberty but has largely been superseded by gonadotrophin releasing hormones. It has proved effective in preventing attacks in patients with hereditary angioneurotic oedema by increasing the synthesis of the complement (C1) esterase inhibitor.

PRECAUTIONS

The successful alleviation of endometriosis and dyspareunia is commonly followed by pregnancy after treatment with danazol has been stopped. Pregnancy should be excluded before danazol is given, as pronounced virilisation of daughters of women given the drug during pregnancy has been reported. It should be used with caution in patients with impaired cardiac, hepatic, or renal function and in patients with other conditions that may be affected adversely by fluid retention—such as epilepsy and migraine. A firm diagnosis and exclusion of malignant disease, particularly in patients with abnormal uterine bleeding, are essential. Until more is known about the long term effects of this agent, treatment should be for the shortest possible time.

ADVERSE EFFECTS

Many of the adverse effects are androgenic in nature and are reversed after treatment has stopped. Weight gain of 1–4 kg occurs in most patients; other common side effects include acne, seborrhoea, decreased breast size, irregular vaginal bleeding, and mild hirsutism. Muscle cramps affect up to a third of patients, and menopausal symptoms, nausea, and rashes occur occasionally. Thrombocytopenia has been reported rarely. Danazol may inhibit the metabolism of some drugs, which may lead to potentiation of the effect of oral anticoagulants or to increased plasma concentrations of carbamazepine and cyclosporin. Side effects are largely dose related and are seldom a problem in patients taking only 200 mg a day.

GESTRINONE

This synthetic steroid (Dimetriose) has similar androgenic, antioestrogenic and antiprogesteronic effects to those of danazol and is also used (2·5 mg twice weekly) in endometriosis. If two or more

293

doses are missed treatment should be discontinued. It may be recommenced following a negative pregnancy test again on the first day of a cycle. Precautions and adverse effects are similar to those for danazol.

ALTERNATIVES TO DANAZOL AND GESTRINONE

Many patients who present with menorrhagia are successfully managed with oral contraceptives or non-steroidal anti-inflammatory drugs, a combination of both, or a progestogen such as norethisterone.

Gonadotrophin releasing hormone analogues

Gonadotrophin releasing hormone agonists or their analogues initially stimulate the release of luteinising hormone, but subsequently inhibit its release during long term (weeks) treatment by desensitising the pituitary. The consequent suppression of sex hormone has been exploited, for example in treating metastatic prostatic cancer by suppressing testosterone. This "medical castration" also underlies the use of these drugs for endometriosis and fibroadenosis of the breast. A number of analogues are now available. Because they are inactivated when taken by mouth delivery is by nasal spray (buserelin and narfarelin) or depot subcutaneous injections (goserelin and leuprorelin). Buserelin (Suprecur) is given as 150 µg into each nostril three times daily while goserelin (Zoladex 3·6 mg) is given subcutaneously into the anterior abdominal wall every 4 weeks. Pregnancy and vaginal bleeding of unknown origin should be excluded before starting therapy. Results to date indicate that these agents are as effective as danazol. As would be expected, adverse effects include hot flushes, diminished libido, and vaginal dryness (hot flushes are more common with depot preparations). Whether osteoporosis is more common during long term treatment remains to be seen, as density of the spine and femoral head fall by about 2% after 6 months' treatment. The results of further, especially comparative, studies are awaited, but efficacy of these hormones seems similar to that of danazol and adverse effects are fewer.

Depot preparations are also used to treat metastatic cancer of the prostate. They prevent androgenic stimulation of the tumour cells and are as effective as bilateral orchidectomy or stilboestrol administration. However, an initial stimulation of testosterone secretion, with a tumour "flare", precedes inhibition, so an antiandrogen such as flutamide should be commenced 3 days before the gonadorelin analogue is administered.

Bromocriptine

Bromocriptine (Parlodel) is an ergot alkaloid, a derivative of lysergic acid that acts as a dopamine agonist. It inhibits both basal and stimulated prolactin secretion from the pituitary. It has some less specific dopamine like actions in other areas in the central nervous system (basal ganglia and vomiting centre) and in blood vessels. These actions underlie the drug's use in Parkinson's disease and explain some of its common side effects such as nausea and hypotension. Bromocriptine is well absorbed and peak concentrations occur after 2 h. It is almost completely metabolised in the liver and excreted in the bile. The effect of a single dose lasts 6–8 h. The use of frequent small doses reduces side effects that are associated with high peak concentrations.

INHIBITION OF LACTATION

Given less than 12 h postpartum bromocriptine (2·5 mg) prevents lactation, without pain or breast engorgement, and restores prolactin to normal concentrations within 48 h. It is superior to all other methods of suppressing lactation, including oestrogens, but is considerably more expensive. Unlike oestrogens, it is also effective in suppressing established lactation and breast engorgement. Bromocriptine (2·5 mg with meals) is usually given twice a day for 2 weeks. Patients should be advised that fertility is rapidly restored: the first ovulation is likely within 4 weeks of delivery, and suitable contraceptives may be needed before the patient leaves hospital.

HYPERPROLACTINAEMIA

This is an important cause of anovulatory infertility, although the mechanism is not fully understood. A few patients with hyperprolactinaemia also have galactorrhoea. If hyperprolactinaemia due to other causes—for example, drugs such as phenothiazine and methyldopa—is excluded the most probable explanation is a chromophobe adenoma of the anterior pituitary. In women this is commonly a microadenoma and may show no sign of local expansion; in men the usual finding is an adenoma large enough to be visible on radiography and causing low gonadotrophin concentrations, hypogonadism, and infertility. Bromocriptine (usually 5–7·5 mg a day) rapidly restores prolactin concentrations to normal, and ovulatory menstruation returns irrespective of the size of the tumour. Some evidence exists that tumours may shrink, particularly in men. Although bromocriptine seems to have no undesirable effects on the outcome of subsequent pregnancies, patients require close supervision as the tumour may expand greatly during pregnancy. Many patients with prolactin secreting tumours have been controlled effectively for several years, but the clinical course and outcome with long term treatment are not known. Patients should be monitored for pituitary enlargement and have gynaecological examination at least yearly. In general, bromocriptine has no established place in managing patients with infertility or impotence if there is no evidence of hyperprolactinaemia.

PARKINSONISM

The overall efficacy of bromocriptine in parkinsonism is similar to that of levodopa (plus decarboxylase inhibitor); few patients who are unresponsive to levodopa respond to bromocriptine. Although the effect of a single dose lasts longer, bromocriptine must be used in high doses (increasing gradually to 10–30 mg three times a day), is more expensive, and has no particular advantages over levodopa. Bromocriptine is usually restricted to patients who have intractable nausea or vomiting with levodopa (nausea with bromocriptine is usually less severe) or to those who show intolerable swings in response (on–off, end of dose akinesia), which often occur after several years' treatment with levodopa. Bromocriptine has two side effects that are largely confined to patients with parkinsonism; dyskinesia (orofacial grimacing and chorea), and hallucinations, particularly visual. The hallucinations may be related to the lysergic acid component of the molecule and may be accompanied by confusion and paranoid delusions.

Two other new dopaminergic drugs—pergolide (Celance) and lysuride (Revanil)—may be used in place of bromocriptine, but all have a similar propensity to cause adverse reactions. Pergolide has a longer duration of effect and may produce a greater reduction in "off" time and end of dose effects than bromocriptine in some patients.

ACROMEGALY

Bromocriptine causes a paradoxical lowering of growth hormone concentrations in most patients with acromegaly. Initial enthusiasm for its use in acromegaly has waned, as the suppression of growth hormone is rarely complete; most patients show only a partial clinical response and then only with doses as high as 20–60 mg a day. It is mainly used for patients who are unsuitable for transsphenoidal operations, as an adjunct to irradiation while awaiting response, and when these forms of treatment have been only partially effective.

Octreotide (Sandostatin) is a synthetic analogue of somastatin, the hypothalamic growth hormone release inhibiting hormone. In preliminary studies it appears considerably more effective than bromocriptine at reducing growth hormone levels. Octreotide is also used to treat gastrointestinal endocrine tumours such as carcinoid and VIPomas. Apart from a transient local reaction at the site of injection, gastrointestinal disturbances and glucose intolerance are the most common adverse effects.

OTHER USES

The use of bromocriptine for conditions such as premenstrual tension, mastalgia, and chronic hepatic encephalopathy has not been firmly established. Patients with benign breast disease who show a cyclical pain pattern may respond to 1·25 mg at bedtime or 2·5 mg twice a day. Bromocriptine does not, however, seem to be quite as effective as danazol for this condition.

ADVERSE EFFECTS

Nausea is a particularly common side effect, and vomiting may occasionally limit the usefulness of bromocriptine. In most patients, however, these symptoms may be prevented by taking the drug with meals and beginning with a low (1·25 mg) dose, which is increased gradually over some days to weeks. Dizziness, postural hypotension, and constipation are other common side effects. Hypotensive reactions may on occasion be severe during the first few days of treatment, and patients operating machinery should be advised accordingly. Gastrointestinal haemorrhage rarely occurs in patients taking high doses (over 10 mg a day) but seems more common in acromegalic patients. Neuropsychiatric side effects are uncommon except in patients with Parkinson's disease.

Other drugs used for parkinsonism

LEVODOPA

Usually given with a peripheral dopa-decarboxylase inhibitor, levodopa remains the best drug for disabled patients. Bromocriptine is reserved for patients who cannot tolerate or have been resistant to levodopa.

SELEGILINE (Eldepryl)

This is a selective inhibitor of monoamine oxidase B and thus reduces the breakdown of dopamine in the brain only. It may also inhibit the re-uptake of dopamine into neurones and exerts a neuroprotective effect. Its main use has been in conjunction with levodopa, when it is particularly useful in reducing "end of dose" deterioration and "off" time by about two thirds. This benefit diminishes after treatment for 1–2 years, but recent studies suggest that selegiline may slow the progression of disease and possibly increase life expectancy for these patients. Some authorities advocate commencing all patients on selegiline (10 mg daily) when the diagnosis is made and continue for as long as possible, introducing levodopa only when symptoms become disabling.

The adverse effects, particularly gastrointestinal, of levodopa may be more pronounced with combined treatment, and the dose of levodopa may need to be reduced. Nausea, vomiting, and dizziness (sometimes with hypotension) occur in up to 20% of patients. Abdominal pain, insomnia, agitation, and confusion may also occur. Dosage is usually 10 mg a day. Selegiline will represent a major advance in the treatment of parkinsonism if the effect on disease progression is confirmed.

Anonymous. Danazol—good mainly for endometriosis. *Drug Ther Bull* 1990;**28**:22–3.

Anonymous. Gonadotrophin releasing hormone analogues for endometriosis. *Drug Ther Bull* 1993;**31**:21–2.

Baker LRI. Prevention of renal osteodystrophy. *Miner Electrolyte Metab* 1991;**17**:240–9.

Burns J, Paterson CR. Single dose vitamin D treatment for osteomalacia in the elderly. *BMJ* 1985;**290**:280–2.

Calne DB. Treatment of Parkinson's Disease. *N Engl J Med* 1993;**329**:1021–7.

Cedarbaum JM. Clinical pharmacokinetics of antiparkinsonian drugs. *Clin Pharmacokinet* 1987;**13**:141–78.

Christiansen C. Hormone replacement and its impact on osteoporosis. *Baillière's Clin Obstet Gynaecol* 1991;**5**:785–960.

Clough CG. Parkinson's disease: Management. *Lancet* 1991;**337**:1324–7.

Delmez JA, Slatopolsky E. Recent advances in the pathogenesis and therapy of uremic secondary hyperparathyroidism. *J Clin Endocrinol Metab* 1991;**72**:735–9.

Dmowski WP. Endocrine properties and clinical application of danazol. *Fertil Steril* 1979;**31**:237–51. (Comprehensive review of basic pharmacology and endocrine effects of danazol. Selection of patients and practical application of treatment are discussed.)

Fraser HM, Waxman J. Gonadotrophin releasing hormone analogues for gynaecological disorders and infertility. *BMJ* 1989;**298**:475–6.

Gateley CA, Mansel RE. Management of cyclic breast pain. *Br J Hosp Med* 1990;**43**:330–2.

Heath DA. Treatment of hypercalcaemia of malignancy. *Baillière's Clin Endocrinol Metab* 1990;**4**:139–45.

Hosking DJ. Advances in the management of Paget's disease of bone. *Drugs* 1990;**40**:829–40.

Mansel RE, Dogliotti L. European multicentre trial of bromocriptine in cyclic mastalgia. *Lancet* 1990;**335**:190–3. (Superiority over placebo established but 29% dropped out while receiving treatment.)

Mansel RE, Wisbey JR, Hughes LE. Controlled trial of antigonadotrophine danazol in painful nodular benign breast disease. *Lancet* 1982;**i**:928–30. (Double blind study reporting objective and subjective improvement and suggesting that 200 mg a day is adequate for most patients.)

Melmed S. Acromegaly. *N Engl J Med* 1990;**332**:966–77.

Parkinson Study Group. Effect of deprenyl on the progression of disability in early Parkinson's disease. *N Engl J Med* 1989;**321**:1364–71. (Deprenyl (selegiline 10 mg) delayed the onset of disability necessitating treatment with levodopa and reduced the risk of having to give up full time employment.)

Paterson CR. Rational prescribing for osteoporosis. *Update* 1993;**46**:909–18.

Russell RGG, Kanis JA. *Tumour-induced hypercalcaemia and its management*. Royal Society of Medicine, 1991.

Weinerman SA, Bockman RS. Medical therapy of osteoporosis. *Orthop Clin N Am* 1990;**21**:109–23.

22 Lipid lowering drugs

PATRICIA O'CONNOR, JOHN FEELY,
JAMES SHEPHERD

Background

Atherosclerotic vascular disease, particularly of coronary arteries, is the main cause of disability and death in the western world. Considerable epidemiological data now establish a direct relation between increased total plasma cholesterol concentrations and the development of atherosclerosis. A similar link has been shown for raised concentrations of individual atherogenic lipoproteins, in particular the low density lipoprotein (LDL) fraction.[1 2] In contrast, a strong inverse relation has been found between high density lipoprotein (HDL) cholesterol concentrations and the risk of coronary heart disease.[3 4] Although it is not certain whether increased triglycerides are an independent risk factor,[5] high concentrations are usually accompanied by low concentrations of HDL, and this may be their link with coronary risk.

Many studies have shown convincingly that dietary and drug induced reductions in cholesterol concentrations are associated with a lower risk of developing coronary heart disease.[6] Evidence also exists not only of a decrease in the rate of progression of atherosclerosis in patients with established disease, especially of the coronary arteries, but also of regression when steps are taken to reduce plasma cholesterol concentrations.[7 8] Regression of xanthomas is commonly seen when patients with familial hypercholesterolaemia have their cholesterol concentrations lowered by drug treatment.[9]

Increasing awareness in doctors and the general population that high plasma cholesterol concentrations are a risk factor for developing coronary heart disease has led to screening for risk factors in the population at large, rather than focusing exclusively on people with established heart disease or a family history of hyperlipidaemia, diabetes, or other conditions related to atherosclerosis.

Hypercholesterolaemia is common and up to a quarter of the British population have total plasma cholesterol concentrations higher than 6·5 mmol/l.[10] British,[11] European,[12] and American[13] expert panels all agree on an ideal total plasma cholesterol concentration of 5·2 mmol/l or less and that people with consistently raised plasma cholesterol concentrations should be treated, especially if other risk factors exist; they have produced comprehensive management guidelines.[11-13]

Triglycerides have a more tenuous link with atherosclerosis. Recurrent acute pancreatitis, however, is a recognised complication of severe hypertriglyceridaemia (> 10 mmol/l) associated with chylomicronaemia. Current recommendations are to maintain total triglyceride concentrations at 2·3 mmol/l or less.[12]

Secondary hyperlipidaemia should be excluded from the diagnoses of all patients presenting with hyperlipidaemia. The more common causative conditions include diabetes, hypothyroidism, and kidney disease. Drug treatment with thiazides, β blockers, oestrogens, or retinoids may also have an adverse effect on serum lipids, and a heavy alcohol intake may raise plasma triglyceride concentrations.

Plasma lipids and lipoproteins

The main lipids are cholesterol, triglyceride, and phospholipids. They are rendered water soluble by their association in macromolecular complexes with proteins formed in the liver and intestine—apolipoproteins. These apolipoproteins are also important as markers for lipid particle recognition by specific receptors in peripheral tissue and particularly on the surfaces of liver cells. This function is highlighted by LDL, the cell uptake and subsequent catabolism of which depends on the interaction of its apolipoprotein (apoprotein B) with specific cell membrane receptors.[14] Three other main lipoprotein fractions exist, which contain varying amounts of cholesterol and triglyceride (table 22.1). High plasma concentrations of these lipoproteins, singly or in combination, form the basis of the Fredrickson classification of hyperlipoproteinaemia. While somewhat outdated, this classification retains some diagnostic and therapeutic usefulness.

Figure 22.1 shows the metabolic interrelation of the plasma lipoproteins. Each day the average Briton eats 120 g of triglyceride and 500 mg of cholesterol. In the intestine these dietary lipids are packaged into large triglyceride rich chylomicrons, which are released into the systemic circulation via the thoracic duct. In the

TABLE 22.1—*Classification (Fredrickson) and characteristics of dyslipidaemias*

Plasmal lipid	Fredrickson type					
	I	IIa	IIb	III	IV	V
Triglyceride	+ + +	N	+ +	+ +	+ +	+ + +
Cholesterol	+	+ +	+ +	+	N/+	+
Lipoproteins raised	Chylomicrons	LDL	LDL VLDL	VLDL remnants Chylomicron remnants	VLDL	VLDL chylomicrons and their remnants

N = Normal; + = mildly raised; + + = moderately raised; + + + = severely raised concentrations.
LDL = Low density lipoprotein; VLDL = Very low density lipoprotein.

bloodstream they are hydrolysed by lipoprotein lipase, which releases triglycerides and generates chylomicron remnants that are taken up by receptors on liver cells. This process of exogenous fat metabolism may contribute to HDL formation. Triglycerides are broken down into free fatty acids and provide an important source of energy. Cholesterol is essential for cell membrane function and synthesis of myelin sheaths and steroid hormones. Most cells can synthesise cholesterol from acetate, and the bulk of cholesterol synthesis and its catabolism takes place mainly in the liver. The enzyme hydroxymethylglutaryl coenzyme A reductase limits the rate of cholesterol biosynthesis, switching on if there is intracellular deficiency and off when stores are replete. Further intake of cholesterol from the bloodstream into cholesterol replete cells can also be regulated by modulating the number of uptake sites (LDL receptors), which are primarily on liver cell membranes.

In the fasting state endogenously produced triglycerides and cholesterol are transported by very low density lipoproteins (VLDL), which are produced by the liver and secreted into the bloodstream. These are predominantly rich in triglyceride. Lipoprotein lipase hydrolyses most of the VLDL triglyceride to form progressively smaller lipoprotein particles called intermediate density lipoproteins (IDL) and ultimately LDL, which contain an increasing percentage of lipids as cholesterol. Some LDL may also be secreted directly by the hepatocytes. Apolipoprotein B100 is the dominant apoprotein on these particles.

LDL is catabolised by two pathways:

1. the major route is via a hepatic and peripheral cell high affinity receptor mediated mechanism[14] that, as noted above, may

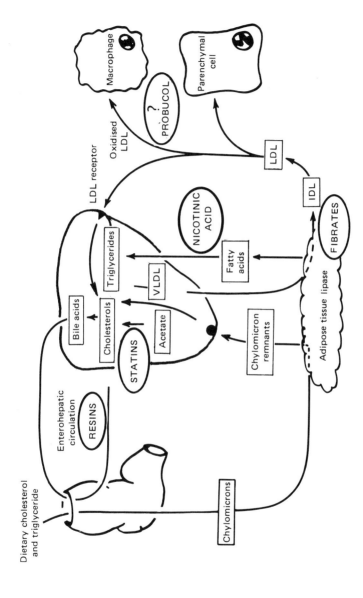

FIG 22.1—Pharmacological modulation of lipoprotein metabolism (LDL = Low density lipoprotein, VLDL = very low density lipoprotein, IDL = intermediate density lipoprotein, HDL = high density lipoprotein. Statins = Inhibitors of hydroxymethylglutaryl coenzyme A reductase.)

be suppressed by the endogenous cellular production of cholesterol; and

2. a minor pathway, via scavenger receptors that are present on macrophages and smooth muscle cells. These receptors take up oxidatively modified LDL and become atheromatous foam cells.

Patients with heterozygous familial hypercholesterolaemia have about half the normal high affinity LDL receptor activity. This consequently limits the receptor mediated liver and peripheral tissue uptake of LDL, which leads to a pronounced rise in total plasma cholesterol concentrations, often to above 10 mmol/l. This accumulated lipoprotein becomes oxidised and is channelled into scavenger macrophages that form foam cells, which contribute to premature atherosclerosis. People with the more rare homozygous familial hypercholesterolaemia are even more incapacitated. As they have essentially no high affinity LDL receptors, they develop very high concentrations of LDL and malignant atherosclerosis in early childhood, and children younger than 10 years occasionally present with myocardial infarction. When LDL is present in excess, some passes through vascular endothelium into the subendothelial space. Monocytes are attracted, particularly if the LDL particles are oxidised, and by engulfing oxidised LDL particles become scavenger macrophages that soon become fat laden foam cells, unable to migrate from the space. They accumulate to form a fatty streak that, when the endothelium layer is breached, forms the basis of an atheromatous plaque.

HDL particles are derived from the liver and intestine during the lipolysis of chylomicrons. A key role of HDL seems to be the reverse transport of cholesterol from peripheral tissues to the liver for subsequent catabolism. This activity is presumably the basis of its antiatherogenic function.

Recent drug development has exploited this fundamental understanding of lipid metabolism with a view to interrupting the pathway at a number of specific sites. Interruption at more than one site forms the basis of combined treatment for more resistant patients (figure 22.1).

Treatment of hyperlipidaemia

The first line treatment of all patients with hyperlipidaemia is generally agreed to be diet and weight control.[12] [13] Such nonpharmacological measures should be continued for several months before considering adding drugs. Concentrations of cholesterol, triglyceride, or both, can be lowered adequately by diet alone in many patients. Some people, however, particularly those with severe hyperlipidaemia, may not respond adequately to dietary intervention. Lipid lowering treatment should be considered only after adequate dietary control has failed (if plasma cholesterol concentrations are higher than 6·5 mmol/l) and is particularly important in people with established coronary heart disease or at enhanced risk of developing the condition because of other risk factors like hypertension or cigarette smoking. Dietary measures should always be continued hand in hand with drugs if they are used.

Drug choice

The dominant abnormality (raised plasma concentrations of cholesterol or triglycerides, or both) usually determines the primary choice of treatment (table 22.2). In some patients combination treatment with small doses of two drugs is more efficacious and causes fewer adverse reactions than the full dose of a single agent.

Table 22.3 shows the main groups of lipid lowering drugs currently available.

TABLE 22.2—*Drug treatment for hyperlipidaemia*

Plasma lipid raised	Lipoprotein accumulation (Fredrickson type)	Treatment		
		First line	Second line	Preferred combination
Cholesterol	LDL (type IIa)	Resin	Statin or nicotinic acid	Resin and statin or resin and nicotinic acid
Triglyceride	VLDL (type IV) Chylomicrons and VLDL (type V)	Fibrate	Nicotinic acid	Fibrate first then add resin or nicotinic acid first then add resin
Cholesterol and triglyceride	(a) VLDL and LDL (type IIb)	Fibrate	Nicotinic acid or statin	Resin and nicotinic acid or resin and fibrate or resin and statin
	(b) VLDL remnants and chylomicron remnants (type III)	Fibrate	Nicotinic acid	—

LDL = Low density lipoprotein; VLDL = Very low density lipoprotein.

TABLE 22.3—*Lipid lowering drugs*

Generic (proprietary) names	Usual change in:		Patient acceptability	Long term safety
	Cholesterol	Triglycerides		
Bile acid binding resins				
Cholestyramine (Questran)	Down 15–30%	Up 5–15%	Poor	Established
Colestipol (Colestid)	Down 15–30%	Up 5–15%		
Fibrates				
Clofibrate (Atromid-S)	Down 5–15%	Down 15–30%	Good	Gall stones
Bezafibrate (Bezalip)	Down 5–15%	Down > 30%		
Gemfibrozil (Lopid)	Down 5–15%	Down > 30%		
Fenofibrate (Lipantil)	Down 15–30%	Down > 30%		Good to date
Nicotinic acid				
Nicotinic acid	Down 15–30%	Down 15–30%	Poor	Established
Acipimox (Olbetam)	Down 5–15%	Down 15–30%	Reasonable	Not established
Probucol (Lurselle)	Down 5–15%	Variable	Reasonable	Not established
Statins				Not established
Simvastatin (Zocor) Pravastatin (Lipostat)	Down > 30%	Down 5–15%	Good	

BILE ACID BINDING RESINS

Bile acid binding resins include *cholestyramine* and *colestipol*. Cholestyramine has been shown to reduce the risk of coronary heart disease, and the long term safety of the drug has been established.[15][16]

The resins bind bile acids in the intestinal lumen and thus interrupt their enterohepatic circulation, greatly increasing the excretion of acidic steroids in the faeces. This drain on the bile acid pool stimulates hepatic synthesis of bile acids from cholesterol. Consequent depletion of the hepatic pool of cholesterol results in production of more LDL receptors on the hepatocytes, which increases LDL cholesterol uptake from the circulation.[17] As this mechanism depends on the presence of functioning LDL receptors, resins are not effective in people with homozygous familial hypercholesterolaemia, although they are the best treatment for the heterozygous condition, in which receptors are deficient rather than absent. It is important to note that these agents stimulate

VLDL production in the liver and may therefore increase triglyceride concentrations. Thus, if used in hypercholesterolaemic patients with marginally or frankly raised VLDL concentrations, such as those with type IIb or type IV hyperlipoproteinaemia, a second agent such as nicotinic acid or a fibrate will be necessary to lower VLDL triglyceride concentrations.

The bile acid sequestrants are marketed as powders that must be mixed with water or fruit juice or sprinkled on food (cholestyramine in 4 g sachets, colestipol in 5 g sachets). The recommendations are to start with a half sachet twice a day to minimise side effects and to increase gradually to a maximum of 24 g (cholestyramine) or 30 g (colestipol) a day. Most patients show a 15–30% reduction in LDL when prescribed about 16 g cholestyramine[18] or about 20 g colestipol[19] a day. Greater reductions may be seen in people who can tolerate the full doses, but many patients cannot tolerate the higher doses because of gastrointestinal symptoms, which include a sensation of fullness, constipation, nausea, and flatulence. Both drugs may interfere with the absorption of other anionic drugs (including digoxin, warfarin, thyroxine, and thiazide diuretics) if they are given with the resins. Other medication should therefore be taken at least 1 h before or 4 h after the bile acid resin. Because they are not absorbed, bile acid resins remain the most suitable treatment for children with heterozygous familial hypercholesterolaemia or women of childbearing age, although they are not recommended for use during pregnancy.

FIBRIC ACID DERIVATIVES

The fibric acid derivatives as a group are effective triglyceride lowering agents. The use of the parent compound *clofibrate* fell abruptly after a primary preventive study showed that it seemed to increase death rates.[20–22] Nevertheless, clofibrate retained a role in the management of type III hyperlipidaemia (dysbetalipoproteinaemia)—a condition in which cholesterol rich VLDL and chylomicron remnant particles accumulate in the plasma.[23] Bezafibrate and gemfibrozil are now increasingly replacing clofibrate for this condition.[24]

Bezafibrate

Bezafibrate has been shown to be an effective lipid lowering drug,[25] but the exact mechanism of its action is not certain. It may

307

be that LDL receptor activity increases because of reduced hydroxymethylglutaryl coenzyme A reductase activity, which results in a fall in plasma LDL concentration, as has been shown in patients with primary hypercholesterolaemia. Restoring the balance of triglyceride to cholesterol in the abnormally triglyceride enriched LDL found in type IIb hyperlipidaemia also possibly restores the normal interaction of the particles with LDL receptors. As with other fibrates, bezafibrate limits the production and promotes the catabolism of VLDL by activating lipoprotein lipase. The activation of lipoprotein lipase may be at the root of the increase in LDL that is seen in type IV patients treated with bezafibrate. Increases in HDL cholesterol have been reported after long term treatment with bezafibrate. The mechanism is thought to result from stimulation of apoprotein AI and AII production.[25] Bezafibrate has also been shown to reduce fibrinogen concentrations, which is also a primary risk factor for the development of atherosclerosis.[26]

The recommended dose is 200 mg three times a day, or 400 mg once a day in the case of the sustained release preparation (Bezalip-Mono).

Adverse effects are rare and mainly gastrointestinal. A myositic syndrome has been reported in patients with poor renal function and is accompanied by increased activity of creatine phosphokinase. Impaired renal function has also been worsened by bezafibrate. Small increases in the lithogenic index of bile have been reported after short term treatment with bezafibrate, but no report of an increased incidence of gall stones has yet appeared. It is important to note that bezafibrate is highly protein bound and may enhance the actions of anticoagulant drugs by displacing them from circulating plasma proteins.

The main limitation regarding recommendations about the use of bezafibrate is the lack of long term studies of its effect on deaths from coronary heart disease. This is important given the divergent results for clofibrate and gemfibrozil. Until results of long term studies are available the preventive role of bezafibrate is under suspicion.

Gemfibrozil

Although structurally different from the other fibrates, gemfibrozil has a very effective plasma triglyceride lowering action. It reduces VLDL and apoprotein B production in the liver and simultaneously stimulates lipoprotein lipase activity, which results in increased clearance of triglyceride rich particles.[27] HDL cholesterol concentrations may also rise, but this is often quite variable.

Gemfibrozil is well absorbed from the gastrointestinal tract. A steady state is achieved within 7–14 days with a twice a day regimen. It may undergo some enterohepatic circulation, although its primary route of excretion is in the urine.[29] The usual dosage is 600 mg twice a day.

Gemfibrozil increases the lithogenic index of bile. Unlike with clofibrate, however, fewer than 1% of patients actually develop gall stones, even after treatment for 2 years.[28] Gemfibrozil is highly protein bound and, as might be expected, enhances the anticoagulant effect of warfarin. It is well tolerated and adverse reactions occur in fewer than 10% of patients.

The main side effects are gastrointestinal—abdominal pain, diarrhoea, and nausea. Rare biochemical abnormalities include increased alkaline phosphatase and transaminase activities. A few cases of severe myositis with increased creatine phosphokinase activities have been described in patients receiving concomitant lovastatin treatment (see below).[29]

Gemfibrozil is indicated in patients with appreciably high serum triglyceride concentrations,[13] particularly those with type III hyperlipoproteinaemia who have not responded to dietary and lifestyle modifications. In patients who present primarily with hypercholesterolaemia its use should be limited to those who show no response to conventional treatment. Combination treatment with another drug such as bile acid binding resin is particularly effective. The response to gemfibrozil is somewhat unpredictable and not all patients respond. Therapeutic trial is therefore recommended for 3–6 months. If no noticeable response has occurred then treatment should be changed. The Helsinki heart study, a primary prevention study in men, showed that 34% fewer men receiving gemfibrozil, compared with placebo, developed coronary heart disease in 5 years.[28]

Fenofibrate

This is an analogue of clofibrate, which has been used in clinical practice in France since 1975. Various trials have shown that it reduces total plasma cholesterol concentrations by 20–25% and reduces high triglyceride concentrations by 40–60%. Concentrations of LDL have been found to fall by 20% in patients with type

IIa hyperlipidaemia and to a lesser extent (6%) in patients with type IIb. In general, HDL rises by 11–15%.[30] [31]

Fenofibrate is absorbed rapidly as a prodrug and maximally when given with food. It is activated by hydrolysis to fenofibric acid in various cells and tissues including red blood cells, the liver, intestine, and kidney. It is highly bound to albumin and has an elimination half life of about 20 h.[32] It is excreted by the kidneys and accumulates in patients with renal impairment. The recommended dose is 100 mg three times a day.[33] Side effects are generally minor and similar to those seen with bezafibrate.

Newer fibric acid derivatives

Newer fibrates such as *ciprofibrate* (Modalim), recently available in the United Kingdom, show promise as effective hypolipidaemic drugs.[14] [16]

NICOTINIC ACID

Nicotinic acid is a commonly used first line agent for hypercholesterolaemia (IIa) and combined hyperlipidaemia (IIb and IV) in the United States.[14] It is a water soluble B vitamin that, when used in pharmacological doses, lowers VLDL and LDL concentrations. The exact mechanism of action is not known. It appears to decrease the formation of triglycerides by reducing the availability of free fatty acids for the hepatic production of VLDL. This in turn leads to a decrease in the production of LDL. Nicotinic acid is the least expensive lipid lowering agent currently available, but is available in 25, 50, and 100 mg tablet preparations only. Patients generally require doses increasing gradually from 100 mg three times a day to 3–6 g (that is, 30–60 100 mg tablets) a day. Nicofuranose (Bradilan) is a compound of nicotinic acid and levulose; 500 mg of nicofuranose is equivalent to 411 mg of nicotinic acid. The recommended dose is 1·5–3 g (6–12 tablets) a day. It should be noted that nicotinamide (niacinamide or nicotinic acid amide) is ineffective in lowering lipid concentrations. Furthermore, use of some sustained release preparations available in the United States has been associated with fulminant liver failure.

Nicotinic acid is well absorbed and is commonly given with or just after meals to reduce gastrointestinal disturbance. The drug is not highly protein bound and the principal route of metabolism is the formation of N-methyl nicotinamide.

Apart from flushing, side effects are uncommon and include raised liver enzyme activities and hyperuricaemia. Glucose intolerance may occur with high doses. Peptic ulcer disease may be activated, and less common side effects include hyperpigmentation of the skin and blurred vision.

Acipimox is a synthetic analogue of nicotinic acid. Like its parent it acts by inhibiting adipose tissue lipolysis.[37] It reduces plasma lipids and lipoproteins and increases HDL in types II, III, and IV hyperlipidaemia (table 22.2).[38] Whereas nicotinic acid may induce transient impairment of carbohydrate tolerance, acipimox seems to exert a favourable effect on glucose tolerance. The usual dose is 250 mg two to three times a day. Acipimox also seems to produce less flushing and gastrointestinal intolerance than nicotinic acid.

When used alone nicotinic acid at a dose of 3–6 g a day can result in a 15–40% decrease in triglyceride and LDL cholesterol concentrations and a rise in HDL cholesterol concentration of about half that value. LDL concentrations in patients with heterozygous familial hypercholesterolaemia have been normalised when nicotinic acid has been used in combination with a bile acid binding resin.[9] Nicotinic acid is also useful in combined hyperlipidaemia.

In a large secondary prevention study, the coronary drug project,[39] administering nicotinic acid to men who had suffered previous myocardial infarction reduced non-fatal myocardial infarctions without affecting total death rates. After a mean follow up of 15 years (that is, 9 years after the end of the trial) the death rate in the men treated with nicotinic acid was significantly lower than that in those given placebo.[39] Although there were limitations in the design of this study, it suggests that overall death rates may be reduced by lipid lowering drugs.

PROBUCOL

Probucol decreases LDL cholesterol concentrations by no more than about 10%. It also causes a reduction of up to 25% in HDL cholesterol concentrations. Despite this, administering probucol to animals has been associated with regression of xanthomas and improvement in coronary artery morphology,[40 41] a finding that seems to run contrary to the suggested protective effect of HDL. The exact mechanism of probucol's action is not known. Probucol has been shown to increase the fractional catabolic rate of LDL in patients heterozygous or homozygous for familial hypercholesterolaemia,[40]

311

which suggests that LDL reduction in this instance is independent of the receptor pathway. Other studies have shown that probucol blocks oxidative modification of LDL and therefore slows down foam cell formation,[42] which could prevent the development of atherosclerosis. Thus probucol may be exerting its anti-atherosclerotic effect independently of lipid reduction.

Probucol is well absorbed. It is lipophilic and is therefore stored in adipose tissue. Detectable concentrations may persist for 6 months after treatment is stopped. It is therefore not recommended for women of childbearing age or children. The dose is 500 mg twice a day. Adverse effects are reported in fewer than 10% of patients, the main problems being gastrointestinal upset with diarrhoea, flatulence, and hyperhydrosis. As prolongation of the QT interval has been noted on electrocardiography, the drug may be contraindicated in patients with ventricular irritability or an initially prolonged QT interval. Until further information is available, probucol is not recommended as a first line agent.

INHIBITORS OF HYDROXYMETHYLGLUTARYL COENZYME A REDUCTASE (STATINS)

About two thirds of body cholesterol is synthesised de novo in the liver and intestine. The rate limiting enzyme in this synthetic pathway is hydroxymethylglutaryl coenzyme A reductase. This key enzyme has recently become the target for pharmacological manipulation, and specific drugs are available that can selectively and competitively inhibit its action, which offers a new approach to treating primary hypercholesterolaemia.

At present three statins (lovastatin, simvastatin, and pravastatin) have been extensively evaluated. *Lovastatin* is currently available in the United States and has been used by over a million patients. Two analogues, simvastatin (Zocor), and pravastatin, have recently been released in the United Kingdom. These drugs act by inhibiting cellular cholesterol production, depleting the intracellular pool of the sterol, and in consequence increasing the expression of LDL receptors. In patients with only half the normal complement of receptors (that is, who are heterozygous for familial hypercholesterolaemia) the increased number of receptors promotes LDL uptake from the bloodstream. The fall in LDL cholesterol in these patients is 30–40%, which often normalises previously high plasma cholesterol concentrations. If a bile acid binding resin is also given LDL cholesterol may be reduced by up

LIPANTHYL® *300*

INDICATIONS THÉRAPEUTIQUES

Ce médicament est un hypolipémiant. Il réduit le taux de lipides (graisses) sanguins.

Ce médicament est préconisé en complément du **régime** alimentaire dans les hyperlipidémies (surcharge en cholestérol et/ou en triglycérides dans le sang) ; un taux élevé de lipides dans le sang est un facteur majeur d'athérome (dépôt de plaques graisseuses sur la paroi des artères).

CONTRE-INDICATIONS

Ce médicament NE DOIT PAS ETRE UTILISÉ dans les cas suivants : - en cas d'insuffisances hépatique ou rénale sévères ; chez l'enfant. - EN CAS DE DOUTE, IL EST INDISPENSABLE DE DEMANDER L'AVIS DE VOTRE MÉDECIN OU DE VOTRE PHARMACIEN.

MISE EN GARDE

Dans le traitement des hyperlipidémies, le respect scrupuleux du régime alimentaire prescrit par le médecin est **indispensable**.

EN CAS DE DOUTE, NE PAS HÉSITER A DEMANDER L'AVIS DE VOTRE MÉDECIN OU DE VOTRE PHARMACIEN.

PRÉCAUTIONS D'EMPLOI

AFIN D'ÉVITER D'ÉVENTUELLES INTERACTIONS ENTRE PLUSIEURS MÉDICAMENTS, IL FAUT SIGNALER SYSTÉMATIQUEMENT TOUT AUTRE TRAITEMENT EN COURS A VOTRE MÉDECIN OU A VOTRE PHARMACIEN. NE JAMAIS LAISSER A LA PORTÉE DES ENFANTS.

AUTRE EFFETS POSSIBLES DU MÉDICAMENT

COMME TOUT PRODUIT ACTIF, CE MÉDICAMENT PEUT, CHEZ CERTAINES PERSONNES, ENTRAINER DES EFFETS PLUS OU MOINS GÊNANTS : troubles digestifs (nausées, gastralgies).

POSOLOGIE ET MODE D'ADMINISTRATION

En moyenne 1 gélule par jour au cours d'un repas.

DANS TOUS LES CAS, SE CONFORMER STRICTEMENT A L'ORDONNANCE DE VOTRE MÉDECIN.

En association avec le régime, ce médicament constitue un traitement symptomatique devant être très prolongé et régulièrement surveillé.

Pour une bonne utilisation de ce médicament, il est indispensable de vous soumettre à une surveillance médicale régulière, celle-ci peut comporter un dosage des lipides.

CONDITION DE DÉLIVRANCE

CE MÉDICAMENT EST INSCRIT A LA LISTE II (TABLEAU C). VOTRE PHARMACIEN NE POURRA VOUS EN DÉLIVRER QUE SUR PRÉSENTATION DE VOTRE ORDONNANCE.

DURÉE DE STABILITÉ

NE PAS DÉPASSER LA DATE LIMITE D'UTILISATION INDIQUÉE EN CLAIR SUR L'EMBALLAGE.

PRÉSENTATION

Boîte de 30 gélules : A.M.M. n ° 328.449.8

Remboursé par la Sécurité Sociale et admis aux Collectivités.

442102 E - Lot 31

CECI EST UN MÉDICAMENT

Ce médicament est un hypolipidémiant. Il est destiné à traiter l'excès de lipides dans le sang (corps gras), notamment de cholestérol, et à prévenir ses conséquences qui peuvent être dommageables pour votre santé. L'hyperlipidémie (excès de lipides) exige de votre part une attention particulière, même si elle ne vous cause pas de troubles apparents. Vous veillerez donc à suivre les recommandations diététiques (régime alimentaire adapté) prescrites par votre médecin et qui aideront ce médicament à agir plus complètement.

1) N'oubliez pas que, pour être efficace, ce médicament doit être utilisé **très régulièrement**, et aussi longtemps que votre médecin vous l'aura conseillé, **même si c'est pour une durée très longue.** En effet, il rétablit dans votre organisme un équilibre que seul le traitement peut maintenir : ne l'arrêtez donc pas de votre propre initiative, quels que soient les résultats de vos analyses de sang.

2) Respectez scrupuleusement : - La dose prescrite, sans l'augmenter, ni la diminuer. - Le nombre de prises et le moment de la prise.

3) **Vous ne devez pas, de votre propre initiative, prendre un autre médicament,** quel qu'il soit, sans l'avis de votre médecin traitant ou de votre pharmacien, car certaines associations médicamenteuses doivent être évitées. Ainsi, même pour des produits que vous utilisez parfois pour des maux que vous connaissez bien, il est préférable d'en parler à votre médecin ou à votre pharmacien.

4) Si vous devez faire appel à un autre médecin, informez-le du traitement que vous suivez actuellement.

5) Toute réaction ou toute manifestation inhabituelles survenant au cours du traitement doivent être signalées à votre médecin.

VOTRE MÉDECIN ET VOTRE PHARMACIEN CONNAISSENT BIEN LES MÉDICAMENTS QUI VOUS SONT PRESCRITS. N'HÉSITEZ PAS A LEUR DEMANDER DES PRÉCISIONS.

| NE LAISSEZ JAMAIS CE MÉDICAMENT A LA PORTÉE DES ENFANTS |

442102 E

Made in France . Imp. Labo. Fournier

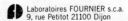

Laboratoires FOURNIER s.c.a.
9, rue Petitot 21100 Dijon

to 50–60%. Nearly all patients with severe hypercholesterolaemia are now amenable to treatment, but those homozygous for familial hypercholesterolaemia, who have no LDL receptors, cannot respond. The effect of statins on triglycerides is variable, although a 5–10% reduction is common and in some studies a small but appreciable increase in HDL of 5–15% has also been reported.

Simvastatin is administered as a lactone and acts as a prodrug requiring conversion to active metabolites in the body. In contrast, *pravastatin* is given in the acid form that is active. The in vitro affinity of simvastatin to hydroxymethylglutaryl coenzyme A reductase seems to be greater than that of pravastatin, but pravastatin seems to be more selective, affecting largely the intestinal and liver enzymes. Nevertheless, in clinical practice both appear to be equally efficacious. Absorption of these drugs is limited to 30–50% of the dose at most. Simvastatin undergoes extensive first pass metabolism. No drug interactions that alter the liver metabolism of the two drugs have been described to date. Clinical experience has shown that combinations of lovastatin with cyclosporin, gemfibrozil, or nicotinic acid can predispose patients to myopathy.[43] Caution is therefore advised when using any of the statins with these agents.

To date statins appear to be free from serious toxicity. Long term safety evaluation is awaited; these drugs should not be used in children or women of childbearing potential. Studies in dogs have suggested that lovastatin in extreme doses may lead to lens opacity, but this has not occurred in humans.[44] No deficiencies of cholesterol based steroid hormones, such as cortisol or sex hormones, have been described during treatment.

Although the elimination half life seems to be short (1–3h), the duration of enzyme inhibition is much longer. Initially statins were given twice a day, but there is now evidence that once a day, particularly at night, may be as effective. This is possibly because cholesterol biosynthesis takes place largely at night. Adverse effects have been relatively few—occasional minor gastrointestinal disturbance in fewer than 5% and rashes in about 1% of patients. Reversible abnormalities of liver function may occur in up to 2% and a rise in muscle creatine phosphokinase activities in about 1% of patients.

Simvastatin and pravastatin are first given at 10 mg a day, and the dose is adjusted according to the response. Most patients require 20–40 mg daily, which may be taken as a single dose with the evening meal. Statins are particularly well tolerated and are the most effective agents to date. If their long term safety is confirmed in large studies they are likely to become first line agents in managing hypercholesterolaemia. They also have a role in patients with combined increases of cholesterol and triglyceride concentrations. Additional data on their impact on coronary disease and death are necessary, however, before the widespread use of statins is contemplated.

OTHER DRUGS

Neither neomycin nor thyroxine is now recommended. Derivatives of ω-3 fatty acids may have some role in the treatment of hypertriglyceridaemia, but their long term efficacy and safety has not been proved and some concern exists about the LDL raising actions of these agents. Several other compounds that reduce sterol absorption from the intestine (sucrose polyester sitosterol, and neomycin analogues) or that inhibit enzymes associated with cholesterol esterification (acyl-cholesterol acyl-transferase inhibitors) are still under investigation.

COMBINED TREATMENT

When a single agent does not produce an adequate reduction in cholesterol or does so only by inducing undesirable side effects, a combination of agents may be efficacious, rational, and well tolerated by patients. The choice is often dictated by synergistic mechanisms, and some examples are shown in table 22.2.

Conclusion

Increasing numbers of highly efficacious and well tolerated lipid lowering drugs are becoming available. Many studies have shown a reduction in the incidence of cardiovascular events in patients treated with lipid lowering agents, but none to date has shown a favourable effect on the overall death rate. Nevertheless, these drugs should be regarded as part of the armoury and must always be combined with dietary treatment. Attention to other risk factors including hypertension, smoking, and diabetes is also clearly indicated.

1 Kannel WB, Doyle JT, Ostfeld AM, *et al*. Atherosclerosis study group. Optimal resources for primary prevention of atherosclerotic diseases. *Circulation* 1984;70:155–205A.

2 Hulley SB, Rhoads CG. The plasma lipoproteins as risk factors: comparison of electrophoretic and ultracentrifugation results. *Metabolism* 1982;**31**:773–7.

3 Gordon T, Kannel WB, Castelli WB, Dawber TR. Lipoproteins, cardiovascular disease and death. The Framingham study. *Arch Intern Med* 1981;**141**:1128–31.

4 Goldbourt U, Holtzman E, Neufeld HN. Total and high density lipoprotein cholesterol in the serum and risk of mortality: evidence of a threshold effect. *BMJ* 1985;**290**:1239–43.

5 Pocock SJ, Shaper AG, Phillips AN, Walker M, Whitehead TP. High density lipoprotein cholesterol is not a major risk factor for ischaemic heart disease in British men. *BMJ* 1986;**292**:515–19.

6 Peto R, Yusuf S, Collins R. Cholesterol lowering trial results in their epidemiological context. *Circulation* 1985;**72**:451. (Abstract No 1083.)

7 Duffield RGM, Lewis B, Miller NE, Jameson CW, Brunt JNH, Colchester ACF. Treatment of hyperlipidaemia retards progression of symptomatic femoral atherosclerosis. A randomised controlled trial. *Lancet* 1983;**ii**:639–42.

8 Brensike JF, Levy RI, Kelsey SF, *et al.* Effects of therapy with cholestyramine on progression of coronary atherosclerosis: results of the NHLBI type II coronary intervention study. *Circulation* 1984;**69**:313–24.

9 Kane JP, Malloy MJ, Tun P, *et al.* Normalisation of low density lipoprotein levels in heterozygous familial hypercholesterolaemia with a combined drug regimen. *N Engl J Med* 1981;**304**:251–8.

10 Ball MJ, Mann JI. Drug treatment for hypercholesterolaemia. *Q J Med* 1986;**232**:733–5.

11 The British Cardiac Society Working Group on Coronary Prevention. Conclusions and recommendations. *Br Heart J* 1987;**57**:188–9.

12 Study Group, European Atherosclerosis Society. The recognition and management of hyperlipidaemia in adults: a policy statement of the European Atherosclerosis Society. *Eur Heart J* 1988;**9**:571–600.

13 National Cholesterol Education Program Expert Panel. Report on detection, evaluation, and treatment of high blood cholesterol in adults. *Arch Intern Med* 1988;**148**:36–69.

14 Brown MS, Goldstein JL, How LDL receptors influence cholesterol and atherosclerosis. *Sci Am* 1984;**251**:58–66.

15 Lipid research clinics program. The lipid research clinics coronary primary prevention trial results. I. Reduction in the incidence of coronary heart disease. *JAMA* 1984;**251**:351–64.

16 Lipid research clinics program. The lipid research clinics coronary primary prevention trial. II. The relationship of reduction in incidence of coronary heart disease to cholesterol lowering. *JAMA* 1984;**251**:365–74.

17 Shepherd J, Packard CJ, Bicher S, Lawrie TDV, Morgan G. Cholestyramine promotes receptor mediated low density lipoprotein catabolism. *N Engl J Med* 1980;**302**:1219–22.

18 Schaefer EJ, Levy RI. Pathogenesis and management of lipoprotein disorders. *N Engl J Med* 1985; **312**:1300–10.

19 Kane JP, Malloy MJ. Treatment of hypercholesterolaemia. *Med Clin North Am* 1982;**66**:537–50.

20 The Coronary Drug Project Research Group. Findings leading to further modifications of its protocol with respect to dextrothyroxine. *JAMA* 1972;**220**:996–1008.

21 Committee of Principal Investigators. A cooperative trial in the primary prevention of ischaemic heart disease using clofibrate. *Br Heart J* 1978;**40**:1069–118.

22 Committee of Principal Investigators. WHO cooperative trial on primary prevention of ischaemic heart disease using clofibrate to lower serum cholesterol—mortality follow up. *Lancet* 1980;**ii**:379–85.

23 Havel R. Familial dysbetalipoproteinemia: new aspects of pathogenesis and diagnosis. *Med Clin North Am* 1982;**66**:441–54.

24 Shepherd J, Packard CJ. An overview of the effects of p-chlor-phenoxy-isobutyric acid derivatives on lipoprotein metabolism. In: Fears R, ed. *Pharmacological control of hyperlipidaemia.* Barcelona, Spain: JR Prous, 1986:135–44.

25 Monk JP, Todd PA. Bezafibrate: a review. *Drugs* 1987;**33**:539–76.

26 Niort G, Bulgarelli A, Cassander M, Pagano G. Effects of short term treatment with bezafibrate on plasma fibrinogen, fibrinopeptide A, platelet activation and blood filterability in atherosclerotic hyperfibrinogenemic patients. *Atherosclerosis* 1988;**71**:113–19.

27 Kesaniemi YA, Grundy SM. Influence of gemfibrozil and clofibrate on metabolism of cholesterol and plasma triglycerides in man. *JAMA* 1984;**251**:2241–7.

28 Frick MH, Ello O, Haapa K, *et al.* Helsinki heart study: primary-prevention trial with gemfibrozil in middle aged men with dyslipidemia. Safety of treatment, changes in risk factors and incidence of coronary heart disease. *N Engl J Med* 1987;**317**:1237–45.

29 Todd PA, Ward A. Gemfibrozil: a review of its pharmacodynamic and pharmacokinetic properties, and therapeutic use in dyslipidaemia. *Drugs* 1988;**36**:314–39.

30 Brown WV, Dujovne CA, Farquhar JW, *et al.* Effects of fenofibrate on plasma lipids. *Arteriosclerosis* 1986;**6**:670–8.

31 Knopp RH, Brown WV, Dujovne CA, *et al.* Effects of fenofibrate on plasma lipoproteins in hypercholesterolaemia and combined hyperlipidaemia. *Am J Med* 1987;**83**(suppl 5B):50–9.

32 Chapman MJ. Pharmacology of fenofibrate. *Am J Med* 1987;**83** (suppl 5B):21–5.

33 Blane GF. Comparative toxicity and safety profile of fenofibrate and other fibric acid derivatives. *Am J Med* 1987;**83** (suppl 5B):26–36.

34 Rouffy J, Chancu B, Bakir R, Dijan F, Goy-Leoper J. Comparative evaluation of the effects of ciprofibrate and fenofibrate on lipids, lipoproteins and apoproteins A and B. *Atherosclerosis* 1985;**54**:273–81.

35 Illingworth DR, Olsen GD, Cook SF, Sexton GJ, Wendel HA, Connor WE. Ciprofibrate in the therapy of type II hypercholesterolaemia—a double blind trial. *Atherosclerosis* 1982;**44**:211–21.

36 Olsson AG, Oro L. Dose–response study of the effect of ciprofibrate on serum lipoprotein concentrations in hyperlipoproteinaemia. *Atherosclerosis* 1982;**42**:229–43.

37 Stirling C, McAleer M, Reckless JPD, *et al.* Effects of acipimox, a nicotinic acid derivative, on lipolysis in human adipose tissue and on cholesterol synthesis in human jejunal mucosae. *Clin Sci* 1985;**68**:83–8.

38 Crepaldi G, Avogaro P, Descovich GC, *et al.* Plasma lipid lowering activity of acipimox in patients with type II and type IV hyperlipoproteinemia: results of a multicenter trial. *Atherosclerosis* 1988;**70**:115–21.

39 Canner PL, Berge KG, Wenger NK, *et al.* Fifteen year mortality in coronary drug project patients: long term benefit with niacin. *J Am Coll Cardiol* 1986;**8**:1245–55.

40 Baker SG, Joffe Bi, Mendelsohn D, Seftel HC. Treatment of homozygous familial hypercholesterolaemia with probucol. *S Afr Med J* 1982;**62**:7–11.

41 Yamamoto A. Matsuzawa Y, Yokoyama S, Funahashi T, Yamamura T, Kishino B. Effects of probucol on xanthoma regression in familial hypercholesterolaemia. *Am J Cardiol* 1986;**57**:29H–35H.

42 Steinberg D. Studies on the mechanism of action of probucol. *Am J Cardiol* 1986;**57**:16H-21H.
43 Grundy SM. HMG-CoA reductase inhibitors for treatment of hypercholesterolemia. *N Engl J Med* 1988;**319**:24–33.
44 Tobert JA. New developments in lipid lowering therapy: the role of inhibition of hydroxy methylglutaryl-coenzyme. A reductase. *Circulation* 1978;**76**:534–8.

23 Anxiolytics and hypnotics

BRIAN R BALLINGER

During the past 30 years benzodiazepines have been widely prescribed to treat anxiety states and sleep disorders. The problem of drug dependence, however, and discussion of alternatives including non-drug methods of management have led to increasing caution in their use. This chapter considers the role of drugs in treating, firstly, anxiety and then sleep disorders.

Anxiolytics

Anxiety is a normal reaction but when severe and disabling it becomes pathological. Phobias are distinguished from anxiety, and some classifications also separate panic attacks. Patients should be assessed carefully to detect associated problems in their lives and to seek evidence of underlying illness, such as depression or organic brain disease, that may present as anxiety: conversely, it should be remembered that some patients presenting with anxiety have an underlying physical illness. Drugs are often not necessary to treat neurotic anxiety, and in many instances a simple form of psychotherapy or sometimes cognitive or behavioural therapy may succeed.

BENZODIAZEPINES

The benzodiazepines have anxiolytic and hypnotic effects, although some have been marketed mainly to treat anxiety. The original benzodiazepine, chlordiazepoxide, has been available for more than 30 years and it has been followed by many others.[1] Although these drugs are not new, it seems appropriate to review their present role in treatment, as advantages such as relative safety in overdose have led to their widespread use. The recently introduced specific benzodiazepine antagonist, flumazenil, may be of use in some cases of overdose. Although the structure of a particular benzodiazepine molecule may influence its activity—for example the 1,5-benzodiazepine, clobazam, may be relatively less sedative than the 1,4-benzodiazepines—in practice the duration of action mainly determines what benzodiazepine to use. The speed of absorption is also relevant, and the high lipid solubility of diazepam may make the effect of a single dose short lived.

Duration of action

Because many benzodiazepines are metabolised in the liver to produce further active forms that are eliminated from the body more slowly than the parent molecule, care has to be taken when assessing information about the duration of action of these drugs. For example, medazepam has an elimination half life of 1–2 h but is metabolised to oxazepam, which has a half life of 6–24 h. Pharmacodynamic studies that record the duration of measurable effects such as sedation are the best source of this information, but because such studies are difficult to undertake a full description is not always available. Prescribers should be alert to the possibility of cumulative hangover effects, especially in elderly people and those whose hepatic function may be impaired. Particular caution is needed with the drugs that have long elimination half lives and those that undergo appreciable oxidative metabolism in the liver (all except temazepam, lormetazepam, oxazepam, and lorazepam).

Dependence

Dependence on the benzodiazepines is now regarded as a serious problem,[2] particularly with longer term treatment and in patients with some types of personality disorder. Benzodiazepines are widely misused by poly-drug users, by injection as well as in tablet form.[3] Patients taking these drugs, even in therapeutic doses, may develop a physical withdrawal syndrome if the drug is stopped. The main symptom of this is anxiety, which usually subsides in 2–4 weeks but sometimes lasts longer, although many patients would have been prone to anxiety before treatment was started. In addition, depression, nausea, depersonalisation, and perceptual changes such as intolerance of loud noises, bright lights, or touch may occur. Insomnia may also be expected but the symptoms are variable. Epileptic seizures, confusion, and visual hallucinations may occur occasionally.

Stopping treatment with short acting benzodiazepines leads to withdrawal symptoms within about 2–3 days, whereas with longer acting drugs there may be a delay of 7 days. Patients being weaned from benzodiazepines need close supervision and support, and the drugs should be withdrawn slowly over weeks or even months. Sometimes β blocking drugs and psychological aids such as relaxation therapy help withdrawal.

Other effects

Drowsiness may be a hazard, particularly when operating machinery or driving, and mental confusion may be precipitated or made worse, particularly in older people. Memory may be impaired and incoordination or ataxia may occur. Loss of control leading to aggressive behaviour or self poisoning is a problem in a few patients.

Age—The production of active metabolites of some drugs depends on oxidative metabolic pathways in the liver, and the elimination of conjugated metabolites depends on renal function. Hepatic and renal functions are known to deteriorate with age and the elderly therefore eliminate benzodiazepines more slowly, which may result in higher peaks of concentration in the body and prolonged duration of action. The aging brain also seems to be more sensitive to the effects of these drugs. For these reasons benzodiazepines usually need to be given to elderly people in smaller doses, and the shorter acting drugs are generally indicated to avoid hangover effects when benzodiazepines are used as hypnotics.

Alcohol—Alcohol and benzodiazepines taken concomitantly may result in greater impairment of psychomotor function than either agent alone. There are many possible explanations for this observation, but acute alcohol intake may inhibit the metabolism of most benzodiazepines, probably excepting those that do not undergo oxidation (see below). The usual effect of the combination of alcohol and benzodiazepines is an increase in the sedative effects of the benzodiazepine, but cases of aggressive behaviour have occurred.

Indications

The decision to start giving benzodiazepines for anxiety should not be taken lightly, and treatment should be limited to patients whose anxiety is causing unacceptable distress.[45] Their use should be avoided for mild anxiety. Treatment should usually be for a limited period only because of the increasing risk of dependence developing and the Committee on Safety of Medicines recommends treatment for 2–4 weeks only. Intermittent flexible dose treatment in which medication is taken occasionally when symptoms are severe, but never continuously, may have advantages. The shorter acting drugs such as oxazepam or lorazepam have sometimes been preferred for acute anxiety, although withdrawal symptoms may be more of a problem with these drugs.

Longer term treatment with benzodiazepines is controversial and many doctors have used it for certain patients with severe neurosis. Given the potential problems of dependence and the present climate of opinion, however, this practice should be avoided except for a few patients already receiving long term treatment whose condition is stable and for whom withdrawal would cause serious problems.

In view of the similarities between benzodiazepines, a limited list of drugs available for NHS prescription has been introduced. It includes diazepam, chlordiazepoxide, lorazepam, oxazepam, and some drugs marketed as hypnotics (nitrazepam, loprazolam, lormetazepam, and temazepam), but changing patients from one drug to another has sometimes proved difficult in practice.

BUSPIRONE

Buspirone is a new drug that is marketed as an anxiolytic; hypnotic or anticonvulsant effects are not claimed for it.[6] It has an entirely different structure from other anxiolytics, and the recommended dose range is 15–30 mg a day in divided doses. It is well absorbed but undergoes extensive first pass metabolism; it is highly protein bound and only 1% is excreted unchanged.

Trials have shown that buspirone reduces symptoms of anxiety, though no more effectively than the benzodiazepines. It is less sedative than diazepam and does not relieve benzodiazepine withdrawal symptoms. Buspirone is not very effective in patients who have not responded to benzodiazepines, and its anxiolytic effect is relatively slow to develop.

Side effects are not usually severe, although gastrointestinal upset, dizziness, and headache have occurred. In contrast to treatment with benzodiazepines, no withdrawal symptoms have been reported on stopping treatment after 6 weeks to 6 months and there is no evidence of tolerance. Buspirone does not seem to have an additive effect with alcohol and has not been shown to impair cognitive function.

Buspirone probably has a limited place in the treatment of anxiety, but its slow action is a disadvantage. The lack of reports of drug dependence is encouraging for longer term treatment, but reports of dependence on other anxiolytics were slow to appear. The absence of sedative effects may be valuable for some patients.

OTHER DRUGS

Barbiturates can no longer be recommended as they are dangerous in overdose, readily cause psychological and physical dependence, and are potent inducers of liver enzymes. *Meprobamate* is less effective than the benzodiazepines and less safe. β *Receptor blockers* such as propranolol have a role in the management of some patients as they control the somatic symptoms of anxiety, such as tremor and palpitations.[7] They are sometimes useful for treating anxiety associated with public speaking and similar activities, but the type of patient who responds to β blockers has not been defined fully.

Small doses of *neuroleptics* such as trifluoperazine have sometimes been used to treat anxiety, and they have the advantage of not causing dependence. The potential hazards of these agents, however, such as tardive dyskinesia, make them unsuitable for the long term treatment of neuroses. The sedative *antidepressants* have an anxiolytic effect and may be useful in managing anxiety when coexisting depressive symptoms justify antidepressant treatment. Tricyclic and similar antidepressants, however, also have a part to play in treating some patients who are liable to recurrent panic attacks and some other people with anxiety states. The antidepressant clomipramine and selective serotonin reuptake inhibitors such as fluoxetine and fluvoxamine are reported to be effective in some sufferers from obsessive compulsive disorder.[8]

Hypnotics

Each patient's condition should be evaluated carefully before a hypnotic is prescribed.[9] Not all people who complain of difficulties in sleeping really have insomnia, and sleep patterns and requirements vary with age and among people. Particular causes of insomnia should be sought, including the use of stimulant drinks such as tea or coffee at bedtime, discomfort, and noise. Painful physical illness or depression may be associated with sleep problems, and these may resolve with appropriate treatment. As with anxiety, psychological methods of treatment have a role in managing insomnia.

Hypnotics should not be given unless insomnia is severe, and their long term use should be avoided as far as possible. The aim should be to give drugs for as short a period as possible, and intermittent use should reduce the risk of dependence. When hypnotics are withdrawn the dose should be reduced gradually.

Benzodiazepines that are promoted for use as hypnotics may be divided into those with short or longer durations of action. Shorter acting benzodiazepines (temazepam, and lormetazepam) are indicated for patients for whom residual effects are undesirable. They are also the most suitable benzodiazepine hypnotics for elderly people, although caution is still required. The very short acting triazolam has been withdrawn because of reports of adverse effects. Longer acting benzodiazepines such as nitrazepam have sometimes been said to be indicated when early morning waking is a problem and some impairment of psychomotor function is acceptable. In very old people drowsiness, confusion, and unsteadiness can be dangerous, and longer acting benzodiazepines should be avoided.

After the regular use of benzodiazepine hypnotics for only a few weeks rebound insomnia can occur when they are stopped. Benzodiazepine hypnotics should not normally be taken for more than 3 weeks and treatment should be intermittent if possible.

ZOPICLONE

A new hypnotic zopiclone (Zimovane),[10] is now available in the United Kingdom. It has similar pharmacological actions to those of the benzodiazepines and it is rapidly absorbed, with a short half life of about 4h. The usual dose is 7·5 mg but a 3·75 mg dose may avoid hangover in some patients. The position about dependence is not clear but rebound insomnia has been reported. It can cause a metallic taste, and occasional neuropsychiatric reactions are recorded. As with the benzodiazepines, its use should be restricted to short term treatment.

OTHER DRUGS

The *barbiturates* can no longer be recommended as hypnotics for the reasons stated above. *Chloral hydrate* is effective and cheap but may cause side effects, including gastric irritation and rashes. Gastric irritation may be reduced by using one of the derivatives such as chloral betaine (Welldorm) or triclofos. *Chlormethiazole* has been recommended for use in the elderly because of its short half life. It often causes nasal and conjunctival irritation when first taken, but this side effect may disappear on continuing its use. Chlormethiazole is less safe in overdose than the benzodiazepines, and reports of dependence are many. It may be helpful in a few elderly patients when other drugs have failed, and it is sometimes used for treatment of withdrawal from alcohol although caution is advised.

Drugs of the *antihistamine* type such as promethazine and trimeprazine have been used as hypnotics, particularly for children, though they have long durations of action and I can see no advantage in their use. Drugs that are not primarily hypnotics may be indicated when insomnia occurs in conjunction with other psychiatric illness. For example, sleep disturbance with depressive illness may respond to the use of sedative antidepressants such as amitriptyline, dothiepin, tradozone, or mianserin, often given as a single dose at night which thus avoids using hypnotics. Sedative *neuroleptics* such as thioridazine may be useful for patients with dementia and nocturnal restlessness if given as an evening dose. Because of potential side effects, however, these drugs should not normally be used as hypnotics unless other indications exist.

Conclusions

After a long period of dominance in the management of anxiety and insomnia benzodiazepines have come under critical review because of the problems of drug dependence, although because of their efficacy and safety in overdose they can still be helpful. Their use in longer term treatment is no longer recommended in most cases, although there are probably a few exceptions. In some conditions antidepressants, β blockers, and other drugs have a part to play, and it is still too early to define the role of the new anxiolytic, buspirone and the new hypnotic, zopiclone. More emphasis should now be placed on managing sleep disorders and anxiety without using drugs.

1 Hockings N, Ballinger BR Hypnotics and anxiolytics. *BMJ* 1983;**286**:1949–51.

2 Lader MH. Benzodiazepine dependence. *Curr Opin Psychiatry* 1988;1:346–9. (Brief review with annotated references.)

3 Sievewright NA, Dougal W. Benzodiazepine misuse. *Curr Opin Psychiatry* 1992;5:408–11.

4 Catalan J, Gath D, Edmonds G, Ennis J. The effects of non-prescribing of anxiolytics in general practice. *Br J Psychiatry* 1984;144:593–602. (Trial comparing counselling with anxiolytics in patients with minor affective disorders and somatic complaints.)

5 Tyrer P, Murphy S. The place of benzodiazepines in psychiatric practice. *Br J Psychiatry* 1987;151:719–23.

6 Goa KL, Ward A. Buspirone: a preliminary review of its pharmacological properties and therapeutic efficacy as an anxiolytic. *Drugs* 1986;32:114–29.

7 Lader MH. Beta-adrenoceptor antagonists in neuropsychiatry: an update. *J Clin Psychiatry* 1988;49:213–23. (This review includes a discussion of the use of β blockers in anxiety disorder, including those characterised by somatic symptoms and performance anxiety.)

8 McDougle CJ, Goodman WK. Obsessive compulsive disorders: pharmacotherapy and pathophysiology. *Curr Opin Psychiatry* 1991;4:267–72.

9 Nicholson AN. Hypnotics: their place in therapeutics. *Drugs* 1988;31:164–76.

10 Zopiclone: another carriage on the tranquilliser train [Editorial]. *Lancet* 1990;335:507–8.

24 Antidepressant drugs

BRIAN R BALLINGER, JOHN FEELY

The classification of depression presents many problems, but many psychiatrists have grouped depressions into psychotic and neurotic (or endogenous and reactive). The new ICD10 classification divides depression into bipolar affective disorder, depressive episodes, recurrent depressive disorders, and persistent mood disorder. Depressive symptoms may also be secondary to other psychiatric illness, such as schizophrenia, or organic syndromes, or may be a side effect of drugs. Antidepressant treatment should usually be considered only after detailed consideration of the nature of the symptoms and causes. Not all patients with depressive symptoms require drugs, and in some people other forms of treatment may be important, such as electroconvulsive therapy, psychotherapy, or cognitive therapy.

Tricyclic antidepressant drugs

Imipramine was the original tricyclic antidepressant and has been used for over 30 years. Most trials have shown it to be superior to placebo, resulting in improvement in about two thirds of cases. *Amitriptyline*, introduced subsequently, was shown to be as effective but more sedative.

The disadvantages of the original tricyclic antidepressants that have become apparent over the years include inefficacy in some cases of depression, slow onset of action, and various side effects, including the commonly occurring anticholinergic side effects, as well as danger when taken in overdose.

A succession of newer tricyclic antidepressants and similar drugs has been introduced, often with claims of speedier action and fewer side effects. They have different degrees of sedative effect but generally seem to have a similar range of activity to each other and to the older drugs. The results of most trials support their claims to be effective antidepressants, although many of the studies have compared them with established agents.

326

Other tricyclic antidepressants include *dothiepin*, which has some sedative action and fewer anticholinergic side effects than amitriptyline. Dothiepin is an effective antidepressant and usually well tolerated. *Clomipramine* has a particularly pronounced effect on the uptake of serotonin, but anticholinergic side effects may sometimes be a problem. It has been used as an intravenous infusion, but there is no evidence that this has any specific advantages. Some evidence exists that clomipramine may also be effective in treating patients with obsessional neurosis, particularly when they have associated depressive symptoms.

Lofepramine (Gamanil) is a more recently introduced tricyclic antidepressant, which may have fewer anticholinergic effects and is probably less cardiotoxic in overdose than amitriptyline, although abnormalities of hepatic enzyme activities have been reported. It is relatively non-sedative.

Amoxapine (Asendis) has recently been introduced in the United Kingdom. It may have fewer cardiovascular side effects than older drugs, but extrapyramidal symptoms and seizures have been reported.

Evidence suggests that most tricyclic antidepressants inhibit the reuptake of noradrenaline and serotonin into neurones. Some drugs—for instance, amitriptyline, imipramine, and clomipramine—act predominantly on the uptake of serotonin, and others—for instance, nortriptyline and desipramine—on noradrenaline. This action is linked to the amine hypothesis of depression, which suggests that symptoms are caused by changes in amine metabolism. It is by no means certain, however, that this is the basis of the antidepressant action of these drugs.

Being lipid soluble, tricyclic drugs are readily absorbed and undergo first pass metabolism in the liver. Their rate of metabolism varies considerably, partly because of genetic polymorphism of drug oxidation (see chapter 1), which results in large variations in plasma steady state concentrations and elimination half lives in patients given the same dose. About 8% of the population are poor hydroxylators and show appreciably higher plasma concentrations, and probably more adverse effects, when given standard doses. Many tricyclics produce demethyl metabolites that are pharmacologically active, and ring hydroxylation leads to inactive metabolites being excreted by the kidneys. Tricyclic antidepressants become distributed widely throughout the body, and as they are 90% protein bound they are not susceptible to active elimination techniques in overdose. Preliminary evidence suggests that plasma concentrations may be higher in elderly people who therefore require lower doses.

New antidepressant drugs resembling tricyclics

Various new antidepressants with different structures have been introduced, but the clinical importance of the structural differences is uncertain. Table 24.1 lists some of these and other agents. In no case has the efficacy of the new antidepressants been shown to exceed that of the tricyclics, but most have fewer anticholinergic side effects than amitriptyline.

Viloxazine is completely absorbed and extensively metabolised in the liver. Unlike the tricyclics, it is not highly protein bound and has a short elimination half life, which has led to the suggestion that it should be given two or three times a day. Viloxazine has little sedative action and few anticholinergic or cardiac side effects. Nausea has been reported as a common side effect and seems to be dose related, which possibly limits the drug's usefulness.

Maprotiline—This "bridged tricyclic" drug shows considerable variation in steady state concentration between people. It seems to be an effective antidepressant and is claimed to have fewer anticholinergic side effects than older drugs, although convulsions and

TABLE 24.1—*Some established tricyclic and new antidepressant drugs*

Approved name	Proprietary names	Elimination half life of active drug (h)	Usual dose range (mg/day)
Amitriptyline	Domical, Elavil, Lentizol, Saroten, Tryptizol	30–45	50–150
Clomipramine	Anafranil	20–40	30–150
Dothiepin	Prothiaden	45–56	75–150
Viloxazine	Vivalan	2–5	150–400
Maprotiline	Ludiomil	30–50	50–150
Mianserin	Bolvidon, Norval	10–17	30–120
Trazodone	Molipaxin	5–8	100–400
Fluvoxamine	Faverin	15	100–300
Fluoxetine	Prozac	24–72*	20
Sertraline	Lustral	26	50–200

Full prescribing instructions should be consulted and lower doses may be appropriate in some elderly patients and higher in refractory depressions.
* Metabolite half life 8–13 days.

skin rashes have been reported. Its fatal toxicity index in overdose does not differ greatly from that of the older drugs. Maprotiline is a sedative antidepressant.

Mianserin is extensively metabolised in the liver, and its profile of action differs considerably from that of the tricyclic antidepressants as it does not block amine uptake. It has negligible anticholinergic side effects and is relatively safe in patients with heart disease. Nevertheless, blood dyscrasias include aplastic anaemia, agranulocytosis and granulocytopenia have been reported, and a full blood count is recommended every 4 weeks during the first 3 months of treatment. Hepatic reactions and arthropathy have also occurred. Mianserin has a pronounced sedative effect and is relatively safe in overdose.

Trazodone is chemically unrelated to other agents, and blocks synaptic serotonin receptors. Trazodone is metabolised in the liver, has a relatively short half life, and is often given in divided doses with the larger portion at bedtime. It is an antidepressant with anxiolytic properties and fewer anticholinergic and cardiac side effects than amitriptyline, although priapism has been reported. Clinical experience indicates that trazodone is a useful agent in some patients.

SELECTIVE SEROTONIN REUPTAKE INHIBITORS

These drugs selectively inhibit the reuptake of serotonin released at nerve terminals but the clinical significance of this action is not clear. They are effective antidepressants with a similar pattern of side effects, particularly nausea, but they may also cause insomnia, tremor, and anxiety. Because they are relatively free from cardiac side effects they may be less toxic than the tricyclics when taken in overdose.

Fluvoxamine (Faverin) selectively inhibits the uptake of 5-HT, and trials suggest that it is an effective antidepressant. It has little sedative action and fewer anticholinergic or cardiac side effects than the earlier tricylic antidepressants. Nausea and vomiting occur relatively commonly, and convulsions have been reported.

Fluoxetine (Prozac) is another inhibitor of 5HT uptake. It is a non-sedative drug that is claimed to have fewer cardiovascular side effects than the older drugs, but nausea and vomiting may occur. This drug is an effective antidepressant and is reasonably well tolerated by most patients. It has a long acting metabolite (norfluoxetine) which means that it should be avoided for at least 5 weeks before starting monoamine oxidase inhibitors. Reports from the United States that it might cause suicide and aggression have not been substantiated.

Sertraline (Lustral) and *Paroxetine* (Seroxat) are other specific serotonin uptake inhibitors. They appear to be as effective in depression as tricyclic antidepressants. Like the other drugs in this class, they have few anticholinergic or cardiac side effects but may cause nausea and vomiting in some patients. Paroxetine has been reported to cause dystonic reactions.

Use of tricyclic and allied antidepressant drugs

Various general considerations apply to the older and newer tricyclic and allied antidepressants.

RESPONSE

These drugs are generally more effective in psychotic (endogenous) depressions, although the results may be less good in patients with prominent delusions. Their antidepressant action does not appear for 1–3 weeks, and further improvement may occur later. The claims that some newer drugs act more quickly have not been fully substantiated.

DURATION OF TREATMENT

When these drugs are effective in treating depression there is evidence that their use should be continued for several months, and trials have suggested that some patients benefit from at least 6 months' treatment. Longer term treatment may prevent depressive episodes in some patients liable to recurrent depression, although lithium is also effective. At the end of treatment the drug may be tailed off gradually and the patient reviewed to detect signs of relapse. Patients with bipolar illness may require treatment with lithium indefinitely.

DOSAGE

Dose requirements and plasma concentrations vary widely between people. Little evidence exists that very small doses of antidepressants should be used in mild depression. Some of the tricyclic antidepressants have similar dose ranges, and doses should be increased over a few days to minimise side effects. Elderly patients generally require smaller doses.

MANNER OF ADMINISTRATION

These drugs are almost always given by mouth, and parenteral administration has no clear advantages. Several trials have shown that administration once a day is as effective as the traditional divided doses, although a few patients tolerate divided doses better. The dose is often best given in the evening, particularly with the more sedative drugs.

PLASMA CONCENTRATIONS

Evidence exists that intermediate plasma concentrations of nortriptyline may be more effective than higher or lower concentrations, and plasma concentrations vary substantially among patients given the same dose. Monitoring services have been introduced in some centres, but it is still not clear whether their routine use would be justified, as a therapeutic range has not been clearly established. They provide a useful index of patient drug compliance in non-responders, although urine testing may be simpler.

SIDE EFFECTS

Side effects have been a serious limiting factor in the use of these drugs, and tend to start before the therapeutic effect is apparent. Side effects include the anticholinergic symptoms such as dry mouth, visual accommodation difficulties, constipation, and hesitant micturition. These are particularly pronounced with amitriptyline but occur in the whole group of drugs and, although a nuisance and occasionally hazardous, may sometimes be a guide to the need to adjust the dose. The problem in their evaluation is that some of the symptoms resemble those of depressive illness. Sedation may be a problem, although this may be minimised by selecting an appropriate drug. Other side effects include precipitation of epilepsy, tremor, nausea, and psychiatric complications including hypomania and confusion. Cardiovascular side effects, including orthostatic hypotension, flattening of the T wave, and conduction defects on the electrocardiogram, have been reported, and occasional sudden cardiac deaths may be a hazard, perhaps

331

particularly with amitriptyline. Cardiac effects may be a major problem in overdose. These drugs should be used with great caution in pregnancy.

DRUG INTERACTIONS

Drug interactions may occur with other sedative drugs, including alcohol. By blocking the uptake of methyldopa, clonidine, and adrenergic neurone blockers such as guanethidine, tricyclics can reverse the antihypertensive effect of those drugs. Neuroleptics such as chlorpromazine inhibit the metabolism of tricyclics, whereas inducers such as antiepileptics lead to lower plasma tricyclic concentrations.

Other antidepressant drugs

Other drugs that differ from the tricyclic and related antidepressants include monoamine oxidase inhibitors, tryptophan, some neuroleptics, lithium, alprazolam, and carbamazepine, the anticonvulsant that has a similar structure to the tricyclics.

Monoamine oxidase inhibitors such as phenelzine, tranylcypromine, and isocarboxazid retain a place in the management of some patients with depression despite the risk of interactions between the drugs and food. Trials of these agents have given variable results, and side effects have led to caution in their use, particularly regarding their hypertensive interactions with certain foodstuffs and drugs (including tricyclic antidepressants). Many psychiatrists believe that monoamine oxidase inhibitors such as phenelzine still have a place in treating depression, particularly in certain patients with "atypical" symptoms including some types of neurotic depression with anxiety and phobic symptoms. They do not seem to be the best agents for most psychotic depressions. A new, reversible, monoamine inhibitor (Moclobemide) is now available. Moclobemide appears to be as effective as tricyclic antidepressants in major depression but there is as yet little to suggest a specific action in "atypical" depression. This drug causes only minimal potentiation of the pressor response to tyramine, so the need for dietary precautions is reduced. It may prove to be a useful agent.

Tryptophan is the precursor of the indolamines, and its use as an antidepressant was suggested by the amine hypothesis of depression. Some trials suggested that it may be effective, but this has not always been confirmed. Several food products containing tryptophan have been removed from the market because of a possible association with eosinophilia and pulmonary infiltrates, and tryptophan is not at present available for prescription in the United Kingdom.

Neuroleptics are mainly used to treat patients with schizophrenia, and depression has been described as a possible side effect of some of them. Nevertheless, flupenthixol (Fluanxol), a thioxanthene derivative, has been advocated as an antidepressant. This is not fully established, but it may be worth trying in certain refractory cases, at a dose range of 1–3 mg a day, although the risk of tardive dyskinesia must not be forgotten.

Alprazolam (Xanax) is a triazolobenzodiazepine that seems to have some antidepressant activity as well as an anxiolytic effect. Its place in treating patients with depression is not really established, and dependence on the drug is possible as it is a benzodiazepine.

Carbamazepine, although primarily an anticonvulsant, has been used to treat patients with affective disorders in recent years. It has some prophylactic action in preventing mania and depression, particularly for illnesses with recurrent short episodes, although its role in managing acute depression is not clearly defined.

Lithium is used particularly in the prophylaxis of manic depressive illness but it also has a role in augmenting tricyclic antidepressants in refractory depression. Regular plasma level checks are essential.

Place of newer antidepressant drugs

The place of newer antidepressants alongside the older agents such as imipramine and amitriptyline has been the matter of some debate. The newer drugs often have fewer anticholinergic and cardiac side effects and are usually safer in overdose. They are less well tried, however, and are not entirely devoid of side effects. There are also some lingering doubts about the relative efficacy of some of them, and the newer drugs are generally more expensive.

The older drugs still have a place in treating patients with depression, but the new agents are now being prescribed more widely and are probably preferable for some patients, such as those with heart disease, many older patients, patients intolerant of the anticholinergic and other side effects of imipramine and amitriptyline, and when there is a risk of suicide.

Anonymous. Mianserin 10 years on. *Drugs ther Bull* 1988;**26**:17–8. (Brief review providing further references to previous work.)

Baldessarini RJ. Current status of antidepressants: clinical pharmacology and therapy. *J Clin Psychiatry* 1989;**50**:117–26. (A review from North America.)

Ballenger JC. The clinical use of carbamazepine in affective disorders. *J Clin Psychiatry* 1988;**49**(suppl 4):13–19. (Reviews available data on clinical effects of carbamazepine for long term and prophylactic treatment of affectively ill patients.)

If at first you do succeed [Editorial]. *Lancet* 1991;**337**:650–1. (Review of specific serotonin re-uptake inhibitors and reversible monoamine oxidase inhibitors.)

Edwards JG. Selective serotonin reuptake inhibitors. *BMJ* 1992;**304**:1644–5.

Ferrier IN, Silverstone T, Eccleston D. Selective serotonin inhibitors: use in depression. *Psych Bull* 1992;**16**:737–9.

Henry JA. The safety of antidepressants. *Br J Psychiatry* 1992;**160**:439–41. (An annotation with references.)

25 Anticonvulsant drugs

D L W DAVIDSON

Considerable experimental study of the mechanisms of epileptoge-
nesis has taken place in recent years using various seizure models.
Greatest interest has focused on the role of the excitatory neurotransmitter, glutamate, the inhibitory transmitter γ aminobutyric
acid (GABA), calcium and sodium channels, and causes of the
changing threshold and spread of seizures in the kindling model.
The new anticonvulsants vigabatrin, lamotrigine, and gabapentin
have emerged and are still finding their place in the management of
epilepsy. While these drugs may be effective as add on therapy
they are expensive, and if there is no clear improvement in seizure
control, adverse effects or quality of life, they should be withdrawn.

As carbamazepine and sodium valproate are the established
drugs, these are discussed (including new formulations) and compared with phenytoin, phenobarbitone, primidone, and ethosuximide. Benzodiazepines are also discussed.

Vigabatrin

Vigabatrin (γ-vinyl-γ-amino butyric acid) is a new anticonvulsant that may find an important place in managing partial seizures.
It irreversibly inhibits GABA transaminase, the enzyme that
catabolises GABA. The resulting increase in synaptic GABA may
be associated with the inhibition of seizures.

PHARMACOKINETICS

The kinetics of vigabatrin are similar in children and adults.
Absorption is rapid, with a peak serum concentration at 1–2 h and
a half life of 5–8 h. Anticonvulsant effects do not, however,
correlate with serum concentrations, and monitoring the concentrations in the blood is therefore not useful. In contrast with older
anticonvulsant drugs, which are metabolised in the liver, vigabatrin is largely excreted unchanged in the urine. Drug interactions

with other anticonvulsants are therefore avoided except for a small fall in serum phenytoin concentrations. Special care is needed in patients with renal failure. Its excretion is slower in the elderly and smaller doses should be used.

USE AND INDICATIONS

Double blind trials have reported better than 50% reduction in seizures in over half the patients with refractory partial seizures. Small numbers may show an increase in seizures; convulsions may occur on withdrawal of the drug, as with other anticonvulsants. An especially important finding is that patients with partial seizures, with or without generalisation, have the best response. If this early experience is confirmed with wider use the drug may find an important place, as at least 40% of patients with partial seizures have incomplete control. There have been reports of improvement in infantile spasms. There is controversial evidence for an optimal daily dose of 2–3 g; some studies have reported improvement up to 4 g daily.

Tachyphylaxis has emerged as a problem in clinical practice with good results initially reported; this declines over a few months in some patients.

ADVERSE EFFECTS

Adverse effects are reported to be mild, reversible, and similar to those for other anticonvulsants—somnolence, confusion, fatigue dizziness, weight gain, and amnesia. Vigabatrin is relatively free of adverse cognitive effects. Improved mood has been reported, as when carbamazepine was introduced, but the mechanism is not clear and full long term cognitive studies have not been undertaken. Agitation and excitement have been noted in children. The most important adverse effect is the production or exacerbation of psychosis, in mild form (increased irritability and mood changes) or as a severe psychosis developing between 5 days and 32 weeks after the start of treatment. Vigabatrin should therefore be started with caution, especially in patients with a history of psychosis, and the possibility of psychosis should be discussed with the patient and/or relatives. The drug must be withdrawn promptly if there is a worsening of the mental state. A small (4%) reduction in haemoglobin concentration and reduction of liver transaminase activity may occur.

Microvacuolation suggestive of intramyelinic oedema has been reported in rodents and dogs treated with high doses of vigabatrin. In humans there is no evidence of abnormality of evoked potentials, or on necropsy or biopsy specimens. Thus, there is no current evidence of a risk to humans, although long term studies have not been reported.

Lamotrigine

Lamotrigine is a novel anticonvulsant drug that emerged from experimental work on antifolate compounds, which may act by reducing the excessive release of the excitatory neurotransmitter, glutamate. It is licenced for the treatment of partial seizures and partial seizures with secondary generalised spread not controlled with other anticonvulsant drugs. There is, however, evidence that it is also effective in absence seizures.

PHARMACOKINETICS

Oral lamotrigine has complete (98%) and rapid absorption with peak levels at about $2\frac{1}{2}$ h. The half life is about 29 h, so a twice daily dosage is satisfactory. It induces its own metabolism to a moderate extent, reducing the elimination half life by about 25%, but as this occurs in the early stages of treatment it is not a clinical problem. Enzyme inducing drugs such as carbamazepine and phenytoin reduce the half life to about 15 h; larger doses may need to be given with these combinations (200–400 mg or more). Sodium valproate inhibits the glucuronidation of lamotrigine, increasing blood levels and lower doses of lamotrigine are required if administered concurrently (100–200 mg). Lamotrigine does not affect the concentrations of other anticonvulsants and is unlikely to affect the metabolism of oral contraceptives. Lamotrigine is about 55% protein bound and has linear kinetics (in contrast to phenytoin) so that blood levels increase progressively with dose. Estimation of serum concentration is not generally available.

USES AND INDICATIONS

Lamotrigine is at present only licensed in the United Kingdom for adults and children over the age of 12 years, although encouraging results have been reported in the treatment of absence attacks, atonic drop attacks, and the Lennox–Gastaut syndrome.

Clinical trials have reported that about 25% of patients with refractory partial, or partial with secondary generalisation, have 50% or more reduction in seizures. A small proportion have complete control. Trials of monotherapy are in progress.

ADVERSE EFFECTS

Drowsiness, dizziness, diplopia, and nausea occur in a small proportion of patients; in one large series about 10% of patients were withdrawn from treatment because of these. About 5% of patients have had to withdraw because of a mild erythematous or maculopapular rash, at times very dramatic as erythema multiforme or part of a Stevens–Johnson syndrome. Some patients report improvement in their mood and mental state. Similar responses have been reported with carbamazepine and it is unclear whether this is a positive psychotropic effect or whether it is related to seizure control or reduction of other anticonvulsants. Psychiatric disturbance has been reported in some patients.

Gabapentin

Gabapentin (Neurontin) is the most recently introduced anticonvulsant drug. Its name arises from a structural similarity to GABA but its mode of action is still unclear; it does not appear to act directly on GABA transmission or metabolism.

PHARMACOKINETICS

Gabapentin is well absorbed after oral administration with a peak concentration in about 3 h. A minor reduction in its absorption has been noted with aluminium/magnesium-containing antacids. The serum levels are linearly correlated with the dosage in the therapeutic range. It does not bind to plasma proteins. A potential advantage, shared with vigabatrin, is its largely renal excretion (80%). It is not metabolised in the liver, and does not interact with other convulsant drugs. The dosage should be reduced in patients with renal impairment, and the manufacturer's data sheet provides a scale of recommended dosages related to the creatinine clearance. There is a small (12%) decrease in the renal clearance of gabapentin caused by cimetidine but this is unlikely to be clinically important.

Gabapentin has a short life of about 6 h, and should be taken three times daily.

Gabapentin has been reported to reduce the number of seizures by more than 50% in 13–29% of adult patients with refractory partial seizures and partial with secondary generalised convulsions. It is not (yet) licensed for children under 12 years. There is a dose related clinical response between 600 and 1800 mg daily, and the drug can be introduced rapidly with 300 mg on day one, 300 mg twice on the second day, and three doses of 300 mg on the third day. Futher increases would depend on the clinical response. The maximum dose is 2400 mg daily. Gabapentin is at present indicated only as add-on therapy in patients whose seizures have not been controlled with standard anticonvulsant therapy such as carbamazepine valproate. Withdrawal should be gradual over a week, in contrast to barbiturates and phenytoin which should be withdrawn much more slowly.

Gabapentin's safety in pregnancy has not been established (although experimental studies show no effects on reproduction) and it should therefore be considered in women who may become pregnant only if there is compelling clinical indication.

ADVERSE EFFECTS

The common side effects are somnolence, dizziness, ataxia, fatigue and nystagmus, occuring in 10–20% of patients. Less common adverse effects, some hardly different from the placebo controlled groups were headache, tremor, diplopia, nausea and/or vomiting, and rhinitis. There have also been rare descriptions of convulsions, pharyngitis, dysarthria, weight increase, dyspepsia, amnesia, nervousness and coughing.

Carbamazepine

Carbamazepine has a tricyclic structure and a poorly understood "membrane stabilising" anticonvulsant effect. It is effective for treating partial seizures and for tonic–clonic seizures (grand mal), whether primary or secondary generalisation from a focal lesion. It is of no value for absence seizures (petit mal).

Oxcarbazine is a metabolite of carbamazepine with anticonvulsant effects, and some trials have reported less adverse effects. It is not, however, licensed in the United Kingdom.

PHARMACOKINETICS

Carbamazepine is variably absorbed from the gut and has a peak serum concentration 4–6 h after a single dose in adults, with an earlier peak in children. This is important as peak concentrations may be associated with transient adverse effects such as "dizziness", blurred vision, and diplopia. The half life is 18–55 h, commonly about 35 h, at the start of treatment but, because carbamazepine induces its own metabolism, in the first 4 weeks of treatment the half life shortens and the dose needs to be increased. It takes about 7 days (four to five half lives) to reach a steady state at the start of treatment. Thus 100–200 mg twice a day may be given at the start of treatment and increased at 1–2 weeks to 200–400 mg daily. Further increments may be required if there are recurrent siezures, with doses up to 1·6 g daily.

Important drug interactions may occur via hepatic metabolism. Serum concentrations of carbamazepine may fall with the introduction of phenytoin or phenobarbitone, which also induce liver enzyme activities. The induction of hepatic enzymes by carbamazepine, as with phenytoin and the barbiturates, may reduce the efficacy of oral contraceptives; an increase in the dose of oestrogen is therefore wise (to at least 50 mg ethinyl oestradiol a day). This contrasts with the lack of effect of valproate on oestrogen metabolism, which means that conventional low dose oral contraceptives are adequate for women taking valproate. Serum concentrations of carbamazepine may be increased by erythromycin or dextropropoxyphene. The plasma binding is 70–80%, less than for phenytoin and valproate, and drug interactions on this basis are seldom important.

SERUM CONCENTRATIONS

The therapeutic range of serum concentrations (table 25.1) should, as with other anticonvulsants, be used only as a guide to treatment. The lower end of the range is poorly defined, as seizures may be controlled at concentrations below the therapeutic range and there is then no indication to increase the dose. The upper level of the range is also poorly defined, as higher serum concentrations have anticonvulsant effects without adverse reactions in some patients. Nevertheless, assays of serum concentrations are a useful guide to compliance, metabolism, or drug failure if seizures continue. Assays are also useful if multiple drugs are used, as the concentrations may change in a complex manner because of drug interactions. There is a linear increase in serum concentration with increasing doses of carbamazepine (in contrast to phenytoin), which may cause toxicity rapidly with small increments in or above the therapeutic range because of the non-linear saturation of phenytoin metabolism.

The main toxic effects are on the central nervous system. Drowsiness may occur, although less commonly than with the barbiturates and phenytoin. Some patients may become more alert and cheerful, though there has been much debate about whether this is from a psychotropic effect of the drug or because of withdrawal of more sedative anticonvulsants and the control of seizures. The use of carbamazepine for stabilising manic–depressive psychosis suggests that the drug does have a psychotropic effect in some patients. This effect contrasts with the depression that may arise with barbiturates.

Dizziness, ataxia, nystagmus, and visual disturbances are other toxic effects; similar adverse effects occur with phenytoin, vigabatrin, and barbiturates. Transient visual disturbances (including diplopia) may occur as the serum concentration rises to a peak: these patients may be better taking the controlled release formulation. Some patients are unduly sensitive to these adverse effects at the start of treatment, but toxicity may be avoided by starting on low doses. Toxic concentrations may be associated with a paradoxical increase in seizures, as with phenytoin. Chronic toxicity, with long term impairment of memory and cognition, behavioural disturbances, cerebellar atrophy and peripheral neuropathy, are most clearly described with phenytoin and the barbiturates, not with carbamazepine or valproate.

Alimentary disturbances are rare. Rashes, mainly maculopapular erythematous eruptions, occur in the early weeks of treatment in 5–10% of patients. Carbamazepine does not produce the coarsening of facial features, acne, and hirsutism that makes phenytoin especially unpopular in young women. Mild changes in hepatic enzyme activity are common but serious hepatic toxicity is rare. Severe bone marrow depression was reported in elderly patients soon after carbamazepine was introduced but has proved to be rare, although mild, reversible and usually unimportant leucopenia is common. Carbamazepine in higher doses has an antidiuretic

TABLE 25.1—*Comparison of oral anticonvulsant drugs*

Anticonvulsant (proprietary name)	Usual daily maintenance dose range	Available preparations (dose)	Optimum serum concentrations μmol/l (μg/ml)	Half life (h)	Common or important adverse effects
Carbamazepine (Tegretol)	Adults 300–1600 mg (start at 100 mg twice a day, increase over 4 weeks) Children 9–20 mg/kg	100, 200, and 400 mg tablets 100 mg/5 ml liquid 200 and 400 mg tablets, controlled release	25–50 (6–12)	25–50 initially 10–30 long term Children 5–30	Drowsiness, dizziness, ataxia, diplopia, rashes, leucopenia heart block, hyponatremia
Clobazam (Frisium)	Adults 10–40 mg at night Children 5–20 mg (over 3 years)	10 mg tablet	Not available	18	Drowsiness, dizziness, confusion, ataxia
Clonazepam (Rivotril)	Adults 1·5–8 mg (start at 0·5 mg twice a day, increase over 4 weeks)	0·5 and 2 mg tablets	Not available	20–60	Drowsiness, ataxia, behaviour disturbance, bronchial hypersecretion in infants
Ethosuximide (Zarontin)	Adults 500–2000 mg (start at 250 mg twice a day) Children 250–1000 mg	250 mg tablet 250 mg/5 ml syrup	300–700 (40–100)	Adults 30–70 Children 30 (variable	Nausea, vomiting, tiredness, dizziness, mood disturbances, leucopenia, rashes
Gabapentin	900–2400 mg	100, 300 and 400 mg capsules	Not available	6	Somnolence, dizziness, ataxia, nystagmus, fatigue
Lamotrigine (Lamictal)	Adults 200–400 mg daily (start on 50 mg or 100–200 mg daily on valproate combination start at 50 mg daily)	25, mg, 50 mg and 100 mg	Not available	29	Drowsiness, dizziness, headache, diplopia, nausea, rash, instability, aggressive and angioedema

Drug	Dose	Formulation	Therapeutic range	Half-life (hours)	Side effects
Phenytoin (Epanutin)	Adults 150–600 mg (start at 100 mg twice a day) Children 5–8 mg/kg	25, 50, 100, and 300 mg capsules/tablets 30 mg/5 ml suspension	40–80 (10–20)	Adults 10–60 Children 5–12	Drowsiness, impaired memory, and attention, ataxia, blurred vision, diplopia, gum hyperplasia, hirsutism, acne, facial coarsening, rashes, sensory neuropathy, liver damage, osteomalacia
Phenobarbitone	Adults 60–240 mg (start at 30 mg) Children 30–180 mg	15, 30, 60, and 100 mg tablets	80–180 (15–40)	Adults 70–120 Children 40–70	Drowsiness, memory impairment, behaviour disorders, hyperactivity
Primidone (Mysoline)	Adults 250–1500 mg (start at 125 mg a day) Children 125–1000 mg	250 mg tablets 250 mg/5 ml suspension	Not available	4–11 (as for phenobarbitone)	As for phenobarbitone, occasionally pronounced at start
Sodium valproate (Epilim)	Adults 200–2000 mg Children 20–30 mg/kg	100, 200, and 500 mg tablets 200 mg/5 ml liquid or syrup	350–700 (50–100)	Adults 6–15 Children 4–14	Drowsiness, confusion, tremor, insomnia, nausea, weight gain, alopecia, bleeding tendency, hepatotoxicity, pancreatitis
Vigabatrin (Sabril)	Adults 2–4 g (start at 500 mg) Children 1 g (age 3–9 years) 2 g (older children)	500 mg tablet	Not available	5–7	Somnolence, fatigue, confusion, dizziness, weight gain, psychosis

action, which produces hyponatraemia, but clinical problems of water intoxication are rare. Regular long term monitoring of the full blood count and concentrations of electrolytes is not required. Increased thyroxine (T4) metabolism after treatment with carbamazepine (as with phenytoin and barbiturates) may result in low concentrations of triiodothyronine (T3), T4, free T4, and free T3, but the concentration of thyroid stimulating hormone is not high and clinical hypothyroidism is rare. Carbamazepine and phenytoin depress the release of thyroid stimulating hormone by the hypothalamus and the pituitary, which complicates the assessment of whether the lethargy, fatigue and constipation are due to hypothyroidism. The free T4 concentration is the best discriminator, and the concentrations of basal thyroid stimulating hormones and thyrotropin releasing hormone should be measured if the T4 concentration is equivocal.

Some patients with epilepsy are hyposexual, probably as a consequence of the epilepsy and/or additional brain damage, though an increase in sex hormone metabolism induced by carbamazepine, phenytoin or the barbiturates is a factor.

CONTROLLED RELEASE CARBAMAZEPINE

Controlled release carbamazepine (Tegretol Retard) reduces the peak dose and the fluctuation in carbamazepine concentrations during 24 h. It may be useful for patients with fluctuating adverse effects (dizziness, diplopia, and drowsiness) and for patients who have difficulty in complying with three or more doses a day, as a twice a day dose is satisfactory.

Sodium valproate

Sodium valproate may act by inhibiting GABA metabolism, reducing excitatory transmission and potassium channels. It has a much broader range of anticonvulsant effects than carbamazepine, phenytoin, vigabatrin or the barbiturates. It is effective against absence attacks (as is ethosuximide (Zarontin)), and also against tonic–clonic, myoclonic, and akinetic seizures. It was initially thought to be less effective against partial seizures than other anticonvulsants, but trials have shown it to be just as effective.

PHARMACOKINETICS

Sodium valproate is rapidly absorbed and has a peak serum concentration 1–4 h after ingestion. It is conjugated in the liver and has a short half life (table 25.1). As it is 80–90% bound to plasma proteins, drug interactions occur from displacement effects: for example, if a patient taking phenytoin with serum concentrations in the therapeutic range starts taking sodium valproate the displacement of phenytoin by valproate may cause phenytoin toxicity. In chronic renal failure the plasma binding of both valproate and phenytoin is decreased. Drug interactions also occur in the liver—for example, valproate may increase serum phenobarbitone concentrations substantially by inhibiting phenobarbitone metabolism. Valproate may also interact with phenobarbitone and with benzodiazepine actions at the GABA-chloride ion iontophore complexes—that is, the putative GABA receptor sites in the brain. Interactions with carbamazepine are seldom clinically important.

SERUM CONCENTRATIONS

Although therapeutic ranges are commonly quoted for valproate (table 25.1), there is no clear relation between serum concentrations and anticonvulsant effects. As the anticonvulsant effect is much longer than its short half life, valproate may be effective in a once or twice a day regimen despite its rapid clearance from the blood.

ADVERSE EFFECTS

An attractive feature of valproate is its relative freedom from sedative, cognitive, and behavioural effects compared with phenytoin, phenobarbitone, and the benzodiazepines: drowsiness, restlessness, and irritability may, however, occur. Dose related reversible postural tremor may also be seen. Oesophageal discomfort and nausea have been reduced with enteric coated formulations. Weight gain is common and is a problem in some patients. Transient alopecia may occur and, curiously, the hair may be curly when it grows again. Although platelet numbers and adhesiveness, and fibrinogen concentrations may be reduced (which produces a mild bleeding tendency), serious haemorrhagic complications are rare. Bone marrow depression is very rare.

Rare idiosyncratic metabolic reactions that produce fatal hepatotoxicity (or even more rarely pancreatitis) are the most serious complications. The hepatotoxicity evolves rapidly, within the first 6 months of treatment, and the most vulnerable patients are children under 3 years old with underlying metabolic disorder, liver disease, major brain damage, or receiving multiple drugs. If the patient develops nausea, vomiting, anorexia, jaundice, drowsiness or loss of control of seizures the drug should be withdrawn promptly. Minor abnormalities of liver function are common (in about 40% of patients) and regular long term monitoring is not helpful, except in high risk patients early in treatment. The hepatotoxicity of valproate contrasts with the rare allergic hepatic damage caused by phenytoin and carbamazepine.

Several metabolic abnormalities have been reported in association with valproate; hyperammonaemia is the most important as it produces impaired consciousness, vomiting and ataxia.

PARENTERAL VALPROATE

Parenteral valproate (Epilim intravenous) is available to maintain medication when it is temporarily impossible to give oral preparations—for example after surgery. The value of parenteral valproate in treating status epilepticus has not been assessed. The dose should be that of the oral medication. To start, parenteral valproate is given as a slow intravenous injection of 400–800 mg (or up to 10 mg/kg) for 3–5 min, followed by an infusion up to a maximum of 2·5 g a day.

CONTROLLED RELEASE VALPROATE

A controlled release formulation of sodium valproate (Epilim Chrono) is now available. It reduces the peak doses and produces a more even plasma level throughout the day. It may be given twice daily. As serum levels are not correlated with the effectiveness in previous studies it is unclear whether the new formulation will alter effectiveness.

Benzodiazepines

The benzodiazepines affect the GABA receptor. Diazepam, clonazepam, nitrazepam, and clobazam all have important anticonvulsant effects.

Intravenous diazepam is useful for status epilepticus, given as an emulsion (Diazemuls) that reduces local thrombophlebitis.

Rectal diazepam (Stesolid) is being increasingly used for patients with a liability to status epilepticus or to serial seizures and may be administered by parents or in special schools and/or training and care centres provided by social work departments. Fears about the practical and medicolegal aspects of administration by non-medical staff demand that the indications are clearly specified by the doctor, and that teachers and care workers are carefully trained in epilepsy and rectal administration. There is a need for national guidelines in its use outwith the NHS. The dose in children aged 1–3 years is 5 mg and 10 mg in older children; the dose in adults is less well established. One study has recently reported better results in 30 mg than 20 mg doses.

Clonazepam may be used parenterally for status epilepticus but has no clear advantage over diazepam. It is a second line anticonvulsant for absence, tonic–clonic, myoclonic, or partial seizures. It is absorbed well after oral administration, has a prolonged half life of 20–60 h, and is metabolised in the liver. Its main advantage is its action against a variety of seizure types but the two main problems are drowsiness and tolerance. The drowsiness, fatigue, and dizziness may be reduced by introducing it gradually. Irritability and behavioural disturbances may occur in children as with barbiturates. Bronchial and salivary hypersecretion may occur with parenteral use.

Clobazam produces less drowsiness than clonazepam although tolerance is still a problem. There is some evidence of its value in preventing menstrual (catamenial) seizures if it is taken for 7–10 days before the onset until the end of the period. Withdrawal seizures may occur. Occasional patients experience long term benefit when receiving regular medication.

Nitrazepam may be used to treat children with refractory absence seizures or myoclonus.

Starting and stopping anticonvulsant treatment

STARTING

There is debate on whether to start a patient on anticonvulsants after a single unprovoked seizure or whether to wait until the liability to seizures has been shown by recurrences (about 80% of seizures are followed by another). The practice most common in the United Kingdom is to start drugs only after two or more unprovoked seizures (excluding alcohol or other drug induced seizures and febrile convulsions): some neurologists would, however, start after a single well defined tonic–clonic seizure occurring without an avoidable precipitant. Patients with photoconvulsive seizures may be free from seizures without taking anticonvulsants after being given advice on avoiding the photic stimuli (sitting at least 10 ft (3 m) away from the television, in some ambient light to reduce contrast, using a small (14 inch) screen and remote control) and covering one eye in situations of flickering light.

STOPPING

There are no precise criteria for predicting which of the 40% of adults and 20% of children will have recurrences when anticonvulsant treatment is withdrawn after 2 years or more free from seizures. The Medical Research Council Antiepileptic Drug Withdrawal study has reported that patients with a long history of seizures before control, myoclonic epilepsy, early morning convulsions, primary tonic–clonic seizures, or focal and/or generalised discharges on electroencephalography have higher risk of recurrence on anticonvulsant withdrawal than others. The need to drive often determines whether to withdraw; people with pressing work or social reasons for driving will not stop taking anticonvulsants.

Choice of anticonvulsant drugs

About 80% of adults presenting with seizures are controlled with monotherapy. Adverse effects and drug interactions increase when two or more anticonvulsants are taken, and the simplest regimen should therefore be used, avoiding combinations if possible. Nevertheless, some patients, especially those with multiple types of seizures, require polytherapy.

Table 25.2 shows the main choices of anticonvulsants. Valproate is the best drug for myoclonic epilepsy. Many studies show that the drugs used for partial and those used for generalised tonic–clonic seizures are of roughly similar effectiveness and there may be little difference between carbamazepine and valproate.

Complete control is obtained in 80–90% of patients with primary generalised seizures but only 30–40% of those with partial seizures. Vigabatrin, lamotrigine, and gabapentin are especially important because they offer the prospect of better control of this most refractory problem. If they also fail then surgery for partial seizures should be considered. The quality of mental function and learning is especially important in children and adolescents, and so carbamazepine, valproate, vigabatrin and lamotrigine should be

TABLE 25.2—*Choice of anticonvulsant drugs (author's choice)*

Type of seizure	First choice (second choice)	Alternatives
Partial (temporal lobe most common), including secondary generalised	Carbamazepine (valproate)	Gabapentin, lamotrigine, vigabatrin, phenytoin, primidone, phenobarbitone, clobazam, clonazepam
Primary tonic–clonic, tonic, or clonic (grand mal)	Valproate (carbamazepine)	Phenytoin, primidone, phenobarbitone, clobazam, clonazepam
Absence (petit mal)	Valproate (ethosuximide)	Clonazepam, nitrazepam
Myoclonus	Valproate (clobazam)	Clonazepam, nitrazepam
Status epilepticus	Intravenous diazepam (intravenous phenytoin)	Chlormethiazole, clonazepam, paraldehyde, thiopentone

used in preference to the older anticonvulsants. The disfiguring effects of phenytoin make it unsatisfactory for young women. The possibility of hepatotoxicity may restrict the use of valproate in children at high risk of liver disease.

In pregnancy, dysmorphism has been associated with barbiturates, the benzodiazepines, and phenytoin. Although initially described as the "fetal hydantoin" syndrome, the broader term "fetal antiepileptic drug syndrome" is better. Valproate has also been associated with a higher than usual (1–2%) risk of spina bifida. The overall risk of malformations, mainly cleft lip and palate, is about 6–7% compared with 3–4% in women not receiving valproate. Carbamazepine appears to carry the least risk. The teratogenic effects of vigabatrin, lamotrigine, and gabapentin are not known. In patients with active epilepsy the risks of uncontrolled seizures are greater than the risk of malformation, and anticonvulsant treatment should be maintained, as monotherapy if possible. α Fetoprotein and ultrasound scanning may be indicated in patients taking valproate to establish whether a neural tube defect is present. As the drug clearance often increases, the serum concentrations of carbamazepine or phenytoin should be monitored and the dose increased accordingly if seizures occur.

Status epilepticus

Intravenous diazepam (Diazemuls) 5–10 mg for adults (0·15– 0·25 mg/kg for children) at a rate of less than 2 mg/min is the best treatment; the dose may be increased up to 20 mg (for adults) if seizures continue and there are no adverse effects. There is some evidence that intravenous diazepam may worsen patients with acute neurological injury by exacerbating respiratory depression: phenytoin would be a better choice for these patients. Rectal administration of diazepam produces peak blood levels only a little later than the intravenous route, and is useful where an injection is not feasible. Clonazepam or lorazepam are used in some centres because they last longer than, and cause less respiratory depression than, diazepam. Clonazepam is an alternative at a dose of 1 mg for adults and 0·5 mg for children given over 30 s. If control is not achieved it is better to change to an alternative regimen than continue with benzodiazepine infusions. There are several choices:

● Intravenous *phenytoin*, 15–18 mg/kg, at a rate of less than 50 mg/min (never intramuscularly) is often effective, and has the advantage that the patient has already received a loading dose for transition to oral medication.

● *Chlormethiazole* has a short half life and rapidly reversible sedative and anticonvulsant effects. It is relatively free from hypotensive and respiratory depressant effects but may potentiate the respiratory depressant effects of barbiturates, phenothiazines, and butryophenones. Local thrombophlebitis may be a problem. Chlormethiazole is best used as a continuous infusion of an 8% solution, given initially as 40–100 ml (320–800 mg) at a rate of 60–150 drops/min, but with the infusion rate adjusted according to response and adverse effects.

● The use of *paraldehyde* has declined, but it may be administered by deep intramuscular injection when intravenous infusion is impossible. Some specialised centres have used intravenous infusions.

● In intensive care units thiopentone can be infused intravenously, using artificial ventilation if necessary. Electroencephalography to monitor the control of seizures is essential.

Chadwick D, ed. *Fourth international symposium on sodium valproate and epilepsy*. London: Royal Society of Medicine, 1989 (International Congress and Symposium Series (ICSS) No 152).

Hopkins A, ed. *Epilepsy*. London: Chapman & Hall, 1987.

Laidlaw J, Richens A, Oxley J. *A textbook of epilepsy*, 4th edn. Edinburgh: Churchill Livingstone, 1992.

Pedley TA, Meldrum BS. *Recent advances in epilepsy*. Edinburgh: Churchill Livingstone, 1983 (vol. 1); 1985 (vol. 2); 1986 (vol. 3); 1988 (vol. 4). (Authoritative essays on various aspects of epilepsy including updates on carbamazepine, valproate, phenytoin, barbiturates, benzodiazepine, and ethosuximide, the toxicity of antiepileptic drugs, and managing status epilepticus.)

Sander JWAS, Hart YM, Trimle MR, Shorvon SD. Vigabatrin and psychosis. *J Neurol Neurosurg Psychiatry* 1991;**54**:435–9.

Remy C, Jourdil N, Villimain D, Favel P, Genton P. Intrarectal diazepam in adult epileptics. *Epilepsia* 1992;**33**:353–8.

26 Other centrally acting drugs

D N BATEMAN, S CHAPLIN

Since the first edition of *New Drugs* several new drugs that act on the central nervous system have been introduced. In this chapter we will consider three groups—the antipsychotics, opioids, and antiemetics. Some of these, including for example the antiemetic domperidone, also exert effects outside the brain. For others, such as the cannabinoid nabilone, the precise mechanism of action remains unclear.

Antipsychotics

The antipsychotic agents are largely drawn from three distinct chemical groups:

- the phenothiazines (for example, chlorpromazine);
- the butyrophenones (haloperidol); and
- the thioxanthenes (for example, flupenthixol).

Sulpiride (Dolmatil) is an example of a fourth group, the benzamides, and has been used extensively in Europe but was introduced into the United Kingdom only recently. In contrast with older drugs, which affect both the D-1 and D-2 subtypes of dopamine receptor, sulpiride is a specific antagonist at postsynaptic D-2 receptors. It also affects presynaptic autoinhibitory dopamine receptors. It is this range of action that distinguishes sulpiride from other neuroleptics but although animal experiments show a different pattern of behavioural effects, clear clinical evidence to support a new effect in humans is still awaited.

SULPIRIDE

Sulpiride is absorbed slowly from the gastrointestinal tract, and its half life is about 10h. The drug seems to be excreted largely unchanged in the urine and faeces. It seems to be as effective as other antipsychotic agents in treating schizophrenia. In patients who show negative symptoms some studies have suggested that sulpiride is more effective than other drugs.

The adverse effects associated with sulpiride are typical of dopamine antagonists and include dystonic reactions, parkinsonism, akathisia, tardive dyskinesia, and galactorrhoea. It is at present not clear whether the pattern of adverse effects is quantitatively as well as qualitatively similar to that of other drugs. The precise role of sulpiride in psychiatry remains unclear, but current evidence does not suggest that it has a great advantage over other neuroleptics.

REMOXIPRIDE (ROXIAM)

Another substituted benzamide, this is a selective dopamine D-2 antagonist. It is well absorbed (bioavailability approaching 100%), with a plasma half life of 6h. Excretion is by both hepatic metabolism (70%) and renal routes. Although it causes extrapyramidal adverse effects, these are less common than with traditional antipsychotics such as haloperidol.[1] There is evidence suggesting a dose–response relationship of benefit in schizophrenia with doses of less than 90 mg per day being less effective than the larger amounts of 150–450 mg once daily usually used.

LOXAPINE (LOXAPAC)

This is a tricyclic dibenzoxepine that has antipsychotic properties. It may have a slower onset of effects than other antipsychotics, as some short term studies (3–4 weeks) suggested that standard antipsychotic drugs were more efficacious, although longer term studies (4–12 weeks) showed that loxapine was comparable with other drugs.[2] Extrapyramidal reactions seem to be common with this drug, and it seems to have no obvious advantages over other standard antipsychotics.

CLOZAPINE

Clozapine (Clozaril) is an old drug originally introduced into clinical study around 1960. It was found to cause agranulocytosis in about 2% of patients treated for 1 year and therefore is a potentially toxic compound. Clozapine has, however, been found to be extremely effective in resistant schizophrenia, improving positive and negative symptoms, and 30% of this group of very difficult patients responded compared with 4% of those treated with chlorpromazine and benztropine.[3] Clozapine also seems to cause fewer extrapyramidal reactions than conventional antipsychotics, which may reflect its pattern of receptor blocking activity as it binds more avidly to D-1 receptors than to D-2 receptors. Further work has also suggested binding at a specific D-4 receptor subgroup.[4]

Clozapine has a bioavailability of about 50% and undergoes extensive first pass metabolism. It has two principal metabolites, the N-oxide and a desmethyl derivative, both of which have some pharmacological activity. The terminal half life is 12–25 h, and the drug is renally eliminated. Slow dose titration is recommended, and once a therapeutic effect has been obtained the dose should be reduced to a maintenance level. Approximately 60% of patients respond.

Close monitoring of patients is clearly required because of the risk of adverse effects in the bone marrow, and clozapine is only indicated for patients who fail to respond to standard antipsychotics or who suffer incapacitating neurological adverse effects with standard treatment. Clozapine is nevertheless an interesting antipsychotic compound, and is currently available in the United Kingdom only via a monitored release system, with patients undergoing regular haematological tests.

Opioids

Several mixed narcotic agonist–antagonist analgesics are now available for treating moderate to severe pain. These drugs act as partial agonists at opioid receptors (they will cause withdrawal symptoms if given to addicts or to patients who have received opiates over a long period). The adverse effects and potential for abuse of opioids that have partial agonist properties vary.[5] *Pentazocine*, though an effective analgesic, was found to exert adverse effects on the heart and central nervous system and to have some potential for causing dependence. *Buprenorphine* seems to be less likely to cause adverse effects, though nausea and vomiting may be troublesome. It has a longer duration of action, but it too seems to have a potential for abuse.

The two most recent additions to this group are nalbuphine and meptazinol. *Nalbuphine* (Nubain) is available only as an injection for subcutaneous, intramuscular, or intravenous use. It undergoes extensive hepatic metabolism and is probably excreted through the bile in the faeces. Its elimination half life is about 5 h. At low doses nalbuphine is comparable to morphine, and analgesia lasts for 4–5 h after intramuscular injection. Unlike morphine, however, increasing doses of nalbuphine seem not to increase analgesia[6]—or respiratory depression—beyond a "ceiling" level. It is less suitable than morphine for managing severe pain.

Nalbuphine causes fewer psychotomimetic effects and has less potential for abuse than pentazocine. Sedation occurred in 30–40% of subjects in clinical trials, and about 10% experienced nausea and vomiting, headache, sweating, and dizziness. Unlike pentazocine nalbuphine does not exert substantial adverse haemodynamic effects, and it may therefore be of value in treating some patients who have heart disease.

Meptazinol (Meptid) injection, like nalbuphine, is licensed for treating moderate to severe pain. Its bioavailability after oral administration is less than 10% because of extensive hepatic first pass metabolism. Meptazinol tablets are licensed for treating moderate pain only. The recommended dose is twice that of the injection, but this provides only 20% as much drug as systemic administration. Although meptazinol is a partial agonist, it also has central cholinergic activity. The importance of this remains unclear. Meptazinol is known to cause a low incidence of adverse cardiac and respiratory effects.

Meptazinol given by injection has a shorter half life than nalbuphine and has therefore been used to treat obstetric pain, when rapid elimination by the mother (half life 2h) and the neonate (half life 3h) is a great advantage. Meptazinol has also been shown in some studies to provide greater analgesia than pethidine, which has a long half life and may therefore cause respiratory depression in the neonate.[7]

After oral administration meptazinol is as effective as pentazocine and co-proxamol in treating moderate pain but, like nalbuphine, it causes fewer psychotomimetic effects and less respiratory depression than pentazocine. It may be less effective than buprenorphine after parenteral administration, but no published trials compare meptazinol with similar agents. Other adverse effects are typical of opioid analgesics and include vomiting, dizziness, sweating, and sedation.[8]

The oral formulation of meptazinol is substantially more expensive than other opioids, but it may be of value in patients who are unable to tolerate the cheaper alternatives or for whom such drugs are contraindicated. Both nalbuphine and meptazinol injections are similarly expensive but offer a fairly low risk of serious adverse effects.

Antiemetic drugs

Nausea and vomiting are common symptoms associated with various systemic diseases, but the main subject of recent interest in antiemetic treatment has been the management of nausea and vomiting caused by cytotoxic drugs. The conventional phenothiazine antiemetic drugs such as prochlorperazine probably owe their effects to a blockade of dopamine receptors at the chemoreceptor trigger zone.

New developments in research into antiemetics include the use of larger doses of metoclopramide than are conventionally given—"high dose" metoclopramide—and the introduction of two new antiemetics that have contrasting pharmacological profiles. *Domperidone* is a dopamine antagonist that affects gut motility. Initial observations in the 1970s that cannabis seemed to have antiemetic potential in patients who were undergoing chemotherapy resulted in the development of synthetic cannabinoids, of which *nabilone* is currently marketed in the United Kingdom. Finally, recognition that high dose metoclopramide was effective because of its agonist effects on a subgroup of 5-hydroxytriptamine receptors (5-hydroxytriptamine-3 receptors) has led to the development of specific agents with those agonist effects but without the dopamine receptor antagonist effects of metoclopramide.

HIGH DOSE METOCLOPRAMIDE

Large doses of metoclopramide were first reported by Gralla and colleagues to be effective in managing vomiting induced by cytotoxic drugs.[9] These workers studied patients who were receiving cisplatin, one of the most potently emetic cytotoxic drugs. Five intermittent bolus doses of metoclopramide given over 8 h to a total dose of around 10 mg/kg body weight greatly reduced vomiting. More recent studies, though confirming metoclopramide to be an effective antiemetic, have often failed to produce the very high response rate described originally. In patients who are receiving cisplatin there is some evidence to suggest that metoclopramide plasma concentrations should be above 800 ng/ml. This can be achieved by giving an intravenous loading dose (3 mg/kg) over 15 min and a subsequent infusion of 3 mg/kg over 8 h.[10] Most oncologists will add other antiemetics when treating patients who are receiving highly emetic regimens, often including steroids (for example, dexamethasone) and a benzodiazepine (lorazepam). With less emetic cytotoxic regimens the most suitable dose of metoclopramide has not been estimated.

The adverse effects of high dose metoclopramide include acute dystonic reactions, particularly in younger patients. These respond to intravenous diazepam or an anticholinergic. Diarrhoea, sedation, and acute restlessness may also occur.

DOMPERIDONE (MOTILIUM)

Domperidone prevents vomiting by antagonising dopamine receptors in the chemoreceptor zone. It penetrates the blood–brain barrier poorly and as a result is associated with a much lower incidence of centrally mediated extrapyramidal adverse effects than other dopamine antagonists such as metoclopramide or prochlorperazine. Occasional cases of dystonia, however, have been reported, and domperidone also causes an increase in the serum concentration of prolactin. Peripherally domperidone directly affects the stomach, increasing gastric emptying and pressure on the lower oesophageal sphincter. The systemic bioavailability of domperidone when given by mouth is around 15%, and the drug undergoes hepatic metabolism.

Domperidone may be of particular use in patients who are at risk of centrally mediated adverse reactions—for example, the young and the elderly, in whom extrapyramidal adverse effects are more common. It has also been found to be valuable in the short term management of patients with parkinsonism who have nausea caused by levodopa or bromocriptine. As domperidone affects gastric emptying it may help some patients who have disorders of upper gastrointestinal motility—for example, diabetic gastroparesis. It is not clear how much of the antiemetic effect of domperidone is due to its gastrointestinal action.

Although early studies of domperidone in managing vomiting induced by cytotoxic drugs gave promising results, particularly in children, the withdrawal of the parenteral preparation—because of concern about cardiac arrhythmias—and the low oral bioavailability have restricted its use for this indication. Domperidone is also available as a suppository, but the bioavailability of this formulation is low.

NABILONE (CESAMET)

Nabilone is a synthetic cannabinoid licensed in the United Kingdom only for treating vomiting induced by cytotoxic drugs, and its supply is restricted to hospitals.[11] It is available only as an oral preparation, and like most cannabinoids it undergoes first pass metabolism by the liver. The precise mechanism of action of cannabinoids as antiemetics is not clear.

Adverse effects, including dysphoria, drowsiness, and dizziness, are common and dose limiting in about one quarter of all patients. These adverse effects are more of a problem in the elderly, who are also susceptible to hypotension. Nabilone has not been formally compared with high dose metoclopramide and is probably less effective. It is, however, an alternative agent that may be of value in patients—for example, the young—who tend to suffer from dystonia if treated with dopamine antagonists. Published studies suggest that it is as effective as oral prochlorperazine, though this has been used at suboptimal doses.

5-HYDROXYTRIPTAMINE-3-ANTAGONISTS

Ondansetron (Zofran) and *granisetron* (Kytril) are both 5HT-3 receptor antagonists licensed for the treatment of nausea and vomiting. They were initially introduced for the management of these symptoms in association with cancer chemotherapy and radiotherapy; because they have no dopamine receptor antagonist action they do not cause extrapyramidal reactions.

Ondansetron is available as both oral and intravenous preparations, whereas granisetron is only available intravenously. Ondansetron is usually given by intravenous infusion or orally thrice daily, whereas a single daily dose of granisetron is often effective. Both drugs are more expensive than traditional antiemetics.

In cisplatin-induced emesis studies suggest that these agents are effective in completely preventing nausea and vomiting in 50–60% of cases, and producing major antiemetic response in over 70% of cases.[12 13] They are even more effective for less emetic chemotherapy regimens, but here the cost–benefit ratio of the more expensive agents do need to be considered. Both these drugs act on the gut, reducing gut motility, and around 7% of patients may suffer constipation. These agents are important advances in the management of vomiting caused by chemotherapy.

More recent studies have shown that ondansetron is effective in treating postoperative vomiting. Nausea and vomiting in this situation are often related to the anaesthetic technique and the role of these agents and their potential to replace established therapies is yet to be clearly established.

SUMATRIPTAN

Sumatriptan (Imigran) is a 5HT-1 receptor agonist which was developed for the management of migraine. 5HT mechanisms are involved in the development of migraine, and this drug has been shown in both experimental animals and humans to alter regional blood flow in the brain by vasoconstriction in the carotid system.

Sumatriptan has been studied in both subcutaneous and oral doses, and has been shown to produce effective release of migraine in 70% of patients when given subcutaneously, compared with 25% with placebo.[14] When given orally efficacy is not as great, response rates being of the order of 50–60%. In some studies recurrence of migraine headache has been clearly documented; following oral dosing this may be as many as 40% of the patients who benefit initially.[15]

Sumatriptan has also been compared with conventional antimigraine treatments, including aspirin and metoclopramide, or ergotamine with caffeine. Sumatriptan was more effective in reducing vomiting, nausea and photophobia than ergotamine, but the recurrence of headache was greater with sumatriptan. When compared with aspirin and metoclopramide, efficacy was not significantly different during the first attack treated (56% sumatriptan, 45% aspirin and metoclopramide), but statistically significant benefit was shown during second and third attacks (58% versus 36%, and 65% versus 34% respectively). Again, recurrence of headache was less frequent following aspirin and metoclopramide than sumatriptan.

The most common adverse effect of sumatriptan has been an injection site reaction, but the effect that has caused most concern is chest pain, and there have been reports of cardiac toxicity, including ventricular arrhythmias and myocardial infarction. This drug is contraindicated in patients with coronary artery disease.

Sumatriptan has a short half life, around 2h, and its bioavailability following oral administration is low at about 15%, but varies between 10 and 26% in individuals. Most of the drug is eliminated by hepatic metabolism.

Sumatriptan is an expensive drug and, in view of the relative frequency of migraine in the community, the economic consequences of its widespread use are considerable. It is therefore important that patients are carefully evaluated before treatment with the drug is commenced.

1 Awad AG, Lappiere YD, Nair NPC, *et al*. The new selective D-2 antagonist, remoxipride, is the treatment of acute schizophrenia—A Canadian multicentre trial. *Schizophrenia Res* 1991;**4**:311–12.

2 Heel RC, Brogden RN, Speight TM, Avery GS. Loxapine: a review of its pharmacological properties and therapeutic efficacy as an antipsychotic agent. *Drugs* 1978;**15**:198–217.

3 Kane J, Honigfeld G, Singer J, Meltzer H, and the Clozaril Collaborative Study Group. Clozapine for the treatment-resistant schizophrenic. *Arch Gen Psychiatry* 1988;**45**:789–96.

4 Van Tol HHM, Bunzow JR, Guan HC, *et al*. Cloning for the gene for human D_4 receptor with high affinity for the antipsychotic clozapine. *Nature* 1991;**350**:610–19.

5 Zola EM, McLeod DC. Comparative effects and analgesic efficacy of the agonist-antagonist opioids. *Drug Intell Clin Pharmacy* 1983;**17**:411–17.

6 Anonymous. Stronger analgesics with low risk of dependence. Buprenorphine, meptazinol and nalbuphine. *Drug Ther Bull* 1985;**23**:45–8.

7 Nicholas ADG, Robson PJ. Double-blind comparison of meptazinol and pethidine in labour. *Br J Obstet Gynaecol* 1982;**89**:318–22.

8 Holmes B, Ward A. Meptazinol. A review of its pharmacodynamic and pharmacokinetic properties of therapeutic efficacy. *Drugs* 1985;**30**:285–312.

9 Gralla RJ, Imri LM, Pisko SE, *et al*. Anti-emetic efficacy of high dose metoclopramide: randomized trials with placebo and prochlorperazine in patients with chemotherapy-induced nausea and vomiting. *N Engl J Med* 1981;**305**:905–9.

10 Taylor WB, Proctor SJ, Bateman DN. Pharmacokinetics and efficacy of high-dose metoclopramide given by continuous infusion for the control of cytotoxic drug-induced vomiting. *Br J Clin Pharmacol* 1984;**18**:679–84.

11 Anonymous. Nabilone and high-dose metoclopramide: anti-emetics for cancer chemotherapy. *Drug Ther Bull* 1984;**22**:9–11.

12 Marty M. Ondansetron in the prophylaxis of anti cisplatin-induced nausea and vomiting. *Eur J Cancer Clin Oncol* 1989;**25** (suppl):541–6.

13 Soukop M. A comparison of two dose levels of granisetron in patients receiving high-dose cisplatin. *Eur J Cancer* 1990;**26** (suppl 1):515–79.

14 Subcutaneous International Study Group. Treatment of migraine attacks with sumatriptan. *N Engl J Med* 1991;**325**:316–21.

15 Oral Sumatriptan International Multiple-dose Study Group. Evaluation of the multiple-dose regimen of oral sumatriptan for the acute treatment of migraine. *Eur Neurol* 1991;**31**:306–13.

27 Non-steroidal analgesic and anti-inflammatory agents

GEORGE NUKI, THOMAS PULLAR

Each year eight million people in the United Kingdom consult general practitioners about rheumatic complaints and 22 million prescriptions for (non-aspirin) non-steroidal anti-inflammatory drugs (NSAIDs) are issued. These are associated with 3500 yellow card reports to the Committee on Safety of Medicines and about 2500 cases of complicated (bleeding or perforated) peptic ulcers, predominantly in people aged over 60. Only a small proportion of these prescriptions, however, are for patients with one of the inflammatory arthritides, such as rheumatoid arthritis or gout, in which the therapeutic superiority of the NSAIDs over simple analgesics is most apparent. In the United Kingdom the number of prescriptions for NSAIDs doubled from 10 to 20 million in the 1970s, and the worldwide market for this class of drugs approached US $2 billion in 1987. More than three quarters of patients receiving these drugs were elderly, when inflammatory joint disease is relatively uncommon. Only in the past 4 years have sales and prescriptions for these drugs begun to decline as a result of public and professional concern regarding their possible risks and benefits.

After the proliferation of new "me too" NSAIDs in the early 1970s the pharmaceutical industry expended much effort to produce drugs with a higher therapeutic ratio (that is, better efficacy with less toxicity) but to date studies have not been large enough to assess the relative risks and benefits of individual agents. Studies of comparative efficacy have been bedevilled by problems with the power of the studies, and postmarketing case control and record linkage studies have not been conducted in large enough populations for firm conclusions to be reached about the comparative safety of individual drugs. Although efficacy and gastrointestinal

tinal toxicity generally go hand in hand, not all of these agents are the same. There is no doubt that they do vary in terms of efficacy and toxicity, and some have a higher than expected incidence of idiosyncratic side effects.

Pharmacology

To a greater or lesser extent all these agents have analgesic, anti-inflammatory, and antipyretic activity. Among a wide range of direct and indirect effects on cellular metabolism, they all inhibit the enzyme cyclo-oxygenase, which results in reduced synthesis of prostaglandins. This is believed to be the basis of the anti-inflammatory effects of these agents and also of their propensity to cause gastrointestinal irritation and, less often, renal impairment or bronchospasm. Gastrointestinal irritation is thought to be caused by the loss of cytoprotective prostaglandins in the gastro-intestinal mucosa. Renal impairment is thought to be the result of reduced synthesis of vasodilatory prostaglandins in patients with compromised renal function whose renal blood flow is under "prostacyclin tone". The mechanism of bronchospasm is not clear, but it is thought to be caused by either the preferential inhibition of the bronchodilatory prostaglandins in susceptible people (with resultant unopposed action of the bronchoconstricting prostaglandins) or by diversion of arachidonic acid metabolites away from prostaglandin synthesis and down the lipoxygenase pathway to produce leukotrienes.

Early attempts to increase the efficacy of these drugs by producing 'dual' inhibitors (inhibitors of cyclo-oxygenase and lipoxygenase) were unsuccessful and the first such drug (benoxaprofen) had to be withdrawn because of serious hepatotoxicity. However, a new generation of 'dual' inhibitors is completing clinical trials and is likely to be launched shortly.

Chemically NSAIDs tend to be carboxylic acid or enolic acid derivatives of several different classes (table 27.1). As a group they are weakly acidic, highly protein bound drugs.

SALICYLIC ACIDS

Aspirin is the oldest and cheapest NSAID. In low doses (300–600 mg) it is an effective analgesic and remains the best drug for many sorts of pain. At the high doses (3·6–4·2 g a day) required to achieve a clinical anti-inflammatory effect in rheumatoid arthritis, up to half the patients will not tolerate simple soluble aspirin for prolonged periods because of dyspepsia (nausea, vomiting, and epigastric pain), occult blood loss, or side effects of the central nervous system (particularly tinnitus). Serious gastrointestinal haemorrhage, hepatotoxicity, and hypersensitivity to aspirin are more remote risks. Patients with severe allergy to aspirin may also react to other NSAIDs. Reye's syndrome may occur in children given aspirin who have a concomitant viral infection, and aspirin is now contraindicated for fever, myalgia, and malaise in children aged under 12 years. It can be used to treat juvenile chronic arthritis, but other NSAIDs such as naproxen or ibuprofen are increasingly being used to treat children with this condition.

The problem of dyspepsia may be reduced in adults by giving aloxiprin or glycinated or enteric coated preparations, but only heavily buffered preparations such as *Alka Seltzer* are associated with reduced faecal blood loss, and these are rapidly excreted by the kidney. *Benorylate* is a paracetamol ester of aspirin that is cleaved to its active constituents in the liver. It is associated with less dyspepsia and blood loss than simple aspirin and may be given in liquid form and twice a day. *Choline magnesium trisalicylate* is a long acting non-acetylated salicylate that may be tolerated better than aspirin, and *salsalate* is a slowly hydrolysed aspirin ester that has a long lasting action and is absorbed only after transit to the small intestine. *Diflunisal* is a non-acetylated, difluorinated salicylate that is marketed as a simple analgesic, but which also has anti-inflammatory effects. There is some evidence to suggest that it has greater potency and better tolerability, as well as longer duration of action, than aspirin.

PROPIONIC ACIDS

Although propionic acids are generally weaker anti-inflammatory agents than aspirin, they are widely regarded as the best drugs for managing patients with inflammatory joint disease because by and large they are the class of NSAID with the lowest incidence of side effects. Comparative trials of *ibuprofen, ketoprofen, fenoprofen*, and *naproxen* have shown that naproxen may be marginally superior, but individual and unpredictable patient preference for one or another propionic acid is more noticeable than consistent differences between the drugs.

Flurbiprofen is more effective than ibuprofen, but its use at the

TABLE 27.1.—*Pharmacology of non-steroidal anti-inflammatory drugs*

Approved (proprietary) name	Dose (mg/day)	Half life (h)	Side effects
Salicylic acids		*Carboxylic acids*	
Soluble aspirin (Solprin, Disprin)	600 × 6	0·25	Tinnitus, deafness, and dyspepsia
Enteric coated aspirin (Nu-Seals)	900 × 4	0·25	
Slow release aspirin (Levius)	1000 × 4	0·25	
Aloxiprin (Palaprin Forte)	1200 × 4	9	
Benorylate (Benoral)	4000 (10 ml) × 2	1	Better gastrointestinal tolerance
Diflunisal (Dolobid)	500 × 2	12	
Salsalate (Disalcid)	1500 × 2	8	
Choline magnesium trisalicylate (Trilisate)	1500 × 2	0·5	
Propionic acids			
Fenbufen (Lederfen)	300 (morning) 600 (night)	10	Occasional dyspepsia, gastrointestinal haemorrhage, and rashes
Fenoprofen (Fenopron)	600 × 4	3	
Flurbiprofen (Froben)	100 × 3	4	Dyspepsia, gastrointestinal haemorrhage, and occasional rashes
Ibuprofen (Brufen)	400–800 × 4	2	
Ketoprofen (Alrheumat)	100 × 2 or 3	2	Occasional dyspepsia, gastrointestinal haemorrhage, and rashes
(Orudis)	100 × 2 or 3		
(Oruvail)	100 × 2		
Naproxen (Naprosyn)	500 × 2	12	
Tiaprofenic acid (Surgam)	200 × 3	2	

	Dose (mg)	Half-life (h)	Side effects
Acetic acids			
Diclofenac sodium (Voltarol)	50 × 2 or 3	2	Dyspepsia, gastrointestinal haemorrhage, haemorrhage, and dizziness
Indomethacin (Indocid)	25–50 × 3	4	Dyspepsia, gastrointestinal ulceration, and haemorrhage
(Indocid-R)	75 × 2	4	Dyspepsia, gastrointestinal ulceration, haemorrhage, headache, and dizziness
Sulindac (Clinoril)	200 × 2	7 (sulphide 18)	Occasional dyspepsia, gastrointestinal haemorrhage, headache, and dizziness
Tolmetin (Tolectin)	400 × 4	5	Dyspepsia, gastrointestinal haemorrhage, headache, and dizziness
Etodolac (Lodine)	200–300 × 2	7	Occasional dyspepsia and gastrointestinal haemorrhage
Anthranilic acids			
Mefenamic acid (Ponstan Forte)	500 × 3	4	Diarrhoea, occasional dyspepsia, gastrointestinal haemorrhage, and rashes
Enolic acids			
Pyrazalones			
Azapropazone (Rheumox)	600 × 2	20	Dyspepsia and gastrointestinal haemorrhage
Phenylbutazone (Butazolidin)	100 × 3	50–100	Dyspepsia, gastrointestinal haemorrhage, fluid retention, stomatitis, and bone marrow suppression
(Butacote)	100 × 3	50–100	
Oxicams			
Piroxicam (Feldene)	20	38	Occasional dyspepsia, gastrointestinal haemorrhage, and rashes
Tenoxicam (Mobiflex)	20	72	
Naphthylalkalones			
Nabumetone (Relifex)	1000 (up to × 2)	24 (active metabolite)	Occasional dyspepsia and gastrointestinal haemorrhage

recommended dose is associated with a higher incidence of gastrointestinal side effects. Ibuprofen is also associated with more gastric irritation when the dose is increased from 1200 to 2400 mg a day. *Tiaprofenic acid* is a more recently introduced agent but, despite initial suggestions based on in vitro and animal studies, its therapeutic ratio is comparable to that of other propionic acid derivatives. *Fenbufen* is a so-called prodrug with no anti-inflammatory activity of its own and a fairly low incidence of gastrointestinal side effects. After absorption it is converted in the liver to an active metabolite (4-biphenylacetic acid) that has a plasma half life of 10 h, which allows the convenience of dosing once or twice a day. Rashes are more common with this agent than with other propionic acids. No good evidence exists that fenbufen has a more favourable therapeutic ratio than other agents, and the strategy of using prodrugs to avoid gastrointestinal toxicity has proved disappointing.

ACETIC ACIDS

Indomethacin, sulindac, tolmetin, and *etodolac* are chemically related cyclic acetic acid derivatives.

Indomethacin

This is one of the more effective agents, but has a high incidence of gastrointestinal side effects including bleeding and ulceration and can also be associated with headaches, confusion, or vertigo in about 15% of patients. The side effects affecting the central nervous system are dose related, so it is always wise to begin with a small dose (25 mg a day) and increase it gradually to 25 mg four times a day or 50 mg three times a day. A 50 mg capsule or a 100 mg suppository at night is often helpful in overcoming early morning stiffness in patients with rheumatoid arthritis, whereas others prefer to use the 75 mg slow release preparation. An enteric coated preparation has recently been licensed.

Sulindac

Sulindac is an indene sulphoxide derivative of indomethacin. It is a prodrug that becomes active only after conversion to a sulphone metabolite in the liver. It is less effective than indomethacin but has relatively good gastric tolerability, although a large recent retrospective analysis of more than 80 000 patients in the United States given one of seven NSAIDs showed that only sulindac was associated with a higher risk of haemorrhage from the upper gastrointestinal tract than ibuprofen. This may have been because sulindac was being used at relatively high dosage and because of enterohepatic recirculation. Some evidence suggests that sulindac may be the NSAID least likely to aggravate mild renal impairment.

Tolmetin

This is a pyrolealkanoic acid with a short half life and a profile of side effects that resembles that of indomethacin.

Etodolac

This is an indole acetic acid. It is highly protein bound and has an elimination half life of around 7h. It seems to be of similar efficacy to the propionic acid derivatives.

Diclofenac

Diclofenac is a phenylacetic acid derivative with a profile of efficacy and gastrointestinal side effects similar to that of the propionic acids.

ANTHRANILIC ACIDS

Mefenamic acid is a relatively weak anti-inflammatory drug with a plasma half life of 4h. Diarrhoea and inflammatory proctitis is a special problem with this agent, and renal insufficiency has been reported in elderly people who have become dehydrated as a result of the diarrhoea. It is one of a number of NSAIDs that has been associated with interstitial nephritis.

PYRAZALONES

Phenylbutazone

This is one of the most potent NSAIDs but also potentially one of the most toxic. In the United Kingdom it is available only on hospital prescription to treat ankylosing spondylitis. In addition to dyspepsia, gastric ulceration, and haemorrhage, renal and hepatic damage have been reported and mouth ulcers and skin reactions may occur (these range from mild erythematous rashes to rare but serious exfoliative dermatitis and toxic epidermal necrolysis). Salt and water retention may be pronounced and should preclude the use of this drug in the elderly or in those with heart disease. Bone marrow suppression was particularly associated with the use of phenylbutazone and its metabolite *oxyphenbutazone* on rare occasions. Agranulocytosis appeared as part of a hypersensitivity reaction, usually in the first 3 months of treatment, while aplastic anaemia was mainly seen in patients aged over 60 who had received at least 6 months' treatment. Although bone marrow suppression was a relatively rare event that occurred only about once in every 3000 patient years of treatment, half of all cases were fatal. Before their use was restricted, phenylbutazone and oxyphenbutazone were responsible for more than a third of all drug induced blood dyscrasias in the United Kingdom and 25–50 deaths a year.

Azapropazone

This drug is free from the risk of bone marrow suppression, but like phenylbutazone it is uricosuric, potentiates the action of warfarin, and gives rise to salt and water retention. In other respects its profile of moderate efficacy and mild gastrointestinal irritation resembles that of the propionic acids.

OXICAMS

Piroxicam

This is a potent and widely used anti-inflammatory agent. It has a plasma half life of about 40 h, which permits the convenience of dosing once a day. The drug is extensively metabolised in the liver and excreted in the urine as glucuronides. Pharmacokinetic studies in the elderly and in patients with renal impairment show no evidence of drug accumulation. Gastrointestinal irritation and occasional rashes are the main adverse effects.

Tenoxicam

Tenoxicam has a similar profile of efficacy and toxicity to piroxicam. It has a long half life (72 h), necessitating administration only once a day. Use in the elderly does not normally require a dose reduction, although patients with impaired renal function should be monitored closely.

NAPHTHYLALKANONES

Nabumetone is the only member of this class to date. It is a non-acidic prodrug that has little cyclo-oxygenase inhibiting activity. It undergoes first pass metabolism to its active metabolite, 6-methoxy-2-naphthyl acetic acid, which is extensively bound to plasma protein and has a terminal elimination half life of about 24 h. This is prolonged in renal impairment and in elderly patients, who have concentrations of the active metabolite one and a half to two times those found in healthy young volunteers. The most commonly reported adverse effects are gastrointestinal but there is some evidence to suggest that this drug has a more favourable therapeutic ratio than acidic NSAIDs.

SIMPLE ANALGESICS

Analgesics without appreciable anti-inflammatory action include peripherally acting agents such as *paracetamol* and centrally acting narcotic analgesics such as *dextropropoxyphene, dihydrocodeine, buprenorphine,* and *pentazocine.* Pentazocine, and combination drugs such as *coproxamol* (paracetamol and dextropropoxyphene) are widely and effectively used to manage pain of many kinds, but centrally acting narcotic analgesics are comparatively ineffective against musculoskeletal pain of all types, and they are strongly contraindicated in patients with chronic rheumatic diseases.

Nefopam is a non-steroidal analgesic that does not inhibit prostaglandin synthesis. It may be useful in patients with musculoskeletal pain, although its use is often limited by nausea. Other side effects include some anticholinergic and sympathomimetic effects. It is contraindicated in patients with a history of convulsions.

Clinical use of NSAIDs

GENERAL PRINCIPLES

As in other areas of therapeutics, a critical approach to the use of these drugs must be taken. Doctors must decide whether the patient's condition is likely to respond, whether the patient has any particular characteristics that are likely to result in an increased incidence of toxicity, and whether the probability of benefit is worth the risk of toxicity. After prescribing the drug the doctor should ascertain whether symptomatic benefit has been achieved, if necessary by temporarily withdrawing the drug. If the drug has helped its efficacy should be checked at regular intervals.

It is generally preferable to start with one of the less toxic (but less effective) drugs such as ibuprofen. For patients with more pronounced inflammation (especially if they are young and otherwise healthy), however, a drug from the middle of the range (such as diclofenac or naproxen) or the top of the range (such as indomethacin) may be used from the start. As well as variation in response among drugs and diseases, there is great variation in response among people treated with the same drug for the same condition. If treatment with one drug at the optimum dose fails several drugs should be tried to identify one suited to that patient: this does not mean, however, that doctors should work through the whole list of over 20 NSAIDs if a patient fails to respond to the first few, perhaps at the expense of instituting other more specific treatment. Doctors should familiarise themselves with three or four of these drugs, preferably some of the older, more established, ones. The choice may be determined by the recommendations of local hospital and practice formularies.

RHEUMATOID ARTHRITIS

Non-steroidal anti-inflammatory drug treatment achieves a high ratio of beneficial to toxic effects in patients with rheumatoid and other types of inflammatory arthritis because these drugs are most effective in the inflammatory arthritides and because the inflammatory arthritides tend to affect younger patients, who are less vulnerable to serious drug toxicity. Few patients with rheumatoid arthritis can be managed successfully without NSAIDs, and one of the "arts" of rheumatology is to find ways of continuing to use them to treat patients who have previously experienced adverse effects. This is usually achieved by choosing a drug of lower efficacy (and toxicity), by using concomitant H_2 receptor antagonists, a prostaglandin analogue (e.g. misoprostol), a H^+/K^+ ATPase inhibitor (e.g. omeprazole), and by the earlier use of a second line or disease modifying drug such as sulphasalazine or gold.

GOUT

NSAIDs are the preferred drugs for treating acute gout. Unlike rheumatoid arthritis, acute gout will respond well to any agent if it is given in adequate dosage early in the course of the attack. Azapropazone, diclofenac, indomethacin, ketoprofen, naproxen, piroxicam, and sulindac have all been shown to be effective. These agents may also be used prophylactically to prevent "break through" attacks of acute gout developing during the first few months of hypouricaemic drug treatment, but small doses of colchicine (0·5 mg twice a day) may be preferable for prophylaxis. Patients with gout should be warned to avoid taking compounds that contain aspirin, which will raise the plasma urate concentration at low doses even though they are uricosuric at larger doses. Azapropazone (600 mg twice a day) has uricosuric as well as anti-inflammatory properties and may be used as a single agent in treating patients with chronic gouty arthritis who require a NSAID, provided that renal function is normal.

OSTEOARTHRITIS

NSAIDs undoubtedly provide symptomatic relief in osteoarthritis, but, as this condition tends to affect elderly people and does not respond as well as the more inflammatory arthritides, great care should be taken in using these drugs for osteoarthritis in the elderly. One large recent study failed to show that ibuprofen was any more effective than paracetamol in patients with knee osteoarthritis. It is therefore sensible to use these drugs only for patients in whom an adequate trial of simple analgesics has been ineffective and for those who have no serious contraindication to treatment with NSAIDs. For most patients with osteoarthritis who do require these agents the choice should probably be restricted to drugs from the mild to moderate end of the efficacy and toxicity range.

Whereas patients with rheumatoid arthritis usually need to take NSAIDs regularly to provide symptomatic relief, for osteoarthritis these agents are best used only as required to supplement a baseline simple analgesic such as regular paracetamol.

SOFT TISSUE RHEUMATISM

Although systemic NSAIDs may provide symptomatic benefit for tenosynovitis, soft tissue injuries, et cetera, local treatment such as local injection of steroids or physiotherapy are probably more appropriate. Topical NSAIDs may be useful in this circumstance and may be associated with less systemic toxicity. The number of such drugs available has increased recently. These characteristically have only marginal efficacy and a relatively large placebo effect. The risk of serious adverse effects is low but systemic toxicity can occur. Topically applied NSAIDs may be

371

worth trying for patients with localised symptoms who cannot tolerate systemic treatment or for whom systemic treatment is not justified.

Fibromyalgia (fibrositis) tends to respond poorly to NSAIDs and may be more amenable to treatment with tricyclic antidepressants or physiotherapy.

NON-RHEUMATOLOGICAL USE OF NSAIDs

Aspirin and ibuprofen are both available over the counter and are used by the general public as analgesics for a wide range of painful conditions. Diclofenac is often prescribed for ureteric colic or after trauma in preference to the opiates. Inhibition of prostaglandin synthesis by NSAIDs is of particular use in treating dysmenorrhoea and the pain associated with bone metastases, two conditions in which prostaglandins are thought to be important mediators. Similarly the anti-inflammatory properties of these drugs are of use in treating pleurisy and pericarditis. Indomethacin and other NSAIDs may also have a role in treating migraine. NSAIDs are very effective when used as antipyretics, although in most cases it is doubtful whether such an effect is desirable. The most important non-analgesic role for NSAIDs is the use of low dose aspirin for myocardial or cerebral ischaemia. Aspirin is unique in that it binds irreversibly to cyclo-oxygenase. The main endothelial cell prostaglandin is prostacyclin, which inhibits platelet aggregation and causes vasodilatation, whereas the main prostaglandin produced by platelets is thromboxane, which is responsible for platelet aggregation. As platelets are unable to resynthesise cyclo-oxygenase, the irreversible inhibition of platelet cyclo-oxygenase by aspirin results in depletion of thromboxane for the life of the platelet, whereas endothelial cells are able to synthesise fresh cyclo-oxygenase and subsequently generate prostacyclin. The net effect is inhibition of platelet 'stickiness'. This produces important therapeutic benefit in unstable angina, after myocardial infarction, and in transient ischaemic attacks.

ADVERSE EFFECTS

In the last decade more NSAIDs have been withdrawn (fenclofenac, indoprofen, flufenamic acid, feprazone, oxyphenbutazone, zomepirac, and osmotically released indomethacin) or had their use restricted (phenylbutazone) because of concern over safety than have been successfully introduced (nabumetone, tenoxicam, etodolac, and acemetacin). This reflects the increased level of concern by the public, doctors, the pharmaceutical industry, and the licensing authorities over the toxicity of this group of drugs. Adverse effects of these drugs fall into two categories—those that are predictable from their pharmacological effect of inhibiting prostaglandin synthesis, and idiosyncratic or unpredictable effects.

Of the predictable effects, gastrointestinal irritation including peptic ulceration is the most common. At any one time up to one third of patients taking these agents have endoscopic evidence of peptic ulceration although many of these ulcers are asymptomatic.

Record linkage studies show that patients taking NSAIDs are twice as likely to develop gastrointestinal haemorrhages or perforated ulcers as controls. The risks are higher in the elderly, in patients with a previous history of gastrointestinal side effects, and in patients also receiving corticosteroids.

Concomitant prescription of the prostaglandin analogue *misoprostol* has been found to reduce appreciably the incidence of endoscopically visible gastric and duodenal ulceration induced by NSAIDs, although the effect on the more rare but more important complications such as major haemorrhage and perforation remains unknown.

It is probably now generally accepted that in the frail elderly, or those with a history of peptic ulceration, misoprostol should be coprescribed. Calendar packs containing misoprostol and naproxen and a single tablet fixed drug combination containing diclofenac and misoprostol are now available for use in this situation. Misoprostol appears from a number of studies to be more effective than H_2 antagonists at preventing peptic ulcers induced by NSAIDs. However, a proportion of people for whom misoprostol is indicated are unable to tolerate it because of diarrhoea and for these individuals an H_2 antagonist might be a suitable alternative. There are no published direct comparisons of misoprostol and H_2 antagonists in the healing of peptic ulcers in patients continuing to use NSAIDs, although their effect would appear to be of a similar magnitude. However, a direct comparison of omeprazole and ranitidine in a subgroup analysis of such patients in a larger study comparing the two drugs in gastric ulcer disease found omeprazole (40 mg daily) to be much more effective than ranitidine. For optimum healing of peptic ulcers in patients who need to continue treatment with NSAIDs omeprazole 40 mg daily is recommended for 4–6 weeks followed by long term treatment with misoprostol.

Renal dysfunction as a result of taking NSAIDs is clinically insignificant in most patients and reverses when treatment stops. Occasionally, however, acute renal failure may ensue. Inhibition of prostaglandin synthesis by these drugs can lead to medullary ischaemia, which may be the basis for the initial lesion in analgesic nephropathy. Salt and water retention may be a clinical problem in patients with pre-existing renal or cardiac impairment. Interstitial nephritis and, more rarely, glomerulonephritis have also been reported.

Bronchospasm, although rare, is difficult to avoid as, in susceptible people, it seems to be an adverse reaction common to all classes of these drugs. Some evidence exists, however, to suggest that azapropazone and nabumetone may not induce bronchospasm in some susceptible patients.

Rapid destruction of the head of the femur ("indomethacin hip") has been ascribed to the inhibition of prostaglandin synthesis by potent NSAIDs, and azapropazone (a weak inhibitor of prostaglandin synthesis) may lack this disadvantage. However, the mechanism and very existence of cartilage and bone hip damage induced by these drugs has been questioned.

While studies in vitro and animal experiments have shown that some NSAIDs stimulate prosteoglycan synthesis while others are inhibitory, there is insufficient clinical data at the present time to justify claims that azapropazone, diclofenac, sulindac or tiaprofenic acid have significant "chondroprotective" effects in clinical practice.

Headache, dizziness, and tinnitus may be associated with several NSAIDs, particularly aspirin, and are related to circulating plasma concentrations. Confusion and psychomotor impairment can also occur, especially with indomethacin, and this can be a particular problem in the elderly. These adverse effects are dose related, although tolerance and cross tolerance may occur. This emphasises the importance of the recommendation that treatment with NSAIDs should be started at a low dose in elderly patients.

Rashes are the most common idiosyncratic side effects of NSAIDs, and their incidence varies from drug to drug. A striking but usually benign cutaneous reaction to fenbufen is the adverse reaction most frequently reported to the Committee on Safety of Medicines.

Bone marrow toxicity is very rare and unpredictable.

Mild and reversible increases in hepatic enzyme activity are common during treatment with NSAIDs in patients with rheumatic diseases. Aspirin, diclofenac, fenoprofen, naproxen, phenylbutazone, and sulindac have all been associated with toxic hepatitis on rare occasions, and reversible cholestatic jaundice can occur with sulindac.

NON-STEROIDAL ANTI-INFLAMMATORY DRUG TREATMENT IN CHILDREN

Aspirin is now generally contraindicated in children because of the possible occurrence of Reye's syndrome. It may be used for patients with juvenile chronic arthritis but naproxen is an excellent alternative. Other agents such as ibuprofen and tolmetin may also be used.

DRUG INTERACTIONS

Protein binding displacement interactions with drugs such as warfarin are of little importance as the increased free fraction is eliminated. This leads to a new steady state in which the total concentration is lower but the unbound (pharmacologically active) concentration is unchanged. If the plasma clearance of the displaced drug is reduced at the same time, however, because metabolism is inhibited by the displacing drug (for example, phenylbutazone inhibits the metabolism of warfarin) or because the displaced drug (such as phenytoin) has saturable metabolism, then an important interaction might occur. Drugs that have been documented as being free from appreciable pharmacokinetic interactions with warfarin include ibuprofen, diclofenac, tolmetin, and indomethacin. The ulcerogenic effect of these drugs, however, puts patients taking warfarin at increased risk.

NSAIDs can appreciably inhibit renal excretion of high dose methotrexate, but this does not seem to be a problem in patients with normal renal function who are taking the doses of methotrexate used for treating patients with rheumatoid arthritis. As NSAIDs may inhibit the renal excretion of lithium when coprescribed plasma lithium concentrations should be monitored closely.

NSAIDs interfere with the antihypertensive effect of various drugs and also the diuretic effects of loop diuretics. In addition, their combination with diuretics in patients with impaired renal function (especially the elderly) may result in an appreciable deterioration of renal function. The combination of indomethacin and triamterene seems to be particularly important in this respect, even in normal people, and should be assiduously avoided. Sulindac may have some advantages over the other NSAIDs in patients with renal impairment or hypertension.

NSAIDs IN PREGNANCY AND LACTATION

Fortunately rheumatoid arthritis often remits during pregnancy, thus removing the need for these drugs. If necessary a short half life drug such as ibuprofen, flurbiprofen, or ketoprofen should be used at the maximum dosage intervals. As a result of their effect on prostaglandin synthesis, all NSAIDs may delay and prolong labour. Aspirin especially may be associated with postpartum haemorrhage and with pulmonary hypertension in the neonate and, if given in the first trimester, with development of oral clefts. Indomethacin may be teratogenic and might also result in neonatal pulmonary hypertension.

During lactation NSAIDs are best avoided. Indomethacin has been reported to cause seizures in one breast fed infant, and toxic concentrations of salicylate may occur in infants whose mothers take high dose aspirin. NSAIDs with a short half life that form inert metabolites (ibuprofen, flurbiprofen, diclofenac) can, however, be safely given to lactating mothers. Ibuprofen is probably the drug whose safe use during lactation is best documented and is the preferred agent if a NSAID is necessary.

Anonymous. Misoprostol for co-prescriptions with NSAIDs. *Drug Ther Bull* 1990;**28**:25–6.

Beardon PHG, Brown SV, McDevitt DG. Gastrointestinal events in patients prescribed non-steroidal anti-inflammatory drugs: a controlled study using record linkage. *Q J Med* 1989;**266**:497–505.

Brooks PM, Day RO. Non-steroidal anti-inflammatory drugs: differences and similarities. *N Engl J Med* 1991;**324**:1716–25.

Fowler PD. Aspirin, paracetamol and non-steroidal anti-inflammatory drugs. A comparative review of side-effects. *Med Toxicol* 1987;**2**:338–66.

Fries JF, Williams CA, Block DA. The relative toxicity of non-steroidal anti-inflammatory drugs. *Arthr Rheum* 1991;**34**:1353–60.

Huskisson EC, ed. Anti-rheumatic drugs I. *Clin Rheum Dis* 1979;**5**:351–733.

Huskisson EC, ed. Anti-rheumatic drugs II. *Clin Rheum Dis* 1980;**6**:463–95.

Kurowski M. *Adverse reactions to non-steroidal anti-inflammatory drugs.* Basle: Birkhauser-Verlag, 1992.

Langman MJS. Peptic ulcer complications and the use of non-aspirin non-steroidal anti-inflammatory drugs. *Adverse Drug React Bull* 1986;**120**:448–51.

Needs CJ, Brooks PM. Antirheumatic medication in pregnancy. *Br J Rheumatol* 1985;**24**:282–90.

Needs CJ, Brooks PM. Antirheumatic medication during lactation. *Br J Rheumatol* 1985;**24**:291–7.

Nuki G. Pain control and the use of non-steroidal anti-inflammatory drugs. *Br Med Bull* 1990;**46**:262–78.

Nuki G. The effects of nonsteroidal anti-inflammatory drugs on cartilage and connective tissue. In: Macleod DAD, Maughan RJ, Williams C, Madeley CR, Sharp JCM and Nutton RW, eds. *Intermittent high intensity exercise*. London: E and FN Spon, 1993: 339–52.

Roth SH. Merits and liabilities of NSAID therapy. *Rheum Dis Clin North Am* 1989;**15**:479–98.

Wilkens RF. The selection of a non-steroidal anti-inflammatory drug. Is there a difference? *J Rheumatol* 1992;**19** (suppl 36):9–12.

28 Controlling symptoms in advanced cancer

T D WALSH, T S WEST

Many patients who have cancer have metastatic disease at diagnosis and cannot be cured by modern cancer treatment, though there are tumours—for example, tumours of the testis, choriocarcinomas, and Hodgkin's disease—that are now curable even at an advanced stage. Some other tumours—for example, in the lung (oat cell), breast, and prostate—may show considerable benefit from chemotherapy or hormonal manipulation. That is why histological proof of diagnosis should always be obtained and management reviewed by an oncologist.

Many patients with cancer present with pain or other symptoms, and for them the need for relief from symptoms occurs throughout the course of the disease and not just in the terminal stages. Patients who are unfortunate enough to have an incurable cancer will often die within 2 years of diagnosis of metastatic disease.

Early in treatment of the disease priority must be given to attempts to obtain a cure. For patients who have advanced cancer, however, the symptoms *are* the illness. A decision must then be made that the disease is incurable and that henceforth the priorities of management must focus on controlling the symptoms. Once this has been decided, medical and nursing care can aim positively at relieving distress. Recognising that "the symptoms are the disease" is an important psychological adjustment for the doctor and the patient. It helps to avoid the "nothing more can be done" syndrome or the continuation of ineffective treatments. Implicit in this decision is tactful honesty and open communication among the patient, doctor, and family.

Principles of controlling symptoms

Studies have repeatedly shown that the control of pain and other symptoms is only too often inadequate. Many doctors (including oncologists) have received no training in caring for dying patients. Some feel helpless and inadequate, with predictable effects on care of the patient. Dying patients are still commonly ignored during ward rounds or placed in a side room.

Success in controlling symptoms lies in time honoured medical care allied with detailed attention to therapeutics. Many doctors who are faced with a patient with advanced cancer abandon the problem solving diagnostic approach that they use in managing other medical disorders, but it is essential to retain such an approach for the optimum management of symptoms. Taking a careful history of the patient's complaints should be followed by a detailed problem oriented physical examination. Invasive diagnostic procedures—for example, taking blood—or other time consuming actions should be kept to a minimum.

Advanced cancer is an acute disease—the clinical picture may change rapidly, so patients must be assessed regularly and plans for treatment and drugs adjusted. First rate nursing care is essential; fortunately, most nurses see this type of work as a professional challenge. Drugs must be constantly reviewed to avoid iatrogenic problems contributing to the patient's misery.

Many of the principles learnt in this type of work are relevant to other incurable diseases—for example, cystic fibrosis and emphysema. We shall not deal with children who have advanced cancer, but the principles and practices are similar to those for adults, with appropriate reductions in drug dosage. Most patients' symptoms can be controlled most of the time by the proper use of a few well known drugs.

Pain

Pain is the most dreaded symptom of advanced cancer. It is due to destruction by the tumour of organs, bones, or nerves and increases in frequency and severity as the disease progresses. Pain is almost always associated with a solid tumour or multiple myeloma, and is uncommon in the lymphomas and leukaemias. Patients commonly have several sites of disease and multiple pains.

The probable cause of each pain should be diagnosed and the greatest attention directed to the pain causing the most distress or incapacity. No patient who has cancer should die in unrelieved pain; the means of obtaining good control of pain are available to any competent medical practitioner.

Pain that is difficult to control occurs in about 5–10% of patients. Emotional and family problems are important. Pain due to extensive bone metastases or pain in young patients may present problems. Such patients may need to be referred to a pain clinic, hospice, or symptom control team.

OPIOIDS

The specific opioid used is often less important than the manner in which it is used. The best results are obtained by giving the drugs orally, tailoring every dose individually to the pain, and giving the drug regularly (usually every 4 h). Dosing round the clock—giving scheduled doses even when there is no pain—is a key concept.

A second key concept in using opioids is the use of "rescue" analgesics for breakthrough pain, in which the patient is instructed to take a predetermined dose of analgesic should pain intervene before a scheduled drug dose is due. The drug used as a rescue can be as simple as paracetamol 500–1000 mg or perhaps 10–25% of the current dose of opioid given by mouth every 4 h. Depending on the circumstances, rescue analgesics can also be given sublingually, rectally, or by injection. The dose of the rescue analgesic is adjusted according to the severity of pain breakthrough. Frequent breakthroughs indicate the need for an increase in the regular dosage of analgesic.

Provided that these simple ideas are followed and explained clearly to the patient, good control of pain can be achieved in most patients. Opioids are most effective against pain of visceral origin and relatively ineffective against pain due to bone metastases or nerve destruction. Opioids must always be accompanied by a regular laxative to prevent the otherwise inevitable constipation.

Morphine

Morphine is the drug of choice for chronic severe pain in advanced cancer. It is flexible and has been in use for a long time. Morphine is used like insulin in diabetes mellitus, except that instead of being tailored to the blood concentration of glucose the dose is tailored to the pain reported by the patient. Morphine in aqueous solution is given every 4 h in five or six doses a day. The early morning (0200) dose is omitted if sleep is not disturbed by pain and provided that the patient wakes free of pain in the morning. A common starting dose is 5–10 mg every 4 h (depending on the patient's previous experience of analgesics and therapeutic response). The dosage is increased in steps (5, 10, 15, 20, 30, 45, 60, 90, 120, 160, or 180 mg every 4 h) until the pain is controlled.

Most patients need one of the smaller doses to control pain. If 30 mg every 4 h is ineffective it is wise to review the diagnosis and treatment to ensure that nothing has been overlooked—for example, non-steroidal anti-inflammatory drugs for painful bone metastases. If doses of 60 mg every 4 h do not provide acceptable relief from pain specialist help should be considered.

Morphine has the advantage that it can also be given sublingually, rectally, or by continuous subcutaneous or intravenous infusion. Intermittent subcutaneous injection should be used only for moderate or severe breakthrough pain in patients who have reached the terminal stage and cannot swallow. Bolus intravenous injections should not be used for routine pain control, as they provide poor relief of pain and give maximum side effects. Every effort must be made to control pain using oral medications.

Alternative routes of administration have to be considered in those who have swallowing difficulties and fluctuating levels of consciousness. Most patients (70%) can continue to take oral drugs to within 72 h of death. Continuous subcutaneous infusion of morphine and other opioids is a useful approach in those who have poor control of pain, are unable to swallow, or suffer from severe nausea or vomiting.

Alternatives to morphine—Heroin and hydromorphone are useful alternative drugs for parenteral use as they are highly potent— that is, they have a greater analgesic effect for each mg administered. They can therefore be given in small volumes, which are less distressing for intermittent subcutaneous or intravenous injection and more convenient for continuous infusion. Heroin, however, has no advantage over morphine in terms of its analgesic efficacy or side effects (table 28.1).

Side effects of morphine—Provided that the oral route and tailored individual doses are used, giving morphine as described above is safe. Respiratory depression is uncommon. Although in advanced disease relief of pain must take priority over concern about possible ventilatory impairment, deliberate overdosing should not be contemplated. Overdosed patients become confused and restless, which distresses staff and other patients. The aim of treatment is to relieve distress, not to create it. It is bad ethics and poor medical practice to overdose dying patients deliberately.

TABLE 28.1—*Recommended alternatives to oral morphine*

Drug	Interval between doses (h)	Tablet	Morphine equivalent (as solution every 4 h)	Comments
Diamorphine (heroin)	4	10 mg (but usually prescribed in an elixir)	10–15 mg	Identical in use with morphine. More soluble
Phenazocine (Narphen)	8	5 mg	20 mg	Useful alternative to morphine. Ceiling effect at 40–50 mg/day
Dextromoramide (Palfium)	2	5 mg (and 10 mg)	15 mg (peak effect)	Too short acting for regular use. Good for "breakthrough pain". Can be given sublingually
Oxycodone pectinate (Proladone)	8	30 mg (suppository)	15 mg	Useful if vomiting occurs and in the home

Taken from: Baines M. *Drug control of common symptoms.* London: St Christopher's Hospice, 1986.

Patients may become physically dependent on opioids—develop a withdrawal syndrome if the drug is abruptly withdrawn—but addiction (drug seeking behaviour) is rare provided that adequate doses of opioids are given. Paradoxically, patients who request increased dosages of analgesics because they are in pain often have their dosage reduced because of ungrounded fears of addiction. Opioids may be withdrawn at any time by reducing the dose in steps similar to the method used for withdrawing corticosteroids. Withdrawal symptoms after accidental withdrawal from oral opioids are surprisingly mild. Naloxone should be used only for specific indications, as it can produce a massive withdrawal syndrome with severe pain breakthrough. Tolerance—a relentless increase in opioid dosage with poor control of pain—is uncommon and its incidence and importance have been exaggerated. It does not prevent good control of pain in most patients who have cancer.

The three common side effects of opioids are constipation, nausea or vomiting, and drowsiness. Constipation is inevitable and must always be anticipated when regular administration of opioids begins. Both nausea or vomiting and drowsiness tend to be mild and transient. They often clear, even with the continued use of morphine, after a few days. An antiemetic—for example, prochlorperazine 5·0 mg orally every 4 h—is often prescribed routinely for a week after morphine is started. Drowsiness is troublesome in only a few patients. It is important to review the treatment to identify other potentially sedative drugs. Excessive sedation may require a reduction in the dosage of morphine; some doctors add a stimulant such as amphetamine.

Severe nausea and vomiting may respond to conventional antiemetics; metoclopramide (given regularly every 8 h) is a good first choice. A change in the way morphine is given may also help. Patients nauseated by liquid morphine may do better with sustained release tablets or vice versa. If fine tuning of the dosage of morphine is required for these problems, however, this is most easily accomplished by using morphine liquid every 4 h.

Sustained release morphine tablets (10, 30, 60, and 100 mg) are now available. This preparation is a considerable practical advance. Once a patient's condition has been stabilised with doses of liquid morphine every 4 h, the dosage is halved and the tablets substituted on a mg for mg basis (20 mg every 4 h = 120 mg/ 24 h = 60 mg of the sustained release tablets every 12 h). The tablets must not be chewed or crushed, as this destroys the sustained release effect and can be dangerous. Some patients need to take them every 8 h, for reasons that are not clear. They are best not used for adjusting morphine dosage and should be avoided for patients who have severe gastrointestinal abnormalities or swallowing difficulties.

NON-STEROIDAL ANTI-INFLAMMATORY DRUGS

Aspirin and related drugs are used in two main ways in treating pain in cancer. Firstly, they seem to have a specific effect on pain caused by bone metastases by interfering with the production of prostaglandin. This is doubly important, as this type of pain responds poorly to opioids. Non-steroidal anti-inflammatory drugs are the best treatment for patients who have diffuse bone metastases and in whom chemotherapy, hormonal treatments, and radiation treatment are ineffective. (In limited painful bone metastases single dose radiation treatment is the first choice and is very effective.) Non-steroidal anti-inflammatory drugs vary in effectiveness, but gratifying responses can be seen within 48–72 h.

Secondly, these drugs have a general non-specific analgesic effect. The combination of one of these drugs and an opioid will provide better pain relief than either drug used alone.

The side effects of non-steroidal anti-inflammatory drugs are well known. For patients who have cancer and who are thrombocytopenic they are best avoided because of the risk of haemorrhage. There is also a confusing number available. It is worth maximising the dosage of individual agents and changing drugs if side effects are a problem or if a poor response is obtained. Aspirin is well tolerated by many patients: naproxen is a suitable alternative. Some degree of trial and error is usual, as responses and side effects vary among different non-steroidal anti-inflammatory drugs.

PSYCHOTROPIC, ANTIEPILEPTIC, AND PSYCHOSTIMULANT DRUGS

Psychotropic drugs have long been used to treat various pain syndromes in malignant and non-malignant disease. Phenothiazines and antidepressants are used alone or in combination. Treatment has been empirical, and specific indications and correct dosages are ill defined. In pain from cancer an opioid sparing action has been claimed for both groups of drugs. There is now evidence that tricyclic antidepressants do have a coanalgesic opioid sparing effect. Curiously, this action does not affect mood.

For the non-specialist who is finding it difficult to control pain in a patient who has advanced cancer, trying an antidepressant is always worth while, as depression is difficult to diagnose in a chronic physical illness. Phenothiazines are sedative, antiemetic, and possibly coanalgesic. They are useful for helping to control anxiety and agitation in the terminal stages.

Pain due to destruction of nerves may respond to antidepressants or antiepileptic agents. Burning pain is said to respond to antidepressants, whereas stabbing pain may respond to phenytoin or carbamazepine. Psychostimulants such as methylphenidate are useful in those complaining of chronic weakness or if there is excessive sedation induced by opioids.

CORTICOSTEROIDS

Corticosteroids seem to help to relieve pain that is caused by the destruction of nerves—for example, damage to the brachial or lumbrosacral plexus. Their mechanism of action is not known. Relief of pain is difficult to separate from their psychostimulating, antianorectic, and strength improving actions, which are all beneficial in advanced cancer. The side effects of corticosteroids are well known and will not be described here. Many patients with advanced cancer will not live long enough to develop serious problems, provided that dosage is carefully monitored. Most patients tolerate moderate doses well—for example, dexamethasone 4–6 mg a day.

Other problems

ANOREXIA

Anorexia is a common but poorly understood complaint. Many find it as distressing as pain. In some patients with cancer it is related to chemotherapy or radiation treatment and if so usually improves once this treatment has been completed. Abnormalities in the sensation of taste are common in patients who have cancer and contribute to the problem.

A dietitian should be consulted about the choice and composition of the diet. A multivitamin tablet should be given daily to those who are unable to eat normally. Megavitamin treatment is best avoided; it is ineffective and can be dangerous. There is no evidence that zinc supplements help. Patients with cancer show a diurnal variation in appetite; their appetite is often best in the morning, and if so appropriate adjustments in the diet should be made. Changes in food preparation or additives help those with abnormalities in taste—for example, reducing salt in cooking if food tastes too salty.

Corticosteroids are very effective against anorexia, and most patients will respond to them. The disadvantage of their use is steroid side effects, which are common, though usually minor. Oral thrush should be routinely looked for and dosage adjusted for the optimum effect at the lowest dose. Alcohol is readily available and is a familiar effective appetite stimulant. Metoclopramide 10 mg orally every 6 h seems specifically to help those who have symptoms of gastroparesis—early satiety—but may help others too. Those who respond will be less anorectic and gain weight. Cyproheptadine may be tried if corticosteroids are ineffective, but its record is unimpressive.

NAUSEA AND VOMITING

Nausea and vomiting are common (60%) symptoms in advanced cancer, mostly in elderly women. Certain diseases are associated with an increased incidence of nausea and vomiting—cancer of the breast, stomach, ovary, and pancreas and leukaemia. The precise cause is often not clear. Among those given opioids vomiting is also more common in women and is more likely to create difficulties in treatment. It is important to exclude common remediable causes such as faecal impaction. Sometimes it may be appropriate to investigate and then attempt to control uraemia or hypercalcaemia or the underlying cause.

Some patients whose vomiting is induced by opioids respond well to metoclopramide, possibly because of its action in helping gastric motility. If vomiting is severe or persistent and unresponsive to single antiemetics a combination of drugs with different sites of action—for example, metoclopramide plus prochlorperazine—should be tried. Cyclizine or an anticholinergic agent such as hyoscine can also be added. This approach is often effective, and there are theoretical reasons to support it.

COUGH AND DYSPNOEA

Dyspnoea is common (> 40%), even in patients without obvious cardiorespiratory disease. In those who have considerable or recurrent pleural effusions and dyspnoea, thoracentesis followed by tetracycline pleurodesis can be performed if the probable survival time of the patient is weeks or months. Morphine in small doses (sustained release morphine 10 mg twice a day) is effective. Dyspnoea due to lymphangitis carcinomatosis is difficult to treat but may respond to a combination of morphine, bronchodilators, and systemic corticosteroids.

Cough is usually treated with codeine when it is an isolated symptom. The opioids are cough suppressants but are best used only if the cough is causing distress—for example, disturbing sleep. There is probably little difference between the opioids in terms of their effectiveness as cough suppressants. Dextromethorphan 15–30 mg orally every 4 h is as effective as codeine and has few side effects; codeine is very constipating. Methadone 5 mg 2 h before retiring is a useful long acting drug for troublesome night time cough.

Steam inhalations help those whose cough is due to difficulty in expectorating sputum. Cough "mixtures" are best avoided; they often contain illogical drug mixtures such as an expectorant plus a cough suppressant. Traditional expectorants are ineffective. Bronchodilators may help cough by stimulating bronchial ciliary activity. Mucolytics—for example, bromhexine 8–16 mg orally every 8 h—reduce the viscosity of sputum. Unfortunately, most coughs in advanced cancer are due to irritant expanding mass lesions. In resistant cases prednisolone 10 mg orally is worth trying every 8 h.

CONSTIPATION

Constipation is common in the elderly, in patients who are bedridden or receiving inadequate diets, and in those taking a variety of drugs (opioids, anticholinergics, sedatives). Regular bowel motions should continue even if there is little dietary intake. An empty rectum does not exclude faecal impaction; if this is suspected the abdomen should be palpated and an abdominal radiograph ordered if there is still any doubt. It is astonishing how often bowel care is mismanaged.

Any patients who have cancer and who have been prescribed a regular opioid should always have a regular laxative started simultaneously. Usually a stool softener suffices. If, despite this, constipation ensues they should be instructed to take as required a stimulant (senna) or osmotic (Milk of Magnesia) laxative. Bulk laxatives—for example, methylcellulose—are often poorly tolerated by patients with cancer.

ITCH

Severe itch is very distressing and in advanced cancer is usually due to cholestasis. Good nursing care and topical treatment of the skin is vital, whatever the cause. Calamine lotion and menthol creams reduce itch by cooling the skin. Antihistamine and phenothiazines are only partly effective, largely because their antipruritic effect is mediated through sedation. Hydroxyzine orally 25–50 mg every 6h is a useful agent.

Cholestyramine 4 mg every 6h is effective for itch caused by incomplete biliary obstruction, but gastrointestinal upset may occur, and it interferes with the absorption of some drugs and the fat soluble vitamins. Dosage should therefore be reduced once a therapeutic response occurs. The itch of lymphomas responds to effective treatment of the lymphoma or, failing that, to non-steroidal anti-inflammatory drugs. Antihistamine ointments are valuable in severe cases. Lignocaine gel applied topically may be tried in intractable cases.

DEPRESSION

Sadness and anxiety are common among patients who have advanced cancer. Severe depression is uncommon, and suicide is rare. About 40% of patients show some evidence of depressive illness. Non-somatic symptoms (particularly feelings of guilt and worthlessness) are helpful in diagnosing depression. Sympathetic support must be offered. Involvement of the family can be therapeutic. Morale is helped by relief of other symptoms and a good patient–doctor relationship. Unspoken fears—for example, about dying—should be gently inquired about.

If an antidepressant is required it is best to start with a low dose—for example, imipramine 12·5 mg at night—as side effects can be a problem. This is particularly true in patients already taking opioids. Whether the natural sadness of the terminally ill responds to drug treatment is not clear. Certainly it is usually eased by an understanding listener.

MALIGNANT BOWEL OBSTRUCTION

Malignant obstruction of the bowel is a common acute or subacute event in cancer of the colon or ovary. "Routine"

TABLE 28.2—*Antiemetic drugs*

| Name | Preparations | | | | Use subcutaneously in syringe driver | Dose (mg)/ 24 h | Comments |
	Tablet	Syrup	Injection	Suppository			
Prochlorperazine (Stemetil)	5 mg 25 mg	5 mg/5 ml	12·5 mg	25 mg (5 mg)	No (skin reaction)	15–50	Effective in many types of vomiting. Minimal sedation
Chlorpromazine (Largactil)	10 mg 25 mg 50 mg 100 mg	25 mg/5 ml 100 mg/ 5 ml	25 mg 50 mg	100 mg	No (skin reaction)	50–150	As prochlorperazine but more sedating
Methotrimeprazine (Nozinan)	25 mg		25 mg		Yes (but some skin reaction)	50–150	Very potent antiemetic and analgesic. Considerable sedation
Haloperidol (Serenace)	1·5 mg 5 mg 10 mg 20 mg	10 mg/5 ml	5 mg 10 mg		Yes	5–20	Minimal sedation. Occasional extrapyramidal side effects
Cyclizine (Valoid)	50 mg		50 mg		Yes	150	Best drug in vestibular induced vomiting. Dry mouth
Metoclopramide (Maxolon)	10 mg	5 mg/5 ml	10 mg (100 mg)		Yes	30–60	Increases gastric emptying. Not sedative. Occasional extrapyramidal side effects
Domperidone (Motilium)	10 mg	5 mg/5 ml		30 mg		30–60	Increases gastric emptying. Not sedative. No extrapyramidal side effects

Taken from: Baines M. *Drug control of common symptoms*. London: St Christopher's Hospice, 1986.

389

nasogastric suction and intravenous fluids are unnecessary in patients who are unfit for surgery. Symptoms can often be managed with oral drugs, especially antiemetics and those that help to control pain from intestinal colic. Sometimes continuous subcutaneous infusion with a syringe driver containing an antiemetic (table 28.2), an opioid for the pain, and an anticholinergic (for example, hyoscine) for the colic will control the symptoms. Faecal impaction must always be excluded.

Terminal phase

The final hours or days of life are indicated by fluctuating consciousness and increasing detachment from the surroundings. Agitation is not uncommon, and pain should be assumed to be the cause in those who are unconscious, and should be treated by analgesic suppository or injections. A distended bladder or impacted rectum should be treated appropriately. If no cause can be found sedation with a phenothiazine can be used to avoid distressing relatives.

Few patients die dramatically, but it is wise to have morphine 10 mg and chlorpromazine 25 mg to hand in a syringe to be given quickly by a nurse (or competent relative if the patient is at home) should there be any dramatic distress or terminal event such as massive haemoptysis. Hyoscine 0·4 mg is a useful addition to help the "death rattle." Most patients prefer to die at home, and their wishes should be respected whenever possible.

Hanks GW, Hoskin PJ. Opioid analgesics in the management of pain in patients with cancer. A review. *Palliat Med* 1987;1:1–25. (Comprehensive and clear review of the opioids and their pharmacodynamics, pharmacokinetics, and clinical use, with clear guidelines for their use in treating chronic cancer pain.)

Mannix KA, Rawlins MD. The management of bone metastases; non-steroidal anti-inflammatory drugs. *Palliat Med* 1987;1:128–31. (Discusses the rationale behind the use of non-steroidal anti-inflammatory drugs and includes a good diagram to illustrate their use in practice.)

Oliver D. The use of the syringe driver in terminal care. *Br J Clin Pharmacol* 1985;20:515–16.

Regnard C. Nausea and vomiting—a flow diagram. *Palliat Med* 1987;1:62–3. (Sets out a clear scheme for diagnosing the cause of nausea and vomiting and lists the preferred antiemetic.)

Saunders CM, ed. *The management of terminal malignant disease.* 2nd ed. London: Edward Arnold, 1984. (Up to date and easy to read book whose 18 authors cover the interests of all those associated with the care of terminally ill patients.)

29 New drug treatments in acne and psoriasis

G M MURPHY, M W GREAVES

Acne vulgaris occurs in at least 90% of adolescents; psoriasis affects about 2% of the population. Established treatments are successful in inducing remission in most cases but management of severely affected patients presents many therapeutic problems. Advances in treatment in recent years have come not only from development of new drugs but also from new regimens for older methods of treatment. Although these treatments have generally proved beneficial, some have introduced unexpected complications. We review in this chapter recent advances in treatment for acne and psoriasis, with comments on associated adverse side effects.

Acne

ANTIBIOTICS

Oral wide spectrum antibiotics are standard treatment for moderate or severe acne. Adequate dosage, for a sufficient period of time, in combination with a topical peeling agent such as benzoyl peroxide or retinoic acid achieves good control of acne in most patients.[1] Oxytetracycline, erythromycin and minocycline are most commonly used. *Propionibacterium acnes* often develops drug resistance; this may account for therapeutic failures in 25% of patients treated. Drug resistance is lowest with minocycline.[2] Although 6 months is the minimum effective period of treatment, the duration of treatment should not be unnecessarily prolonged.

Topical antibiotics are generally less effective than their oral counterparts but are adequate for mild acne and have the advantage of avoiding systemic side effects,[3] though drug resistance remains a problem. Adequate comparative studies with benzoyl peroxide and retinoic acid have not been performed but topical antibiotics are useful for patients who are intolerant to benzoyl

391

peroxide or retinoic acid. Lotions containing tetracycline 0·22% (Topicycline), clindamycin 1·0% (Dalacin T) and erythromycin 2% (Stiemycin) are now available. Combination of zinc with erythromycin reduces bacterial resistance (Zineryt). Azelaic acid (Skinoren), a natural product of *Pityrosporum ovale*, has recently been shown to be an effective topical treatment for acne. It has a considerable antimicrobial effect against *Propionibacterium* spp. and seems to be as effective as benzoyl peroxide and retinoic acid without causing their irritant side effects.[4]

HORMONAL TREATMENT

Acne depends on the action of androgens on sebaceous glands to develop. Plasma concentrations of circulating androgens may be normal or increased. Hormonal manipulation is frequently successful in women who fail to respond to antibiotics, and is especially indicated in women who require oral contraception. Cyproterone acetate is an antiandrogen with both central and peripheral activity. Diane (cyproterone acetate 2 mg combined with ethinyloestradiol 50 μg) was recently replaced by Dianette (cyproterone acetate 2 mg ethinyloestradiol 35 μg), to reduce the risk of thromboembolism: both are effective antiacne preparations, with the additional advantage of ensuring contraception. Diane induces longer lasting remission of acne than oxytetracycline.[5]

Possible side effects (which are less likely with Dianette) may include menstrual disturbance, weight gain, breast tenderness, hypertension and mood changes. Cyproterone has been shown to cause feminisation of the male fetus in animal studies. Spironolactone, which also possesses antiandrogenic activity and is moderately effective in acne[6] avoids the problems associated with oestrogen administration in older women, though concern has been expressed regarding carcinogenicity in mice. The most common side effects include disturbance of menstruation and breast tenderness.

Long acting synthetic peptide analogues of gonadotrophin releasing hormone are currently being assessed for effectiveness in the polycystic ovary syndrome and show promise in the treatment of severe recalcitrant nodulocystic acne in women. The pituitary gland usually responds to the pulsed release of luteinising hormone releasing hormone from the hypothalamus: synthetic gonadotrophin releasing hormone analogues given as a nasal spray or depot injection lead, after initial stimulation, to a lack of response by pituitary gonadotrophins. Acne conglobata responds to buserelin,[7] administered by nasal spray: goserelin,[8] a new preparation given by monthly depot injection, although not yet assessed in acne, may ultimately prove superior. Analogues of gonadotrophin releasing hormone are also efficient oral contraceptives without the attendent problems of oestrogen administration and may prove to be useful in difficult acne in women. Cyclical administration is recommended for women, to avoid menstrual irregularities. Hypo-oestrogenism, reduced libido, and flushing are the main side effects of long term administration.

RETINOIDS

The management of severe acne has been revolutionised by the development of the synthetic vitamin A derivative, isotretinoin (Roaccutane).[9][10] It has a dramatic effect on the production of sebum, reducing the size of sebaceous glands by 90% in the first month of treatment. Inhibition of sebaceous gland activity is the main reason for its efficacy. Isotretinoin also affects keratinisation of the hair follicle, resulting in reduced formation of comedones, and has immunological effects that may suppress inflammation. A dramatic reduction in oiliness of the skin is apparent within a month of starting treatment, although patients should be warned that initially nodulocystic acne may be exacerbated. A 4 month course of treatment leads to a considerable reduction in the number and size of lesions. The benefit continues after treatment has stopped, leading in most instances to 80% improvement by about 2 months afterwards. Relapse rates are low and, although some patients require more prolonged treatment or second courses, many are apparently completely cured. Isotretinoin is available through hospitals and is usually prescribed at 0·5–1·0 mg/kg body weight. It should be taken during or after meals as this doubles its bioavailability. It is bound to plasma proteins and theoretically could influence the activity of concurrently administered plasma bound drugs, although this does not appear to be a problem in practice. It may cause an increased concentration of serum lipids and if so a low fat diet should be advised. Isotretinoin should not be given to patients with pre-existing hyperlipidaemia or cardio-vascular disease: the activity of transaminases may increase, and hypercalcaemia may occur. Rarely, lesions similar to pyogenic granuloma occur when treating cystic acne, but these generally resolve with continuation of therapy; severely affected patients

393

may also require systemic steroids until the lesions resolve in order to minimise scarring. The half life of isotretinoin is at most several days; oral contraception should be continued for 1 month after stopping treatment, as it is highly teratogenic. Table 29.1 lists other side effects of retinoids.

TABLE 29.1—*Side effects of the retinoids*

Mucocutaneous	*Musculoskeletal*
Cheilitis	Arthralgia
Dryness of mucous membranes	Disseminated idiopathic skeletal
Epistaxis	hyperostosis
Blepharoconjunctivitis	Premature fusion of epiphyses
Dermatitis	Muscle stiffness
Palmoplantar desquamation	
Photosensitivity	*Miscellaneous*
Paronychia, shedding of nails	Teratogenicity
Diffuse hair loss	Hepatotoxicity
	Hyperlipidaemia
Ophthalmological	
Papilloedema, intracranial	
hypertension	
Night blindness	

Psoriasis

No treatments for psoriasis are curative, but there have been important recent advances in suppressive treatment.

TOPICAL TREATMENT

Standard topical treatments for psoriasis include tar and dithranol. These preparations, especially when given in combination with ultraviolet B are usually effective and are the mainstay in the management of most patients with chronic plaque psoriasis. They are, however, irritant, messy to apply and stain skin, hair and clothes.

One useful variant of dithranol treatment has been "short contact" dithranol treatment[11] with cosmetically acceptable preparations formulated in cream bases. High concentration dithranol (2–4%) is applied to the lesions for 20–60 min and then washed off. It is convenient for use at home, is associated with less staining and inflammation than overnight regimens and achieves greater compliance by patients.

Vitamin D (calciferol) is produced in the skin by the action of ultraviolet B on 7-dehydrocholesterol to form provitamin D_3, a thermally unstable molecule. Isomerisation of double bonds converts this to vitamin D_3, which either enters the circulation or is photoisomerised in the skin to other products such as lumisterol or tachysterol. Vitamin D_3 undergoes further transformation in the liver to 25-hydroxycholecalciferol$_3$ (a biologically inactive form), followed by hydroxylation in the kidney to calcitriol (1,25-dihydroxyvitamin D_3). In the past decade it has been appreciated that receptors for this molecule are expressed by keratinocytes, activated T and B lymphocytes and dermal fibroblasts.[12 13] Studies in vitro of cultured human keratinocytes showed inhibition of proliferation in the presence of 1,25-dihydroxyvitamin D_3 and stimulation of terminal differentiation.[14] Open studies of oral and topical 1,25-dihydroxyvitamin D_3 show effectiveness in psoriasis, and more recently double blind controlled trials of calcipotriol (a topical analogue of calcitriol)[15] indicate that it is at least as effective as moderately potent topical steroids[16] and superior to short contact dithranol.[17] As yet adequate long term comparative studies of safety and relapse rates have not been published. Systemic disturbance of calcium metabolism does not seem to have been a problem, at least during limited periods of treatment. Calcipotriol is an effective, cosmetically acceptable (though mildly irritant) new method of treating chronic plaque psoriasis. Efforts are currently directed towards evaluating topical calcipotriol in combination with other treatments for recalcitrant psoriasis.

Biologically active amounts of the 5-lipoxygenase product leukotriene B_4 are present in psoriatic lesional skin,[18 19] suggesting that lipoxygenase products may be important in the pathogenesis of psoriasis, probably acting synergistically with other mediators.[20] Topical application of lonapalene (RS-43179) a dimethoxynaphthalene derivative and selective 5-lipoxygenase inhibitor, has been shown to be an effective, though occasionally irritant, topical treatment for chronic plaque psoriasis.[21] Reduction in leukotriene B_4 (but not arachidonic acid or 12-hydroxyeicosatetraenoic acid) preceding clinically evident improvement has been demonstrated in lesional skin treated by lonapalene, suggesting that the mode of action may be by selective inhibition of the 5-lipoxygenase pathway.[22] These findings also support a pathogenetic role for 5-

395

lipoxygenase products in psoriasis. Therapeutic prospects for systemic or less irritant topical 5-lipoxygenase inhibitors are therefore encouraging.

PHOTOTHERAPY

Ultraviolet B (280–315 nm) radiation therapy has been used successfully for treatment of psoriasis for many decades. Improved ultraviolet B sources such as UV21 and UV6 fluorescent tubes have been developed that produce more of the therapeutic ultraviolet B, and much less of the non-effective but erythemogenic ultraviolet C (< 280 nm) wavelengths. Open sources such as mercury vapour lamps emit an unacceptable amount of ultraviolet C, and provide undesirable amounts of ultraviolet scatter to staff working with the unit. Narrow band TL01 lamps are experimental but appear effective for treatment of psoriasis. Emitting light at 311 (± 1) nm, these lamps should be less carcinogenic than conventional broad band ultraviolet B lamps, but animal experiments seem to show the opposite. More studies need to be completed to fully assess the worth of such lamps in the management of psoriasis.

PHOTOCHEMOTHERAPY

Oral psoralen (8-methoxypsoralen or 5-methoxypsoralen) and ultraviolet A (PUVA) treatment is now well established and effective for chronic plaque psoriasis though visits to hospital several times each week are required until remission is achieved. The British Photodermatology Group has recently issued guidelines for the safe use of PUVA therapy.[23] Skin cancer is a possible complication, especially with higher total doses of ultraviolet A.[24]

Advances in PUVA include optimising dosage and reducing the numbers of treatments required to clear psoriasis, thereby reducing carcinogenic risk.[25] It is now recommended that a total dose of 1000–15 000 J/cm^2 (or more accurately, because of difficulties in standardisation of ultraviolet A measurements, that a maximum of 200 treatment sessions) should not be exceeded.[23] Combination regimens have therefore been adopted to minimise PUVA doses. Of the combination treatments studied, PUVA plus retinoids, PUVA plus methotrexate, and PUVA plus ultraviolet B are most frequently used.[26] New soft gelatin capsules of liquid 8-methoxypsoralen give more rapid absorption and higher plasma concentrations than the crystalline preparations currently on the market.[27]

5-Methoxypsoralen is a useful alternative, and is associated with fewer phototoxic side effects and a lower incidence of nausea or vomiting.

Bath PUVA has been in regular use in Scandinavia for many years with apparently excellent results; trimethylpsoralen 50 mg in 100 ml ethanol is added to a bath containing 150 l water. The patient bathes for 15 min, and then immediately undergoes ultraviolet A radiation. Photosensitivity is maximal immediately after bathing and is about 15 times greater than after oral psoralens. It remains high for 15 min but declines rapidly thereafter. Doses of ultraviolet A must be decreased appropriately and the minimal phototoxic dose should be assessed. Systemic absorption of psoralen is low and obviates the need to wear sunglasses.[28]

RETINOIDS

Etretinate (Tigason), a second generation monoaromatic retinoid, has been used in the United Kingdom since 1979.[29] Licensed for prescription only in hospitals, it is a useful agent in hyperkeratotic, hyperproliferative skin disorders, such as psoriasis. Its mode of action is not fully understood. In psoriatic skin, mitosis is reduced and acanthosis is diminished but the importance of etretinate's immunological influence remains unclear.

Etretinate is effective in generalised pustular psoriasis and in a chronic disabling form of pustular psoriasis, palmoplantar pustulosis; severe chronic plaque psoriasis and erythrodermic psoriasis also respond, but less dramatically. Unfortunately relapse rates are high once treatment is stopped.

The response to etretinate is often incomplete, and combination treatments are therefore used. A combination of etretinate with PUVA allows reduction in the total dosage of ultraviolet A required to clear psoriasis. This, combined with the apparent antitumour effect of retinoids, may reduce the carcinogenic risk of psoralens and ultraviolet A but this has not yet been proved. Some centres have used etretinate–ultraviolet B combination therapy successfully. Reports of enhancement of the effects of topical corticosteroids, dithranol, and methotrexate abound and studies are in progress to assess these combined regimens. Dosage of etretinate is usually 0·5–1·0 mg/kg body weight per day. As the secretion of bile salts leads to increased solubility, the absorption of etretinate is enhanced when it is taken with fatty food. Therapeutic effects are apparent within 1–2 weeks, with full benefit obvious by about 5 weeks. Hyperlipidaemia and hepatotoxicity may occur. Etretinate is deposited in adipose tissue, from which it is eliminated very slowly, the half life ranging from 80 to 170 days. The drug is highly teratogenic and any woman of child bearing age must take adequate contraception while on treatment and for 2 years after it ceases (see table 29.1). Acetretin (Neotigason), the active metabolite of etretinate, is as effective as etretinate,[30] and has recently been licensed for use. Recommended daily dosage is 0·5 mg/kg, adjusted on the basis of clinical response. Although water soluble and therefore rapidly eliminated, acetretin undergoes biotransformation in the body to etretinate, which has been detected in the plasma of some patients on this drug, therefore the guidelines with regard to etretinate and oral contraception should be followed.

IMMUNOSUPPRESSANTS

Methotrexate is a well tried, effective and (in many patients) non-toxic drug for treatment of severe psoriasis resistant to, or intolerant of, topical treatment, retinoids and PUVA. Hepatotoxicity is its chief drawback, necessitating regular liver biopsies to detect early signs of hepatocellular damage. Hydroxyurea and azathioprine are occasionally used but are less effective. *Razoxane* was highly effective in patients for whom methotrexate was deemed unsuitable but as the incidence of acute myeloid leukaemia was unexpectedly high[31] it is no longer used.

Cyclosporin A is a cyclic polypeptide of low molecular weight isolated from soil fungus. Since its introduction in 1976, oral administration has been used to prolong the survival of renal, bone marrow and liver allografts. Although its mode of action is complex, it acts by arresting division of T lymphocytes in the G0 or in the early G1 phase of the cell cycle, and inhibits at a pretranslation level the generation of interleukin-2. The end result is complex but reversible inhibition of T cell responses to interleukin-2. Cyclosporin is effective in moderate to severe psoriasis in low dosage (less than 5 mg/kg/day).[32 33] Potentially serious side effects include irreversible nephrotoxicity and hypertension, both of which are dose related. In order to prevent nephrotoxicity an initial estimation of the glomerular filtration rate should be carried out: if this is normal then the serum creatinine should be used to monitor renal function. Two baseline serum creatinine levels should be obtained before starting treatment and should be repeated every 4 weeks. A rise of 30% above baseline should prompt a reduction in cyclosporin dosage. Hypertension should be treated by nifedipine. Because of the impairment of immunosurveillance caused by cyclosporin, the drug is contraindicated in patients with a history of any form of malignancy.

Other immunosuppressive drugs with a mode of action similar to that of cyclosporin, including FK 506 and rapamycin, are currently undergoing clinical evaluation but at the time of writing show no distinctive advantages over cyclosporin.

In patients who are intolerant to cyclosporin and other potentially toxic antipsoriatic systemic drugs, *oral sulfasalazine* may be useful. Recent trials have provided encouraging results in plaque type psoriasis and a recent double blind study[34] showed a clear benefit over placebo, with a very low incidence of side effects.

The pathogenetic and therapeutic roles of interferons in psoriasis are currently under investigation. Interferon γ and lesser amounts of interferon α have been found in fluid from suction blisters raised on psoriatic lesions.[35] Abnormally high levels of interferon like activity have also been found in the sera of patients with psoriasis.[36] The interferons possess a broad spectrum antiproliferative action, which includes an effect on human keratinocytes.[37] Cultured keratinocytes from psoriatic plaques respond by reduction of proliferation when exposed to interferon γ,[37] and it has therefore been suggested that the pathogenesis of psoriasis may relate to down grading of the sensitivity of keratinocytes to this agent.[38] Interferon γ administered systemically appeared to partially resolve psoriatic lesions in open studies over an 8 week period.[39 40] Interferon α in high dosage may exacerbate psoriasis,[41] but low dosage appeared effective in one patient and without benefit in one other.[42] Patients experience occasionally incapacitating influenza like symptoms during treatment with interferon, a major drawback to this treatment, the role of which remains to be established.

Conclusions

The last few years have produced various new effective drugs and several with potential applications that remain to be fully assessed before their place in the management of acne and psoriasis is established. Although isotretinoin may cure acne, we still need treatments with fewer side effects. Psoriasis is a genetically determined disease, but we do not know what determines its clinical expression and existing treatments aim at suppressing the disease and inducing prolonged remission. The newer antipsoriatic drugs are important not only because of improved management of psoriasis but also because analysis of their modes of action may shed new light on the cellular and molecular basis of this disabling disease and their links with the underlying genetic abnormality.

1 Cunliffe WJ, Clayden AD, Gould D, Simpson NB. Acne vulgaris—its aetiology and treatment. A review. *Clin Exp Dermatol* 1981;6:461–9.

2 Eady EA, Cove JH, Holland KT, Cunnliffe WJ, Cove JH. Superior antibacterial action and reduced incidence of bacterial resistance in minocycline compared to tetracycline-treated acne patients. *Br J Dermatol* 1990;122:233–44.

3 Eady EA, Holland KT, Cunliffe WJ. Should topical antibiotics be used for the treatment of acne vulgaris? *Br J Dermatol* 1982;107:235–46. (This is a review of the role of topical antibiotics in the management of acne.)

4 Norris J, Cunliffe WJ, Burke B. Azelaic acid really does work in acne: A double blind national and international study. *Br J Dermatol* 1987;117(suppl 32):34–5.

5 Greenwood R, Brummitt L, Burke L, Cunliffe WJ. Acne: Double blind clinical and laboratory trial of tetracycline, oestrogen-cyproterone acetate and combined treatment. *BMJ* 1985;291:1231–5.

6 Muhlemann MF, Carter GD, Cream JJ, Wise P. Oral spironolactone: An effective treatment for acne vulgaris in women. *Br J Dermatol* 1986;115:227–32. (A doube-blind controlled trial.)

7 Waxman J, Rustin MHA, Perry L, Kirby JDT. Acne conglobata responding to buserelin, a gonadotrophin-releasing hormone analogue. *Br J Dermatol* 1983;109:679–81. (A case report.)

8 Thomas EJ, Jenkins J, Lenton EA, Cooke ID. Endrocrine effects of Goserelin, a new depot luteinising hormone releasing hormone agonist. *BMJ* 1986;293:1407–8.

9 Bollag W. Vitamin A and retinoids: From nutrition to pharmacotherapy in dermatology and oncology. *Lancet* 1983;i:860–3. (This paper reviews the history of the development of the retinoids and outlines future areas of research.)

10 Strauss JS, Rapini RP, Shalita AR, *et al.* Isotretinoin therapy for acne: Results of a multicentre dose response study. *J Am Acad Dermatol* 1984;10:490–6.

11 Statham BN, Ryatt KS, Rowell NR. Short contact dithranol therapy—a comparison with the Ingram regime. *Br J Dermatol* 1984;110:703–8.

12 Stumpf WE, Sar M, Reid FA, *et al.* Target cells for 1,25-dihydroxyvitamin D_3 in intestinal tract, stomach, kidney, skin, pituitary and parathyroid. *Science* 1979;206:1180–1190.

13 Holick MF, Smith E, Pineus S. Skin as the site of vitamin D synthesis and target tissue for 1,25-dihydroxyvitamin D_3. *Arch Dermatol* 1987;123:1677–83a.

14 Smith EL, Walworth NC, Holick MF. Effect of 1,25-dihydroxyvitamin D_3 on the morphologic and biochemical differentiation of cultured human epidermal keratinocytes grown in serum-free conditions. *J Invest Dermatol* 1986;86:709–14.

15 Kragballe K, Beck HI, Sogaard H. Improvement of psoriasis by a topical vitamin D₃ analogue (MC 903) in a double blind study. *Br J Dermatol* 1988;**119**:223–30.

16 Cunliffe WJ, Berth Jones J, Claudy A, *et al.* Comparative study of calcipotriol (MC 903) ointment and betamethasone 17-valerate ointment in patients with psoriasis vulgaris. *J Am Acad Dermatol* 1992;**26**:736–43.

17 Berth Jones J, Chu AC, Dodd WAH, *et al.* A multicentre parallel-group comparison of calcipotriol ointment and short-contact dithranol therapy in chronic plaque psoriasis. *Br J Dermatol* 1992;**127**:266–71.

18 Brain S, Camp R, Dowd P, *et al.* The release of leucotriene B₄-like material in biologically active amounts from the lesional skin of patients with psoriasis. *J Invest Dermatol* 1984;**83**:70–3.

19 Grabbe J, Czarnetzki BM, Mardin M. Chemotactic leucotrienes in psoriasis. *Lancet* 1982;**ii**:1464.

20 Greaves MW, Camp RDR. Prostaglandins, leucotrienes, phospholipase, platelet activating factor and cytokines: an integrated approach to inflammation of human skin. *Arch Dermatol Res* 1988;**280**(suppl):S33–S41.

21 Lassus A, Forsstrom S. A dimethoxynaphthalene derivative (RS-4317 gel) compared with 0·025% fluocinolone acetonide gel in the treatment of psoriasis. *Br J Dermatol* 1985;**113**:103–5.

22 Kobza Black A, Camp R, Cunningham F, *et al.* The clinical and pharmacological effect of lonapalene (RS-43179), a 5-lipoxygenase inhibitor, applied topically in psoriasis. *Br J Dermatol* 1988;**119** (suppl 13):33.

23 British Photodermatology Group. Guidelines for PUVA. *Br J Dermatol* 1993 (in press).

24 Stern RS, Laird N, Melski J, *et al.* Cutaneous squamous-cell carcinoma in patients treated with PUVA. *N Engl J Med* 1984;**310**:1156–61.

25 Carabott FM, Hawk JLM. PUVA therapy of psoriasis: An improved dose schedule. *Photochem Photobiol* 1986;**43**:23S. (An abstract outlining the proposed schedule.)

26 Morison WL. PUVA combination therapy. *Photodermatology* 1985;**2**:229–36. (A review of combination treatments.)

27 Sullivan TJ, Walter JL, Kouba RF, *et al.* Bioavailability of a new oral methoxsalen formulation. A serum concentration and photosensitivity response study. *Arch Dermatol* 1986;**122**:768–71.

28 Fischer T. Advantages of Bath PUVA. *Semin Dermatol* 1985;**4**:297–9. (Details of the method are outlined.)

29 Kingston TP, Matt LH, Lowe NJ. Etretin therapy for severe psoriasis. Evaluation of initial clinical responses. *Arch Dermatol* 1987;**123**:55–8.

30 Orfanos CE, Stadler R, Gollnick H, Tsambos D. Current developments in oral retinoid therapy with three generations of drugs. *Curr Probl Dermatol* 1985;**13**:33–49.

31 Horton JJ, Caffrey EA, Clark KGA, *et al.* Leukaemia in psoriatic patients treated with Razoxane. *Br J Dermatol* 1984;**110**:633–4.

32 Ellis CN, Fradin MS, Messana JM, *et al.* Cyclosporine for a plaque-type psoriasis. Results of a multi-dose double blind trial. *N Engl J Med* 1991;**324**:277–84.

33 Griffiths CEM, Powles AV, Leonard JN, *et al.* Clearance of psoriasis with low dose cyclosporin. *BMJ* 1986;**293**:731–2. (An uncontrolled study of 10 patients.)

34 Gupta AK, Ellis CN, Siegel MT, *et al.* Sulfasalazine improves psoriasis: a double blind analysis. *Arch Dermatol* 1990;**126**:487–93.

35 Bjerke JR, Livden JK, Degree M, *et al.* Interferon in suction blister fluid from psoriatic lesions. *Br J Dermatol* 1983;**108**:295–9.

36 Diezel W, Waschke SR, Sonnichsen N. Detection of interferon in the sera of patients with psoriasis, and its enhancement by PUVA treatment. *Br J Dermatol* 1983;**109**:549–52.

37 Yaar M, Karassik RL, Schnipper LE, Gilchrest BA. Effects of alpha and beta interferons on cultured human keratinocytes. *J Invest Dermatol* 1985;**85**:70–4.

38 Nickoloff BJ, Mitra RS, Fisher GS, Voorhees JJ. Altered responsiveness of psoriatic keratinocytes to gamma interferon. *J Invest Dermatol* 1988;**90**:592.

39 Morhenn VB, Pregerson-Rodan K, Mullen RH, *et al*. Use of recombinant interferon gamma administered intramuscularly for the treatment of psoriasis. *Arch Dermatol* 1988;**123**:1633–7.

40 DiGiovanna JJ, Toombs EL, Peck GL. Gamma interferon therapy of psoriasis. *J Invest Dermatol* 1988;**90**:554.

41 Quesada JR, Gutterman JU. Psoriasis and alpha-interferon. *Lancet* 1986;**i**:1466–8. (Report of three cases.)

42 Harrison PV, Peat MJ. Effect of interferon on psoriasis. *Lancet* 1986;**ii**:457–8.

30 Antibacterial drugs

ROGER FINCH

This chapter will focus on agents effective in the management of bacterial infections. The major innovations in antibiotic treatment since this subject was last reviewed have been largely dominated by the availability of an increasing number of fluoroquinolones and novel macrolide agents. Among the β lactams there have been further additions to the β lactamase stable cephalosporins in the form of cefixime for oral administration; several others are at an advanced stage of development. In addition, the β lactamase inhibitor tazobactam has been licensed in combination with piperacillin.

Cephalosporins

ORAL AGENTS

Cefadroxil

This oral cephalosporin has a range of activity similar to that of cephalexin, cephradine, and cefaclor, though cefaclor is more active against *Haemophilus influenzae*. Cefadroxil has a slightly longer half life of $1\frac{1}{2}$ h and is recommended for twice daily administration, though the justification for doses twice a day is controversial, as many other oral cephalosporins with half lives of about 1 h are given four times a day. The antibacterial activity of the oral cephalosporins remains modest compared with that of other drugs, though they are used widely, especially in general practice.

Cefuroxime axetil

This is an oral prodrug of cefuroxime. Its broader range of activity, including greater stability to β lactamase inactivation, have promoted its use in treating infections of the lower respiratory tract and other infections in which ampicillin or amoxycillin are no longer effective because of drug resistance, as is the case with *H influenzae* and many strains of *Moraxella catarrhalis*.

Cefixime

Cefixime is another broad spectrum oral agent highly active against streptococci (including pneumococci), but in common with all cephalosporins is inactive against enterococci. Its activity against *Staphylococcus aureus* is inadequate for clinical use. In contrast, it is extremely resistant to hydrolysis by many Gram negative β lactamases and therefore is active against neisseria, *H influenzae* and Gram negative enteric bacteria. It is inactive against *Pseudomonas* spp. Its half life of 4 h permits once or twice daily administration according to the severity of the target infection. Its main indications are in the treatment of upper and lower respiratory and urinary tract infections in community practice. Less than 20% of the oral dose is recoverable in the urine, which reflects the relatively poor bioavailability of the extended spectrum oral cephalosporins, including cefuroxime axetil. This is responsible in part for a relatively high incidence of gastrointestinal side effects, including the potential for *Clostridium difficile* associated gut complications.

Other oral cephalosporins in advanced stages of development include cefetamet pivoxil, cefpodoxime proxetil and ceftibuten: the first two agents are esters of the parent parenteral compound. These agents are all highly stable to a range of β lactamase enzymes, but suffer from lower activity against *Staph aureus* than the earlier oral cephalosporins. Their indications are likely to be similar to other β lactamase stable oral cephalosporins.

PARENTERAL CEPHALOSPORINS

The extended spectrum cephalosporins currently marketed (cefotaxime, ceftizoxime, ceftriaxone, and ceftazidime) present further difficulties to prescribers trying to discriminate between the various merits of this group of antibiotics. Cefotetan is marketed in many countries but remains unlicensed in the United Kingdom. Table 30.1 summarises the main points of difference in activity and pharmacokinetic behaviour of these compounds.

Cefotaxime (Claforan)

This was the first extended spectrum cephalosporin to be introduced; it has become widely used to treat serious sepsis such as intra-abdominal infection, including urinary and biliary infections and infections associated with the gut, infections of the lower

TABLE 30.1—*Comparison of antimicrobial and pharmacokinetics of extended spectrum cephalosporins, aztreonam, and imipenem*

Drug	Minimum inhibitory concentration (mg/l) against 90% of each strain tested (MIC_{90})							Pharmacokinetics	
	Staphylococcus aureus	*Streptococcus pyogenes*	*Haemophilus influenzae*	*Escherichia coli*	*Klebsiella pneumoniae*	*Pseudomonas aeruginosa*	*Bacteroides fragilis* spp *fragilis*	Half life (h)	C_{max}† (mg/l)
Cefuroxime	2·0	0·05	0·5	2·0	2·0	>64	≥64	1·2	110
Cefixime	16	0·25	0·25	0·25	1·0	32	≥64	3·5	5·5*
Cefotaxime	2·0	0·05	0·01	0·6	0·6	>64	≥64	1·1	50
Ceftizoxime	1·0	0·05	0·03	0·25	0·1	≥64	≥64	1·7	90
Cefsulodin	6·0	2·0	24	>64	>64	8	>100	1·6-1·9	65
Ceftazidime	12	0·3	0·06	0·5	0·5	4	>100	1·8	85
Ceftriaxone	6·0	0·03	0·01	1·0	0·1	≥64	>100	8·0	150
Cefotetan	8	2	4	0·12	0·07	>64	4	3·0-4·6	140
Imipenem	0·1	0·01	0·1	0·4	0·4	12·5	0·2	1·0	60
Aztreonam	>100	>100	0·1	0·2	0·8	25	>100	1·7	125

C_{max} = Maximum concentration achieved in serum
*After an oral dose of 400 mg.
†After intravenous dose of 1 g by bolus injection.

respiratory tract, and, more recently, meningitis in childhood. It is highly active microbiologically and is also stable to many of the β lactamase enzymes produced by Gram negative enteric bacteria. Despite broad spectrum activity, however, it is only modestly active against *Staph aureus*, *Pseudomonas aeruginosa*, and anaerobic bacteria, making it an inappropriate first choice for the treatment of infections with those organisms. In common with all cephalosporins, cefotaxime lacks activity against enterococci and *Listeria monocytogenes*, which is an occasional cause of meningitis.

Superinfection with enterococci and *P aeruginosa* have made prescribing these potent cephalosporins more complicated. Resistance to the drugs has generally not been a problem, though occasional strains of enterobacter, serratia, citrobacter, and indole positive proteus have developed resistance through inducible enzymic inactivation. Cefotaxime is metabolised to the microbiologically active desacetyl cefotaxime, which has a longer half life. Reduction of the dose is therefore necessary only in severe renal insufficiency (glomerular filtration rate ⩽ 10 ml/min), unlike the reductions required with other cephalosporins.

Ceftizoxime (Cefizox)

This drug is similar to cefotaxime in antibacterial activity and has a slightly longer half life but is not metabolised.

Ceftazidime (Fortum)

Ceftazidime also possesses broad spectrum activity but is more active against *P aeruginosa* and less active against *Staph aureus*. Indications for its use are similar to those for cefotaxime, but its greater activity against *P aeruginosa* has led to it being used in pulmonary exacerbations of cystic fibrosis and in febrile neutropenic patients who have a haematological malignancy and in whom *P aeruginosa* may be pathogenic. Under these circumstances it is prudent to combine ceftazidime with an aminoglycoside, though success has also been reported when the drug has been used alone or in combination with another β lactam compound. *Cefsulodin* (Monaspor) is a narrow spectrum cephalosporin with antipseudomonal activity, which is the primary reason for its use, though it has been used less widely than other agents.

Other extended spectrum cephalosporins include *ceftriaxone*, *cefpirome*, and *cefepime* (the last two are unlicensed at the time of writing).

Ceftriaxone (Rocefin)

This agent differs from the above cephalosporins because of its prolonged half life of about 8 h. It has proved to be effective against a wide range of serious infections when administered either once or twice a day. It is remarkably effective against gonorrhoea, for which a single dose of 250 mg is curative.

Ceftriaxone has been extensively used outside the United Kingdom in the treatment of bacterial meningitis. It is active against most pathogens responsible for this disease, with the exception of *Listeria monocytogenes*. In particular, it achieves very high concentrations in the cerebrospinal fluid in relation to target pathogens, which is now known to be critical to a satisfactory outcome. Similarly, the rapid emergence of pneumococci with reduced susceptibility or frank resistance to penicillin in many parts of southern Europe has resulted in ceftriaxone becoming the drug of choice for the treatment of pneumococcal meningitis. Its relative insolubility in bile occasionally results in the rapid formation of biliary concentrations; these are rarely of clinical significance and disappear with time. It has also proved valuable in managing the chronic manifestations of Lyme disease.

Cefepime and cefpirome

Cefepime and cefpirome are potent, broad spectrum, β lactamase stable, injectable cephalosporins with good activity against both Gram positive and Gram negative pathogens likely to be encountered in high dependency units dealing with serious hospital and community acquired infections. Significant anaerobic activity is lacking.

Monobactams

The monobactams are a new class of antibiotic originally derived from *Chromobacterium violaceum* but now synthesised chemically; they are unique among the β lactam group in that their structure consists of a single β lactam ring (figure 30.1). Manipulation of the side chains is fairly simple and produces many compounds, including some suitable for oral use.

The first monobactam to be licensed was *aztreonam*, which is characterised by high activity limited to Gram negative enteric bacilli. It is administered parenterally. The main indications for its use are serious infections associated with hospitals and those originating from the urinary, biliary, gastrointestinal, and female genital tracts. Of interest is the comparative lack of hypersensitivity reactions to aztreonam and in particular an appreciable lack of cross hypersensitivity to penicillins or cephalosporins. This suggests that the sensitising component of the β lactam molecule resides in either the thiazolidine or dihydrothiazine ring attached to the β lactam ring (figure 30.1). The lack of useful activity against Gram positive or anaerobic organisms requires aztreonam to be given with other agents when the nature of the infection remains uncertain or when a mixed infection is present.

Carbapenems

IMIPENEM

Imipenem, formerly known as N-formimidoyl thienamycin, is an extremely potent, broad spectrum β lactam antibiotic. Its range of activity includes staphylococci, *P aeruginosa*, *L monocytogenes*, and enterococci as well as bacteria susceptible to the extended spectrum cephalosporins discussed above. Against many anaerobic pathogens, including *B fragilis*, it is as active as metronidazole.

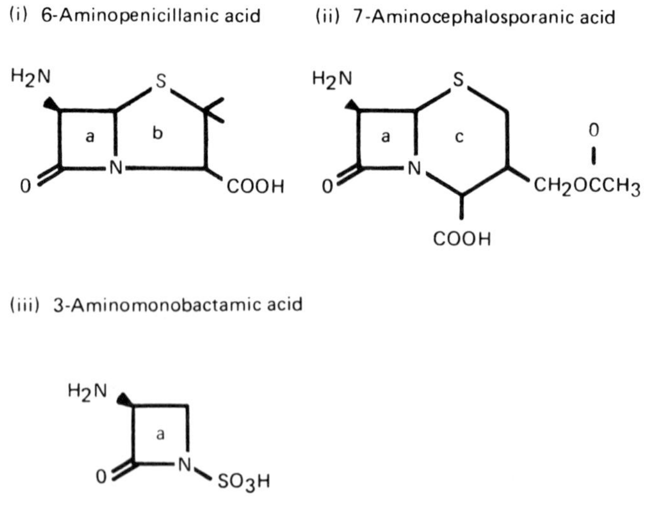

(i) 6-Aminopenicillanic acid   (ii) 7-Aminocephalosporanic acid

(iii) 3-Aminomonobactamic acid

FIG 30.1—Structure of: (i) penicillins; (ii) cephalosporins; (iii) monobactams (a = β lactam ring; b = thiazolidine ring; c = dihydrothiazone ring).

Pseudomonas spp. other than *P aeruginosa* tend to be less susceptible, as is *Enterococcus faecium* and staphylococci resistant to methicillin. Unfortunately, imipenem proved to be nephrotoxic in laboratory animals, whereas in humans, though it was not demonstrably nephrotoxic, urinary recovery was much reduced owing to inactivation by the renal tubular brush border enzyme dehydropeptidase I. An innovative solution to the problem has been the development of *cilastatin*, a reversible inhibitor of dehydropeptidase I that protects against nephrotoxicity in animals and degradation of the drug in humans and has matched pharmacokinetics, thus allowing coadministration with imipenem.

IMIPENEM-CILASTATIN

Imipenem-cilastatin has proved to be effective in treating a wide range of serious infections in hospital patients including empirically treating febrile neutropenic patients who have a haematological malignancy. Side effects have included hypersensitivity reactions, common to all β lactam antibiotics, gastrointestinal intolerance, and phlebitis. Diarrhoea or colitis due to *Clostridium difficile* has also occurred. In a few patients myoclonus, confusion, and seizures have been reported. Resistance has been seen in *P aeruginosa* during treatment and deserves further monitoring.

MEROPENEM

Meropenem differs from imipenem in possessing increased activity against *P aeruginosa*. It is also more active than imipenem against some Gram negative pathogens. It is strikingly resistant to many plasmid and chromosomally mediated β lactamases. Unlike meropenem it is not inactivated by renal dehydropeptidase I. Although currently unlicensed, its range of indications is likely to be very similar to those of imipenem.

Formulations containing β lactamase inhibitors

Resistance to the β lactam antibiotics is largely mediated by enzymic inhibition. A variety of β lactamase inhibitors have been developed, which include clavulanic acid, sulbactam and (most recently) tazobactam. Although possessing antimicrobial activity in their own right, this is clinically inadequate. Their major function lies in their ability, when coadministered with a β lactam antibiotic, to restore activity to these agents by virtue of their broad spectrum activity against many common β lactamases.

Clavulanic acid is an antibiotic that lacks clinically useful activity but is a potent inhibitor of many β lactamase enzymes responsible for bacterial resistance to the β lactam antibiotics. It is available as a formulation with amoxycillin for oral and parenteral use (Augmentin) and has recently been licensed as a combination with ticarcillin (Timentin).

AMOXYCILLIN-CLAVULANIC ACID

Amoxycillin-clavulanic acid (co-amoxiclav) is active against staphylococci, streptococci, anaerobic bacteria, and Gram negative enteric organisms such as *Escherichia coli*, proteus, klebsiella, and *H influenzae*, including strains that produce β lactamase and are resistant to amoxycillin. *Pseudomonas* spp. are resistant. It has proved to be effective in treating infections of the upper and lower respiratory tracts and urinary, biliary, and female genital tracts. It has also been used to treat intra-abdominal sepsis as well as being effective prophylactically for operations, as the formulation is active against anaerobes, including *B fragilis*.

TICARCILLIN-CLAVULANIC ACID

This is a formulation containing 3 or 5 g ticarcillin together with 200 mg clavulanic acid. As with amoxycillin-clavulanic acid, both components have matched pharmacokinetics. The range of activity is greater than that of amoxycillin-clavulanic acid and includes activity against *P aeruginosa*, though strains in which the mechanism of resistance is due to impermeability of the bacterial cell wall are not affected. In clinical use ticarcillin-clavulanic acid provides a further broad spectrum parenteral agent and, though it is active against *P aeruginosa*, serious infections caused by this organism are best treated with ticarcillin-clavulanic acid in combination with an aminoglycoside.

SULBACTAM

Sulbactam inhibits β lactamases of *Staph aureus*, Gram negative enteric bacteria, *H influenzae* and *Bacteroides* spp. In combination with ampicillin in a ratio of 2:1 (ampicillin:sulbactam) it has indications similar to co-amoxiclav. Prominent among its side effects is diarrhoea, which is common to most β lactamase inhibitors.

TAZOBACTAM

Tazobactam is the most recent β lactamase inhibitor to be used in combination with the established ureidopenicillin, piperacillin. This has recently been licensed for the treatment of a wide range of serious infections, including neutropenic infections when combined with an aminoglycoside. The usual dose is tazobactam 0·5 g in combination with piperacillin 4 g administered thrice daily. The formulation provides useful activity against *Staph aureus*, *H influenzae*, and most Enterobacteriaceae, but with little enhancement in activity against *Pseudomonas* spp.

Quinolones

The quinolones are an established and rapidly expanding group of antibiotics. *Nalidixic acid* was the forerunner of these agents and was introduced over 20 years ago, though modest activity and poor tissue pharmacokinetics have restricted its use to treating infections of the urinary tract; bacterial resistance and gastrointestinal side effects are other problems associated with its use. Related compounds have included oxolinic acid and acrosoxacin (Eradacin). *Oxolinic acid* is also used to treat infections of the urinary tract but offers no advantage over nalidixic acid, whereas *acrosoxacin* is systemically active but limited to the oral treatment of gonorrhoea.

The quinolones are also active against a wide range of bacterial gut pathogens, and experience suggests that they have a selective role in treating serious forms of campylobacter, shigella, and salmonella infections, though further information is awaited.

Much interest in recent years has focused on the fluoroquinolones, which include ciprofloxacin, enoxacin, norfloxacin, ofloxacin, lomefloxin, and pefloxacin. These drugs are characterised by high potency and broad spectrum activity especially against Gram negative enteric bacteria, though activity against staphylococci and streptococci is more modest (table 30.2). Pneumococci, and in particular *B fragilis*, are far less susceptible. Other agents at an advanced stage of development include fleroxacin and sparfloxacin.

CIPROFLOXACIN

Ciprofloxacin is the most active agent in vitro and can be given parenterally and orally. It is particularly active against Gram

TABLE 30.2—*Comparison of antimicrobial activity and pharmacokinetics of fluoroquinolones*

Drug	Minimum inhibitory concentration (mg/l) against 90% of each strain tested (MIC$_{90}$)							Pharmacokinetics		
	Staphylococcus aureus	*Streptococcus pneumoniae*	*Haemophilus influenzae*	*Escherichia coli*	*Klebsiella pneumoniae*	*Pseudomonas aeruginosa*	*Bacteroides fragilis* spp *fragilis*	Half life (h)	C$_{max}$ (mg/l)	Oral dose (mg)
Ciprofloxacin	0·5	2	0·05	0·015	0·25	1	8	3·9	2·5	500
Enoxacin	2	16	0·25	0·25	2	2	12	6·2	3·7	400
Lomefloxacin	2	16	0·03	0·25	2	8	32	8·0	3·2	400
Norfloxacin	2	16	0·12	0·012	1	2	32	3·5	1·5	400
Ofloxacin	0·5	2	0·03	0·06	1	4	4	7·4	5·6	400
Pefloxacin	0·5	8	0·06	0·25	2	2	8	11·3	5·8	400

C$_{max}$ = Maximum concentration

negative bacilli. The drug achieves modest but adequate serum concentrations in many body tissues and seems to be preferentially concentrated in sites such as the lungs and prostate and also within phagocytic cells. In clinical trials this agent has proved to be particularly effective in treating complicated and uncomplicated infections of the urinary tract, intra-abdominal sepsis, and infections of the lower respiratory tract, although failures have been reported against pneumococcal disease. Gonococcal infections, including those resistant to penicillin, respond very rapidly to ciprofloxacin.

Ciprofloxacin has been used in the oral treatment of infective exacerbations of cystic fibrosis of the lung when *P aeruginosa* has been present, and response rates comparable to those achieved with parenteral treatment have been reported. Resistance to the drug during treatment has been noted most frequently in pathogens such as *P aeruginosa*, *Staph aureus*, and *Staph epidermidis*.

Ciprofloxacin has been well tolerated, though occasional patients have developed headache, confusion, irritability, and anaphylactic reactions. Divalent cationic antacid preparations can impair quinolone absorption from the gut, owing to the action of ciprofloxacin on the hepatic cytochrome *P*-450 enzyme system, thus increasing serum concentrations of theophylline and the risk of toxic side effects, including seizures. Ciprofloxacin should be used with caution in patients taking theophylline. It is also contraindicated in pregnancy, and its use in children should be limited to those who have strong medical indications, as alterations to articular cartilage have been observed in puppies.

ENOXACIN

Enoxacin is also licensed for treating urinary tract infections, skin and skin structure infections, urethral and endocervical gonorrhoea, and shigellosis. Acute urinary tract infection responds to three days' treatment, whereas more complicated infections require 7–14 days' treatment. Chancroid is also susceptible. Adverse reactions to enoxacin are similar to those caused by ciprofloxacin and include an interaction with theophyllines.

NORFLOXACIN

This is largely active against Gram negative enteric organisms. It is administered only by mouth and is rapidly excreted in the urine in high concentrations. Its major indication is in the treatment of urinary tract infection although it has found some use in managing severe shigellosis and in the prophylaxis of traveller's diarrhoea.

LOMEFLOXACIN

Lomefloxacin shows similar, although slightly lower, microbiological activity to other currently available fluoroquinolones. It is inactive against pneumococci and anaerobic bacteria and less active against *Pseudomonas* spp. Its main indications are for the treatment of complicated and uncomplicated urinary tract infection, and infective exacerbations of chronic bronchitis. Its minimal interaction with theophylline is an advantage, although photosensitivity reactions are of concern.

OFLOXACIN

This is available in both oral and parenteral formulations. On balance, its microbiological activity is comparable to that of ciprofloxacin when allowance is made for the superior kinetics of ofloxacin. Its major indications are the treatment of urinary and respiratory tract infections. It is administered once or twice daily according to the severity of the infection. It is also effective in gonococcal and non-gonococcal genital infections. Ofloxacin does not appear to interact with theophylline or caffeine.

Glycopeptides

The currently available glycopeptides include *vancomycin* and *teicoplanin*. The former has been available for many years and has been widely used for the treatment of serious Gram positive infections among high risk patients such as those in haematology/ oncology and intensive care units. The major target pathogens are *Staph aureus*, including methicillin resistant strains, coagulase negative staphylococci and enterococci resistant to ampicillin. Many of these infections occur in relation to a variety of intravascular devices such as central venous lines and Hickman catheters. The concerns over vancomycin nephrotoxicity and ototoxicity have been ameliorated, although not completely eliminated, with the cleaner formulation, and hence the importance of therapeutic drug monitoring to maintain adequate yet safe serum concentrations; this is particularly important in renal insufficiency. Vancomycin should be infused slowly over 1 h to avoid the sudden release of histamine, which can cause flushing and occasional vascular instability (described as the red man syndrome). Oral vancomycin 125 mg every 6 h remains the drug of choice for *Clostridium difficile* colitis, although metronidazole is often effective and preferred by some. Teicoplanin has certain advantages over vancomycin in that it is administered once daily, appears relatively free of nephrotoxicity and ototoxicity and does not induce histamine release. Initial difficulties with regard to establishing the most appropriate dose and the laboratory determination of susceptibility appear to have been clarified. It has similar indications to vancomycin.

Macrolides

Erythromycin has dominated the macrolide class of agents. Globally other compounds such as *spiramycin* and *josamycin* are in use. These macrolides offer a limited spectrum of activity against staphylococci, streptococci and pneumococci, with variable activity against *H influenzae*. Their spectrum also encompasses atypical lower respiratory tract pathogens (chlamydia, coxiella and mycoplasma) as well as *Legionella* sp. Erythromycin has been particularly popular in the treatment of childhood infections; syrup formulations are widely used. It is also popular in those hypersensitive to β-lactams for the treatment of upper and lower respiratory tract infections. Erythromycin remains an alternative to tetracycline for the treatment of non-gonococcal genital infections. The major adverse experience with erythromycin is in relation to gastrointestinal intolerance, particularly nausea, vomiting and epigastric discomfort. This reflects the prokinetic activity of this class of agents and occurs with parenteral as well as the various oral formulations.

Several new compounds have emerged and include *clarithromycin, azithromycin* and *roxithromycin*. These possess a similar spectrum of activity to erythromycin. Clarithromycin has enhanced activity against *H influenzae*, which is further enhanced by its hydroxy metabolite. Azithromycin presents novel pharmacokinetic characteristics with a half life of 36–50 h. Serum concentrations are

415

extremely low but tissue concentrations, including intracellular uptake, are relatively high. The indications for this agent are similar to those for other macrolides but with the potential advantage of short course therapy in several situations. Treatments of 3–5 days are effective in upper and lower respiratory tract infections, while single dose therapy is effective in chlamydial genital infections. Its efficacy in pneumonia has yet to be proven, where concerns that bacteraemic infections may not respond to the relatively low blood levels must be addressed. Roxithromycin is comparable to erythromycin but with major improvements in its absorption and tolerance.

Future developments

Many new compounds are at various stages of development; licensing can be anticipated in the area of oral and injectable cephalosporins, as discussed earlier. Likewise, interest in the macrolides continues with agents such as dirythromycin. Among the quinolones agents such as sparfloxacin, tosufloxacin, difloxacin, and fleroxacin are at an advanced stage of development. Improvements in old molecules such as the tetracyclines is anticipated, while the expansion in the availability of the quinolones will continue to dominate antibacterial developments. Changes in patent protection laws are likely to maintain the high cost of injectable agents and hence it is important to emphasise rational prescribing based on clear definitions of infection with regard to the use of these agents. Efficacy and safety remain the most important criteria for acceptance of a new agent, with issues such as pharmacokinetic differences, microbiological spectrum, and frequency of administration of secondary importance.

Acar JF, Neu HC. Gram-negative aerobic bacterial infections: a focus on directed therapy, with special reference to aztreonam. *Rev Infect Dis* 1985;7 (suppl):537–843. (Reviews the development of the monobactams and in particular aztreonam. Its pharmacokinetics, safety, and low immunogenicity are reported. Experience in treating infections of the respiratory tract, those associated with obstetric and gynaecological problems, intra-abdominal sepsis, infections of the urinary tract, and infections in neutropenic patients are reported.)

Brown EM, Hamilton-Miller JMT, Spencer RC, Daly PJ. Cefpirome: a novel extended spectrum cephalosprin. *J Antimicrob Chemother* 1992;29(suppl A):1–104. (This supplement reviews in vitro pharmacokinetics and clinical data on the broad spectrum β lactamase stable injectable cephalosporin.)

Campoli-Richards DM, Monk JP, Price A, Benfield P, Todd FA, Ward A.

Ciprofloxacin. A review of its antibacterial activity, pharmacokinetic properties and therapeutic use. *Drugs* 1988;**35**:373–447. (A comprehensive review of the preclinical, clinical efficacy and safety data of this most widely prescribed fluoroquinolone.)

Conference. Clavulanate/β-lactam antibiotics: further experience. *J Antimicrob Chemother* 1989;**24** (suppl B):1–226.

Cooper TJ, Ladusans E, Williams PEO, Polychronopoulos V, Gaya L, Rudd RM. A comparison of oral cefuroxime axetil and oral amoxycillin in lower respiratory tract infections. *J Antimicrob Chemother* 1985;**16**:373–8. (Experience with cefuroxime axetil in the treatment of infection of the lower respiratory tract is reported, including comparative data with oral amoxycillin. The drug was shown to be effective and well tolerated.)

Davey PG, Emmerson AM, Grüneberg RN, Daly PJ. Teicoplanin: laboratory and clinical developments. *J Antimicrob Chemother* 1991;**27** (suppl B):1–73. (A useful collection of papers on the in vitro activity, disposition, and in particular the clinical performance, of this new glycopeptide.)

Finch RG, Speller DE, Daly PJ. Clarithromycin: new approaches to the treatment of respiratory tract infection. *J Antimicrob Chemother* 1991;**27** (suppl A):1–124. (Clarithromycin is representative of the new class of macrolide. It has enhanced activity, improved pharmacokinetics and appears well tolerated. The papers in this supplement provide a useful summary of its performance to date.)

Geddes AM, Stille W. Imipenem: the first thienamycin antibiotic. *Rev Infect Dis* 1985;**7** (suppl 3):353–536. (The antibacterial activity of imipenem, its pharmacokinetics in association with cilastatin, and an assessment of its clinical efficacy and safety in the treatment of a wide range of serious hospital infections are reported.)

Greenwood D, Finch RG. Piperacillin/tazobactam: a new β-lactam/β-lactamase inhibitor combination. *J Antimicrob Chemother* 1993;**31** (suppl A):1–124. (Papers are presented on the activity of tazobactam in restoring the activity of piperacillin through β lactamase inhibition. A useful set of clinical papers assesses the performance of this formulation.)

Harding SM, Williams PEO, Ayrton J. Pharmacology of cefuroxime as the 1-acetoxyethyl ester in volunteers. *Antimicrob Agents Chemother* 1984;**25**:78–82. (A pharmacokinetic study of the oral administration of cefuroxime axetil in healthy volunteers. Bowel flora were also monitored during treatment.)

Leigh DA, Ridgway GL, Leeming JP, Speller DCE. Azithromycin (CP-62,993): the first azalide antimicrobial agent. *J Antimicrob Chemother* 1990;**25** (suppl A):1–126. (Azithromycin is unusual among the new macrolides in possessing a remarkably long half life. The papers presented in this supplement summarise experience to date in treating a range of common community infections.)

Neu HC, Phillips I. Cefotaxime. *J Antimicrob Chemother* 1984;**14** (suppl B):1–338. (Provides a comprehensive review of the microbiological activity and pharmacokinetic behaviour of cefotaxime in various populations and also discusses the clinical use of the drug in meningitis, haemodialysis, gonorrhoea, and infection of the urinary tract as well as the prophylactic use of cefotaxime in a broad range of operations.)

Phillips I, Reeves D, Lewis D. Enoxacin in antimicrobial therapy: a look forward. *J Antimicrob Chemother* 1984;**14** (suppl C):1–94. (Reviews the in vitro activity, pharmacokinetics, and early clinical data of enoxacin in the treatment of infections of the respiratory tract and gonorrhoea.)

Phillips I, Wise R. The role of cefadroxil in oral antibiotic theory. *J Antimicrob Chemother* 1982;**10** (suppl B):1–161. (Reviews the antibacterial activity, pharmacokinetics, tissue penetration, and clinical experience of cefadroxil in the treatment of respiratory, urinary, ear, nose, and throat, skeletal, skin, and soft tissue infections.)

417

Phillips J, Pechere JC, Davies A, Speller D. Roxithromycin: a new macrolide. *J Antimicrob Chemother* 1987;**20** (suppl B):1–183. (The in vitro performance and pharmacokinetic behaviour of this new macrolide are complemented by a series of clinical studies assessing its efficacy and safety.)

Richards DM, Brogden RN. Ceftazidime. A review of its antibacterial activity, pharmacokinetic properties and therapeutic use. *Drugs* 1985;**29**:105–61. (A critical assessment of the in vitro activity, mode of action, pharmacokinetics, and therapeutic use of ceftazidime in infections of the respiratory and urinary tracts, septicaemia, infections of the skeleton, skin, and soft tissues, and gynaecological and intra-abdominal sepsis. It also reviews experiences of treating patients with cystic fibrosis.)

Sattler FR, Weitekamp MR, Ballard JO. Potential for bleeding with the new beta-lactam antibiotics. *Ann Intern Med* 1986;**105**:924–31. (Reviews the problem of impaired haemostasis in patients receiving cephalosporins, especially those agents possessing the methylthiotetrazole side chain.)

Scandinavian Study Group. Imipenem/cilastatin versus gentamicin/clindamycin for treatment of serious bacterial infections. *Lancet* 1984;**i**:868–71. (Randomised study of imipenem/cilastatin compares gentamicin/clindamycin in the treatment of a wide range of serious infections. The study showed superior clinical and bacteriological efficacy and safety for imipenem/cilastatin.)

Stratton CW, Anthony LB, Johnston PE. A review of ceftriaxone: a long-acting cephalosporin. *Am J Med Sci* 1988;**296**:221–2. (A useful summary of the microbiology, pharmacokinetics and clinical application of this potent broad spectrum long acting cephalosporin.)

Symposium. Focus on ofloxacin—a new 4-quinolone antimicrobial agent. *J Antimicrob Chemother* 1988;**22** (suppl C):1–175. (Ofloxacin has become the second most widely prescribed quinolone. These papers summarise its performance against common and some less common target infections. Its safety is also discussed.)

Symposium. Clinical pharmacology and efficacy of cefixime. *Ped Infect Dis J* 1987;**6**:949–1009. (The distribution of cefixime with various tissues and target sites are presented, together with an assessment of its performance, especially in the area of upper and lower respiratory tract infections.)

Wolfson JS, Hooper DC. Norfloxacin: a new targeted fluoroquinolone antimicrobial agent. *Ann Intern Med* 1988;**198**:238–51. (Norfloxacin has found particular use in the management of urinary tract infections. This article summarises published experience to date.)

31 Drug overdosage and poisoning

L F PRESCOTT

Drug overdosage remains a common medical emergency and a considerable burden on the health services. Management of the severely poisoned patient depends primarily on intensive supportive treatment, and in the past decade this has improved as a result of continued progress in the techniques of resuscitation and intensive care. Management has also improved with better understanding of mechanisms of toxicity and wider appreciation of the importance of pharmacokinetic principles in the rational use of specialised methods of enhancing the elimination of drugs from the body. Unfortunately, specific antidotal treatment is available for very few of the drugs commonly taken by self poisoners, and there have been few recent developments of note on this topic. Further advances have been made in analytical methodology, but the service role of the hospital laboratory remains largely restricted to the emergency identification and measurement of agents for which specific treatment is available and when measures for active removal of the drug are being considered. Regrettably, not all changes have been for the better. The units used for reporting drug concentrations must now be checked very carefully because, without consultation, many hospital laboratories have changed to molar SI units to measure drug concentrations, and this has caused dangerous and unnecessary confusion.

Changes in the pattern of self poisoning

Most adults who take overdoses do so on impulse at a time of crisis (often while under the influence of alcohol), and the drugs taken are those that come immediately to hand. These are usually prescribed drugs, and as prescribing fashions change over the years, so do the patterns of drugs used for self poisoning. Overdosage with benzodiazepines is at last declining, and most serious

419

poisonings now entail non-prescription or narcotic analgesics, tricyclic antidepressants, or a miscellany of less commonly taken drugs including major tranquillisers, β blockers, anticonvulsants, theophylline, and quinine. Over the counter analgesics deserve special mention because they are freely available and there have been important changes in their use over the years. Paracetamol is by far the most popular drug in this group, and consequently it is used for self poisoning much more often than aspirin or ibuprofen. Salicylate intoxication is uncommon but the incidence of ibuprofen overdosage is increasing rapidly although it is still low.

Household and industrial products are used for intentional poisoning less often than drugs, but agents such as methanol, ethylene glycol, pesticides, and herbicides can cause serious toxicity. Toddlers and young children are still often poisoned accidentally, but they rarely come to great harm. They tend to go for relatively non-toxic substances that they find around the house, and although brightly coloured tablets and capsules are irresistible, the amounts taken are usually small.

Over the years, the trend has been towards the introduction of safer drugs that produce less acute toxicity. As a result, proportionately fewer poisoned patients now require ventilation and the full resources of intensive care. Indeed, self poisoning is relatively safe (otherwise it would not be so popular), and the overall death rate in hospital patients is about 0·5%. A fatal outcome is more likely in the elderly and in patients with serious pre-existing disease.

Intensive supportive treatment

The management of seriously poisoned and unconscious patients is based on conservative intensive supportive treatment with good nursing care, close attention to the adequacy of ventilation, cardiovascular support, and correcting abnormal acid–base, electrolyte, and fluid balance. Careful observation and monitoring is mandatory, and potentially serious complications such as repeated convulsions, pneumonia, and renal failure should be anticipated and treated promptly. Meddlesome medical interference is a major hazard for the patient. Other drugs must be avoided unless absolutely necessary, and there is no case for the prophylactic use of antibiotics.

Cardiac arrhythmias are common but seldom life-threatening.

The temptation to rush in with cardiotoxic antiarrhythmic drugs solely on the basis of an alarming electrocardiogram must be firmly resisted unless common sense measures such as correcting acidosis, hypoxia, and electrolyte abnormalities have failed and the rhythm disturbance is seriously compromising cardiac output. Hypotension is another common complication of poisoning, caused by myocardial depression or impaired autonomic peripheral vascular reflexes. The vasodilatation resulting from the latter reduces the venous return to the heart and increases the vascular volume so that there is relative hypovolaemia. Assisted ventilation may also reduce the cardiac output. A fall in systolic blood pressure to 80 mmHg or so in a previously healthy young or middle aged person is rarely of consequence if peripheral perfusion and urine output are maintained. The cardiac output can usually be improved by raising the foot of the bed and if necessary by administering a plasma expander and monitoring the central venous pressure. More severe hypotension with oliguria may respond to intravenous infusion of dopamine.

Reduction in gastrointestinal absorption

Gastric aspiration and lavage with a wide bore tube is probably the most reliable method for removing unabsorbed drug or poison. Most overdoses seem to be absorbed with surprising rapidity, however, and although gastric lavage is usually performed only within 4 h of ingestion, obtaining a gratifying return of tablet material is rare. The need for routine gastric lavage is being questioned and it now tends to be used more selectively for patients who are thought to have taken a potentially lethal overdose. Gastric lavage is hazardous if the protective pharyngeal reflexes are obtunded and if corrosives or hydrocarbons have been taken. It is also traumatic for young children. An increasingly popular alternative is induction of emesis with syrup of ipecac, and this is usually effective within 15–20 min. Other emetics such as salt and copper sulphate solutions should never be used as they can cause fatal toxicity if retained. The relative efficacy of gastric lavage and induced emesis in removing unabsorbed drug remains a subject for debate, and neither can be relied on to empty the stomach completely.

Oral activated charcoal is often recommended in the hope that it will prevent further absorption by binding unabsorbed drug in the gastrointestinal tract. Activated charcoal is a powerful non-specific adsorbent that can appreciably reduce the absorption of most drugs if taken at the same time. Unfortunately, it has little or no effect when its administration is delayed for more than about 1 h, which is usually the case in poisoned patients referred to hospital. The increasing use of slow release products may cause problems as absorption may be delayed and prolonged. Once past the pylorus drugs cannot be retrieved, but absorption may be reduced by accelerating gastrointestinal transit with whole gut lavage using large volumes of saline. There is no other indication for the use of cathartics or laxatives in poisoned patients.

Enhancing drug removal from the body

Most poisoned patients recover satisfactorily with conservative supportive care, and relatively few indications exist for using techniques to enhance drug elimination. These include repeated administration of oral activated charcoal, forced alkaline diuresis, haemodialysis, peritoneal dialysis, haemoperfusion, plasmapheresis, and exchange transfusion. Fortunately, a better understanding of the relevant physiological and pharmacokinetic principles has led to a more selective and realisti. approach to using techniques to enhance drug elimination. The clearance of drugs by peritoneal dialysis is very low, and the fraction of the total amount of drug in the body that can be removed by plasmapheresis and exchange transfusion is usually very small. Consequently there are few, if any, indications for the use of these methods. However, several drugs and poisons can be removed effectively by haemodialysis and haemoperfusion. These measures may occasionally be indicated in very severely poisoned patients who do not respond to conventional treatment within a reasonable time and whose survival is otherwise in doubt. They may also be necessary in seriously ill patients with complications such as pneumonia or renal failure.

REPEATED ORAL ACTIVATED CHARCOAL ADMINISTRATION

The most important recent advance in techniques for enhancing drug removal is the repeated oral administration of adsorbents such as activated charcoal and exchange resins. These act by irreversibly binding drugs that undergo enterohepatic circulation and are secreted into the intestine in bile, and also drugs that diffuse passively from the circulation into the intestinal lumen. The latter mechanism is undoubtedly the most important. A high concentration gradient for diffusion is maintained because the drug is immediately removed by the charcoal, and transfer across the gut wall is a continuous process. The gastrointestinal clearance of drugs by this mechanism is limited by their lipid solubility and plasma protein binding, the splanchnic blood flow, and the adsorptive capacity of the charcoal. Whether or not the overall rate of drug removal from the body increases appreciably depends on the gastrointestinal clearance relative to the normal clearance by other routes.

The therapeutic objective is to fill the intestine with charcoal and to promote peristalsis to avoid stagnation and saturation with endogenous compounds. A dosage schedule used commonly is 50–75 g charcoal in a slurry with water given every 4 h until the patient recovers. Repeated oral charcoal can appreciably enhance the removal of many drugs including phenobarbitone, diphenyl-hydantoin, carbamazepine, theophylline, digoxin, quinine, dapsone, and salicylate. With some drugs (such as phenobarbitone) repeated oral charcoal is much more effective than conventional forced alkaline diuresis, and at least as effective as haemoperfusion, whereas with others (such as diphenylhydantoin and quinine) it is more effective than any other method of removal. It is not useful for treating patients poisoned with tricyclic antidepressants and benzodiazepines.

Although repeated oral charcoal administration is a simple, safe, cheap, and effective means of enhancing drug removal, there are problems with its use. It is black, messy, and unpleasant to take, it cannot be given to patients who are nauseated or vomiting, and the charcoal itself may induce vomiting. It must be given to unconscious patients by nasogastric tube, and prior endotracheal intubation is advisable. Great care must be taken to avoid the aspiration of charcoal into the lungs for, although it is supposedly inert, fatal pulmonary aspiration has been reported.

FORCED ALKALINE DIURESIS

Forced alkaline diuresis is now indicated only for moderate and severe intoxication with salicylate, phenobarbitone, and a few other acidic compounds such as 2,4-dichlorophenoxyacetic acid and chlorpropamide. These agents are all excreted largely

423

unchanged by the kidney, and their clearance depends largely on urine pH. The relation between the renal clearance of a drug such as salicylate and urine pH is logarithmic, whereas the relation with flow rate is not. Theoretically, its clearance would increase 1000-fold with a change in urine pH from 5 to 8. Producing maximally alkaline urine is therefore much more important than attempting to force diuresis. Forced acid diuresis is a more hazardous procedure; it is of no value in treating patients with quinine poisoning, and there is no convincing clinical evidence to justify its use in any other form of poisoning.

Forced diuresis should not be undertaken lightly. Administering large volumes of fluid may cause disturbances of electrolyte balance, fluid overload, and pulmonary and cerebral oedema. Particular hazards exist for the elderly and patients with impaired cardiac or renal function.

HAEMODIALYSIS AND HAEMOPERFUSION

The removal of many drugs and poisons can be enhanced appreciably by haemodialysis and charcoal or ion exchange resin haemoperfusion. Haemoperfusion is usually the preferred method as it is simpler and usually more effective than haemodialysis. Nevertheless, haemodialysis is preferred for removing compounds of low molecular weight, such as methanol and salicylate, and the associated abnormalities of acid–base and electrolyte balance can be corrected at the same time.

The efficacy of these procedures in enhancing the removal of drugs from the body depends on achieving an extracorporeal clearance that approaches or exceeds the endogenous clearance of the compound. The extracorporeal clearance depends on the blood flow rate and the fraction extracted by the procedure. The latter in turn depends on factors such as the extent of binding of the drug to plasma proteins, its affinity for adsorbents (haemoperfusion), and molecular size (haemodialysis). In practice the most effective removal is of drugs that are not strongly protein bound and have a small volume of distribution and a low endogenous clearance rate.

Drug clearance often falls progressively during haemoperfusion because of saturation of the charcoal, and treatment is normally limited to about 6 h. The poison should be identified and the amount estimated before treatment, as not all compounds can be removed. Haemodialysis is ineffective in removing paraquat, and haemoperfusion does not increase usefully the elimination of agents such as quinine, atropine, camphor, and diphenylhydantoin. The complications of haemodialysis and haemoperfusion include hypotension and thrombocytopenia, and these invasive procedures can only be carried out in specialised units.

HAEMODYNAMIC SUPPORT

Many drugs are lethal because they cause severe cardiovascular and respiratory depression. If the patient reaches hospital alive ventilation is simple, but life cannot be sustained for long if the cardiac output is grossly reduced. Furthermore, attempts to clear the drug by haemodialysis or haemoperfusion may fail because an adequate blood flow through the device cannot be obtained. In such circumstances cardiac output is unlikely to be increased by pacing or administering inotropes, and the use of an intra-aortic balloon pump (or even cardiopulmonary bypass) should be considered to support the circulation and promote elimination of the drug before cardiogenic shock becomes irreversible.

Specific treatment

Although there are relatively few indications for specific antidotal treatment, it is important that these are recognised and that treatment is instituted without delay.

N-ACETYLCYSTEINE FOR PARACETAMOL POISONING

Sulphydryl compounds have been used to prevent hepatic necrosis after paracetamol overdosage for more than 15 years, and intravenous N-acetylcysteine is established as the preferred treatment. At one time oral methionine was advocated, but any form of oral treatment is unreliable because of the early onset of vomiting in most patients with severe paracetamol poisoning.

Intravenous N-acetylcysteine is very effective if given within 8–10h of the ingestion of paracetamol. Only a small minority of patients is at risk of severe liver damage, however, and as using N-acetylcysteine is not entirely without risk the need for treatment should always be established, if possible by emergency estimation of the plasma paracetamol concentration. Treatment is indicated when the concentration is above a line on a semilogarithmic graph joining concentrations of 200 mg/l at 4h and 30 mg/l at 15h after ingestion. The protective effect of N-acetylcysteine falls off progressively when treatment is delayed more than 10h, and no properly controlled studies have been reported to show that it has any useful effect after 24h. Because of this critical time limit, treatment should never be delayed more than 8h while awaiting the laboratory result. If the patient subsequently turns out not to have been at risk it is simple to discontinue treatment. Initial fears that late treatment with N-acetylcysteine might be harmful to patients with impending severe liver damage have not been realised. Although appreciable benefit is unlikely after 15h, there is no contraindication to treatment up to 24h, and this would certainly be justifiable in patients who present late with high plasma paracetamol concentrations.

As intravenous N-acetylcysteine is used extensively to treat patients with paracetamol poisoning, it is not surprising that there have been reports of adverse reactions. Most of these "anaphylactoid" reactions have been mild and transient, and effects such as mild hypotension and flushing can probably be regarded as normal pharmacological responses. Other reported adverse effects include tachycardia, urticaria, and bronchospasm. Fatalities have occurred, but these have usually been associated with gross overdosage of the N-acetylcysteine. Many of the reports of reactions to N-acetylcysteine resulted from circumstances in which there were no indications for its use in the first place.

N-Acetylcysteine can protect against many forms of glutathione dependent toxicity, including that produced by alkylating agents, heavy metals, and some halogenated hydrocarbons. As expected, it does not prevent hepatic necrosis caused by carbon tetrachloride.

FLUMAZENIL FOR BENZODIAZEPINE POISONING

The benzodiazepines probably lead the field of drugs taken by self poisoners, and the introduction of flumazenil, a specific benzodiazepine antagonist, is an important new development in specific antidotal treatment. When taken in overdosage on their own, the benzodiazepines rarely cause serious or life threatening toxicity. They potentiate the effects of other central nervous system depressants, however, and may contribute appreciably to respiratory depression and hypotension after multiple drug overdosage, particularly in the elderly and patients with pulmonary disease. In such circumstances reversal of the benzodiazepine component by flumazenil might be beneficial, but otherwise there are few indications for its use in poisoned patients.

DRUG OVERDOSAGE AND POISONING

The depressant effects of the benzodiazepines are reversed almost immediately after intravenous injection of an adequate dose of flumazenil. Its duration of action is usually brief, it is eliminated rapidly and has a half life of about 1 h: repeated doses or continuous intravenous infusions are usually necessary to maintain arousal. Flumazenil seems to be well tolerated, but it may precipitate a withdrawal reaction in patients who are dependent on benzodiazepines and it might cause convulsions and cardiac arrhythmias.

HYPERBARIC OXYGEN FOR CARBON MONOXIDE POISONING

Carbon monoxide is a major metabolic poison that can cause serious and irreversible cerebral damage. There may be delayed neuropsychiatric sequelae, even in patients who seem to make a rapid and complete recovery. Although intentional carbon monoxide poisoning is rare, accidental exposure may occur whenever carbonaceous fuels are incompletely burned and it is an important cause of illness and death after fires. Immediate treatment consists of removing the patient from the site of exposure and administering maximum concentrations of oxygen. In recent years there has been increasing evidence that recovery is more rapid and the incidence of late complications appreciably reduced by treatment with hyperbaric oxygen, even when this is delayed. This form of treatment should be considered for every patient with moderate to severe carbon monoxide poisoning, and information concerning the availability of facilities in Britain can be obtained from local poisons information bureaux (telephone numbers are inside the front cover of the *British National Formulary*).

DANTROLENE FOR MALIGNANT HYPERTHERMIA

Overdosage with amphetamines, monoamine oxidase inhibitors, or combinations of phenothiazines, butyrophenones, or lithium may cause a syndrome that resembles malignant hyperthermia. This is often delayed in onset and is characterised by coma, hyperpyrexia, tachycardia, hyperventilation, and generalised muscle rigidity. Muscle damage may result in hyperkalaemia, myoglobinuria, and renal failure. Without treatment the prognosis is poor, but intravenous dantrolene is usually rapidly effective in abolishing muscle rigidity and the associated abnormalities.

HEAVY METAL POISONING

Established treatment for patients with acute and chronic

intoxication with heavy metals includes sodium calcium edetate (for lead poisoning), D-penicillamine (for copper or lead), and dimercaprol (for mercury, arsenic, gold, et cetera). Recent studies suggest that other thiols such as 2,3-dimercaptosuccinate may be at least as effective and safer than the agents currently in use.

Fab ANTIBODIES FOR DIGOXIN OVERDOSAGE

Serious and life threatening intoxication with cardiac glycosides can be dramatically reversed by the administration of Fab fragments of digoxin specific antibodies raised in sheep ("Digibind"). The fragments have a greater affinity for digoxin than for its binding sites in the myocardium and other tissues, and they are less immunogenic than the complete IgG antibody. Intravenous administration of the Fab fragments usually leads to rapid reversal of cardiotoxicity and other complications such as hyperkalaemia. This is associated with a rapid rise in the plasma concentration of inactive protein bound digoxin and a dramatic fall to a very low concentration of free digoxin. The required dose of Fab fragments of antibody to digoxin is equivalent to about 60 times the total amount of digoxin in the body, and this can be estimated from the body weight and plasma digoxin concentration. Serious adverse effects have not been reported, but plasma potassium concentrations should be monitored carefully as hypokalaemia may occur. Treatment is very expensive and should be reserved for serious life threatening intoxication. The availability of digoxin specific Fab antibody fragments has revolutionised the management of patients poisoned with cardiac glycosides, and the development of similar specific immunotherapy for the safe effective treatment of patients intoxicated with other lethal poisons would be a major step forward.

Anonymous. Emergency drugs: agents used in the treatment of poisoning. *BMJ* 1984;**289**:742–8. (Comprehensive list of agents that might be used to treat poisoned patients, based on advice in the appendix to DHSS circular HN (78) 23. Includes indications, modes of action, presentation, and sources of supply.)

Brogden RN, Goa KL. Flumazenil: a preliminary review of its benzodiazepine antagonist properties, intrinsic activity and therapeutic use. *Drugs* 1988;**35**:448–67.

Fournier L, Thomas G, Garnier R, *et al*. 2, 3-Dimercaptosuccinic acid treatment of heavy metal poisoning in humans. *Med Toxicol Adverse Drug Exp* 1988;**3**:499–504. (Treatment of 14 patients with lead, arsenic, or mercury poisoning.)

Neuvonen PJ, Olkkola KT. Oral activated charcoal in the treatment of intoxications: role of single and repeated doses. *Med Toxicol Adverse Drug Exp* 1988;**3**:33–58.

Norkool DM, Kirkpatrick JN. Treatment of acute carbon monoxide poisoning with hyperbaric oxygen: a review of 155 cases. *Ann Emerg Med* 1985;**14**:1169–71. (Review of treatment of large number of patients.)

Prescott LF. Drug overdosage and poisoning. In: Speight TM, ed. *Avery's drug treatment*. 3rd ed. Auckland: ADIS Press, 1987;283–302. (Review of pharmacological basis of treating poisoned patients, including specific treatment and use of special techniques for enhancing drug elimination.)

Prescott LF. Paracetamol overdosage: pharmacological considerations and clinical management. *Drugs* 1983;**25**:290–314. (Detailed review of mechanisms of paracetamol hepatoxicity and clinical management of overdosage including use of specific treatment.)

Proudfoot AT. *Diagnosis and management of acute poisoning*. Edinburgh: Blackwell Scientific, 1982. (Authoritative concise guide to managing poisoned patients based on extensive personal clinical experience.)

Stolshek BS, Osterhout SK, Dunham G. The role of digoxin-specific antibodies in the treatment of digitalis poisoning. *Med Toxicol Adverse Drug Exp* 1988;**3**:167–71.

Vale JA, Meredith TJ, eds. *Poisoning—diagnosis and treatment*. London: Update Books, 1981:1–220. (Practical account of diagnosing and treating patients with clinically important drug overdosage and poisoning.)

Index